ADVANCES IN Surgery

Editor-in-Chief
John L. Cameron, MD

ELSEVIER

PHILADELPHIA LONDON TORONTO MONTREAL SYDNEY TOKYO

ADVANCES IN
Surgery

VOLUMES 1 THROUGH 42 (OUT OF PRINT)

VOLUME 46

VOLUME 45

10. Pancreatic Necrosectomy *by Jordan R. Stern and Jeffrey B. Matthews*

11. The Impact of Health Care Reform on Surgery *by Donald D. Trunkey*

12. Glucose Elevations and Outcome in Critically Injured Trauma Patients *by Joseph J. DuBose and Thomas M. Scalea*

13. Advances in the Surgical Management of Gastrointestinal Stromal Tumor *by Umer I. Chaudhry and Ronald P. DeMatteo*

14. Choledochoceles: Are They Choledochal Cysts? *by Kathryn M. Ziegler and Nicholas J. Zyromski*

15. What Does Ulceration of a Melanoma Mean for Prognosis? *by Glenda G. Callender and Kelly M. McMasters*

16. Influence of Surgical Volume on Operative Failures for Hyperparathyroidism *by Barbara Zarebczan and Herbert Chen*

17. Perioperative Normothermia During Major Surgery: Is It Important? *by Nestor F. Esnaola and David J. Cole*

18. Surgical Management of Hereditary Nonpolyposis Colorectal Cancer *by Matthew F. Kalady*

19. How to Change General Surgery Residency Training *by Steven C. Stain*

20. Recent Advances in the Diagnosis and Treatment of Gastrointestinal Carcinoids *by Joseph Valentino and B. Mark Evers*

21. The Past, Present, and Future of Biomarkers: A Need for Molecular Beacons for the Clinical Management of Pancreatic Cancer *by Jonathan R. Brody, Agnieszka K. Witkiewicz, and Charles J. Yeo*

22. Robotic-Assisted Major Pancreatic Resection *by H.J. Zeh III, David L. Bartlett, and A. James Moser*

23. Immunotherapy for Metastatic Solid Cancers *by Simon Turcotte and Steven A. Rosenberg*

24. Prophylaxis for Deep Vein Thrombosis and Pulmonary Embolism in the Surgical Patient *by Taki Galanis, Walter K. Kraft, and Geno J. Merli*

VOLUME 44

1. Single-Port Laparoscopic Surgery *by Anthony Y. Tsai and Don J. Selzer*

19. The Role of PET Scanning in Pancreatic Cancer *by Oscar K. Serrano, Muhammad A. Chaudhry, and Steven D. Leach*

20. Reoperative Surgery for the Zollinger-Ellison Syndrome *by Stephen R. Grobmyer and Steven N. Hochwald*

21. Computerized Physician Order Entry System in a Surgical Practice *by William M. Stone*

VOLUME 43

1. Natural Orifice Translumenal Endoscopic Surgery: Current Status *by Denise W. Gee and David W. Rattner*

2. The Accuracy and Role of Cross-sectional Imaging in the Diagnosis of Acute Appendicitis *by Joshua D. Hawkins and Richard C. Thirlby*

3. Management of Pancreatic Serous Cystadenomas *by Jennifer A. Wargo, Carlos Fernandez-del-Castillo, and Andrew L. Warshaw*

4. Stem Cells and the Liver: Clinical Applications in Transplantation *by Jayme E. Locke, Michael J. Shamblott, and Andrew M. Cameron*

5. Is Intermittent Vasculogenic Claudication Still a Nonsurgical Disease? *by Spence M. Taylor*

6. Changes in Operative Case Experience for General Surgery Residents: Has the 80-Hour Work Week Decreased Residents' Operative Experience? *by John C. Kairys, Paul J. DiMuzio, Albert G. Crawford, Daniel J. Grabo, and Charles J. Yeo*

7. Laparoscopic Pancreatic Resections *by Attila Nakeeb*

8. The Role of Perioperative Hyperglycemia in Postoperative Infections *by Selwyn O. Rogers, Jr. and Michael J. Zinner*

9. Can Ileal Pouch Anal Anastomosis Be Used in Crohn's Disease? *by Myles R. Joyce and Victor W. Fazio*

10. Are Airbags Effective in Decreasing Trauma in Auto Accidents? *by Regan F. Williams and Martin A. Croce*

11. Posterior Retroperitoneoscopic Adrenalectomy *by Glenda G. Callender, Debra L. Kennamer, Elizabeth G. Grubbs, Jeffrey E. Lee, Douglas B. Evans, and Nancy D. Perrier*

Vice President, Continuity Publishing: Kimberly Murphy
Editor: Yonah Korngold

Editorial Office:
Elsevier
1600 John F. Kennedy Blvd,
Suite 1800
Philadelphia, PA 19103-2899

International Standard Serial Number: 0065-3411
International Standard Book Number: 978-1-4557-7272-8

Printed and bound by CPI Group (UK) Ltd, Croydon, CR0 4YY

Transferred to digital print 2012

ADVANCES IN
Surgery

CONTRIBUTORS

DANIEL E. ABBOTT, MD, Assistant Professor, Department of Surgery, Pancreatic Disease Center, University of Cincinnati Medical Center, Cincinnati, Ohio

SYED A. AHMAD, MD, Associate Professor, Department of Surgery, Pancreatic Disease Center, University of Cincinnati Medical Center, Cincinnati, Ohio

USAMA AHMED ALI, MD, Department of Colorectal Surgery, Digestive Disease Institution, Cleveland Clinic, Cleveland, Ohio

ELIZABETH A. ARENA, MD, Department of Surgical Oncology; Gastrointestinal Research Program, John Wayne Cancer Institute, Saint John's Health Center, Santa Monica, California

ANU BEHARI, MS, Additional Professor, Department of Surgical Gastroenterology, Sanjay Gandhi Post-Graduate Institute of Medical Sciences (SGPGIMS), Lucknow, Uttar Pradesh, India

JAIME BENARROCH-GAMPEL, MD, MS, Department of Surgery, The University of Texas Medical Branch, Galveston, Texas

JAI BIKHCHANDANI, MD, Chief Resident, Surgery, Department of General Surgery, Creighton University Medical Center, Omaha, Nebraska

ANTON J. BILCHIK, MD, PhD, Department of Surgical Oncology; Gastrointestinal Research Program, John Wayne Cancer Institute, Saint John's Health Center, Santa Monica; California Oncology Research Institute, Los Angeles, California

PATRICK L. BOSARGE, MD, Assistant Professor, Section of Trauma, Burns, and Surgical Critical Care, Department of Surgery, The University of Alabama at Birmingham, Birmingham, Alabama

ELLIOT L. CHAIKOF, MD, PhD, Chairman, Roberta and Stephen R. Weiner Department of Surgery; Surgeon-in-Chief, Beth Israel Deaconess Medical Center; Johnson and Johnson Professor of Surgery, Harvard Medical School, Boston, Massachusetts

CALLISIA N. CLARKE, MD, Resident, Department of Surgery, Pancreatic Disease Center, University of Cincinnati Medical Center, Cincinnati, Ohio

DEMETRIOS DEMETRIADES, MD, PhD, FACS, Professor of Surgery, Director of Trauma, Emergency Surgery and Surgical Critical Care, Division of Trauma and Acute Care Surgery, LAC and USC Medical Center, University of Southern California, Los Angeles, California

FREDERICK THURSTON DRAKE, MD, MPH, Resident Physician and Research Fellow, Department of Surgery, University of Washington, Seattle, Washington

SARA FERNANDES-TAYLOR, PhD, Department of Surgery, University of Wisconsin School of Medicine & Public Health, Madison, Wisconsin

CELESTE C. FINNERTY, PhD, Associate Director of Research, Shriners Hospitals for Children; Institute for Translational Sciences, Sealy Center for Molecular Medicine; Associate Professor, Department of Surgery, University of Texas Medical Branch, Galveston, Texas

ROBERT JOSEPH FITZGIBBONS Jr, MD, Professor of Surgery, Chief General Surgery, Department of General Surgery, Creighton University Medical Center, Omaha, Nebraska

DAVID REED FLUM, MD, MPH, FACS, Professor of Surgery, Adjunct Professor in Health Services and Pharmacy; Associate Chair for Research, Department of Surgery, University of Washington, Seattle, Washington

DAVID YU GREENBLATT, MD, MSPH, Department of Surgery, University of Wisconsin School of Medicine & Public Health, Madison, Wisconsin

DAVID N. HERNDON, MD, FACS, Chief of Staff and Director of Research, Shriners Hospitals for Children; Professor, Department of Surgery and Jesse H. Jones Distinguished Chair in Burn Surgery, University of Texas Medical Branch, Galveston, Texas

GEORGE W. HOLCOMB III, MD, MBA, Surgeon-in-Chief and Katharine Berry Richardson Professor of Pediatric Surgery Director, Department of Surgery, Center for Minimally Invasive Surgery, Children's Mercy Hospital, Kansas City, Missouri

VINAY K. KAPOOR, FACS, FACG, FRCS, Professor, Department of Surgical Gastroenterology, Sanjay Gandhi Post-Graduate Institute of Medical Sciences (SGPGIMS), Lucknow, Uttar Pradesh, India

K. CRAIG KENT, MD, Department of Surgery, University of Wisconsin School of Medicine & Public Health, Madison, Wisconsin

JEFFREY D. KERBY, MD, PhD, Professor, Section of Trauma, Burns, and Surgical Critical Care, Department of Surgery, The University of Alabama at Birmingham, Birmingham, Alabama

MARY E. KLINGENSMITH, MD, Professor of Surgery and Vice Chair for Education, Department of Surgery, Washington University School of Medicine, St Louis, Missouri

GEOFFREY W. KRAMPITZ, MD, General Surgery Resident, Stanford University School of Medicine, Stanford, California

SEAN JOSEPH LANGENFELD, MD, Assistant Professor of Surgery, Department of Surgery, University of Nebraska Medical Center, 983280 Nebraska Medical Center, Omaha, Nebraska

ANDY M. LEE, MD, Department of Surgery, Beth Israel Deaconess Medical Center, Harvard Medical School, Boston, Massachusetts

FRANK R. LEWIS, MD, Executive Director, American Board of Surgery, Philadelphia, Pennsylvania

RODNEY J. MASON, MD, PhD, Associate Professor of Clinical Surgery, Department of Surgery, University of Southern California, Los Angeles, California

JEFFREY A. NORTON, MD, The Robert L. and Mary Ellenburg Professor in Surgery, Chief of Surgical Oncology and General Surgery, Stanford University School of Medicine, Stanford, California

DMITRY OLEYNIKOV, MD, Professor of Surgery, Department of Surgery, University of Nebraska Medical Center, 983280 Nebraska Medical Center, Omaha, Nebraska

THEODORE N. PAPPAS, MD, Distinguished Professor of Surgical Innovation, Chief, General and Advanced Gastrointestinal Surgery, Interim Chair, Department of Surgery, Vice Dean for Medical Affairs, Duke University School of Medicine, Durham, North Carolina

TAYLOR S. RIALL, MD, PhD, Department of Surgery, The University of Texas Medical Branch, Galveston, Texas

JOHN E. SCARBOROUGH, MD, Associate Professor, Department of Surgery, Duke University School of Medicine, Durham, North Carolina

SHAWN D. ST. PETER, MD, Professor of Surgery, Program Director, Pediatric Surgery and Surgical Scholars Director, Department of Surgery, Center for Prospective Clinical Trials, Children's Mercy Hospital, Kansas City, Missouri

JEFFREY J. SUSSMAN, MD, Associate Professor and Chief of Surgical Oncology, Department of Surgery, Pancreatic Disease Center, University of Cincinnati Medical Center, Cincinnati, Ohio

PEDRO G.R. TEIXEIRA, MD, Fellow, Surgical Critical Care, Division of Trauma and Acute Care Surgery, LAC and USC Medical Center, University of Southern California, Los Angeles, California

JON S. THOMPSON, MD, Shackelford Professor of Surgery, Chief of General Surgery, Department of Surgery, University of Nebraska Medical Center, 983280 Nebraska Medical Center, Omaha, Nebraska

JON D. VOGEL, MD, Colorectal Surgery Residency Program Director, Department of Colorectal Surgery, Digestive Disease Institution, Cleveland Clinic, Cleveland, Ohio

CONTENTS VOLUME 47 • 2013

Duodenal Switch for Morbid Obesity: Is it Safe?

Rodney J. Mason

Is Propranolol of Benefit in Pediatric Burn Patients?

Celeste C. Finnerty and David N. Herndon

Advances in Surgery 47 (2013) 1–27

ADVANCES IN SURGERY

Repair of Giant Ventral Hernias

Jai Bikhchandani, MD*, Robert Joseph Fitzgibbons Jr, MD

Department of General Surgery, Creighton University Medical Center, 601 N 30th Street, Omaha, NE 68131, USA

Keywords

• Giant ventral hernia • Incisional hernia • Component separation • Loss of domain

Key points

- Repair of huge ventral hernias is technically challenging for the surgeon and a major operation for the patient and should be performed by experienced surgeons in centers that are used to caring for patients who are commonly massively obese, with significant comorbidities.
- Preoperative medical optimization of patients is an important part in the overall management of these large hernias.
- Conventional component separation with retromuscular mesh repair is the workhorse operation, which successfully deals with many giant ventral hernias, but multiple alternative strategies must be available to address situations in which myofascial elements are completely deficient or there is significant loss of domain.
- The complexity of this surgery is reflected by recurrence rates ranging from 10% to 30% and wound complication rates as high as 40% to 50% in experienced centers.

INTRODUCTION

Approximately 1 million abdominal wall hernia repairs are performed in the United States each year [1]. Of these operations, roughly 69% are groin, 15% umbilical, 9% incisional, and 7% are miscellaneous, (eg, Spigelian, lumbar, traumatic). The term ventral is most commonly used to describe collectively those hernias that occur outside the groin and is the convention that is used in this article. It is estimated that about 5% of the population develop a ventral hernia at some time in their life. Most hernias are small and can be managed in general practice using standard techniques. However, there is a subset of these patients who develop enormous hernia sacs. These hernias are usually described as giant ventral hernias. Other synonyms used in the literature for giant ventral

*Corresponding author. *E-mail address*: jai_9c@yahoo.com

0065-3411/13/$ – see front matter
http://dx.doi.org/10.1016/j.yasu.2013.02.008

hernia are large, massive, huge, or complex ventral hernia. Sometimes, the whole visceral contents herniate into the hernia sac outside the abdominal cavity (Fig. 1). These hernias are usually associated with loss of domain, because the abdominal cavity proper shrinks with the visceral contents lying chronically outside it. If an attempt is made to force these extra-abdominal viscera into the native abdominal cavity, there can be severe respiratory and cardiovascular compromise, causing the abdominal compartment syndrome.

Repair of huge ventral hernias with significant loss of domain is technically challenging, with high mortality, morbidity, and recurrences rates [2,3]. Moreover, these hernias are often associated with overlying skin ulceration, persistent infection, enterocutaneous fistulas, diverting stomas, and morbid obesity. Many of these hernias have been repaired multiple times, and each repair has failed, distorting the anatomy of the abdominal wall further. This article focuses on the management of these complex huge ventral hernias and the newer advances in abdominal wall reconstructions.

SURGICAL ANATOMY

The root cause of a ventral hernia is failure of key anatomic elements to contain intra-abdominal viscera within the abdominal cavity. Repair of ventral hernias requires a thorough understanding of the anatomy of the abdominal wall [4]. The abdominal wall is made up of the centrally located rectus abdominis muscles and the 3 lateral muscles: the external oblique, internal oblique, and transversus abdominis. The linea alba is the midline confluence of the aponeuroses of these muscles.

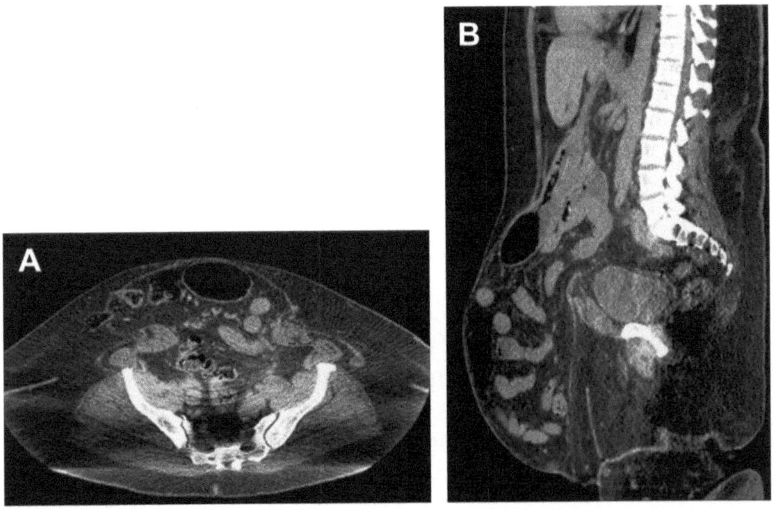

Fig. 1. (*A, B*) Computed tomography scan (*axial and sagittal view*) of a patient with giant ventral hernia. Note that a significant amount of the intra-abdominal viscera including the stomach is in the hernia.

The external abdominal oblique muscle (Fig. 2) is the most superficial of the 3 lateral abdominal muscles. The external abdominal oblique arises from the posterior aspects of the lower 8 ribs and interdigitates with both the serratus anterior and the latissimus dorsi at its origin. The direction of the muscle fibers varies from nearly horizontal in its upper portion to oblique in the middle and lower portions. The horizontal fibers, which originate posteriorly, insert onto the anterior portion of the iliac crest. The obliquely arranged anteroinferior fibers of insertion fold on to themselves to form the inguinal ligament. The remaining portion of the aponeurosis inserts into the linea alba after contributing to the anterior portion of the rectus abdominis sheath. The middle layer of the lateral abdominal group is the internal abdominal oblique muscle (see Fig. 2). This muscle primarily arises from the iliac fascia along the iliac crest and forms a band of iliac fascia fused with the inguinal ligament. The uppermost fibers course obliquely toward the distal ends of the lower 3 or 4 (floating) ribs. The muscle fibers of the internal oblique fan out, following the shape of the iliac crest, so that the lowermost fibers are directed inferiorly. The aponeurosis of the internal oblique (Fig. 3A) above the level of the umbilicus splits to envelop the rectus abdominis, then reforms in the midline to join and interweave with the fibers of the linea alba. Below the level of the umbilicus (see Fig. 3B), the aponeurosis does not split but rather runs anterior to the rectus muscle, continues medially as a single sheet, joins the anterior rectus sheath, and contributes to the linea alba. The aponeurotic portion of the internal oblique is widest at the level of the umbilicus. The transversus abdominis muscle arises from the fascia along the iliac crest and inguinal ligament and from the lower 6 costal cartilages and ribs, where it interdigitates with the lateral diaphragmatic fibers. The muscle bundles of the transversus abdominis for the most part run horizontally. However, the lower medial fibers may continue in a more inferomedial course toward the site of insertion on the crest and pecten of the pubis. The aponeurosis of the transversus abdominis joins the posterior lamina of the internal abdominal oblique, forming above the umbilicus a portion of the posterior rectus sheath. Below the umbilicus, the transversus abdominis aponeurosis is a component of the anterior rectus sheath. The gradual termination of aponeurotic tissue on the posterior aspect of the rectus abdominis forms the arcuate line of Douglas.

The rectus abdominis forms the central and anchoring muscle mass of the anterior abdomen. The rectus muscle arises from the fifth to the seventh costal cartilages and inserts on to the pubic symphysis and pubic crest. Each rectus muscle is segmented by tendinous intersections at the levels of the xiphoid process and the umbilicus and at a point midway between these 2. The lateral edge of the muscle is demarcated by a slight depression in the aponeurotic fibers, corresponding to the lateral edge of the rectus muscle; this depression is the semilunar line. It marks the site of initial lateral insertion of the aponeurotic tendons of the lateral abdominal muscles.

The composition of the rectus sheath varies depending on axial level of the abdominal wall [5]. The anterior sheath superior to the umbilicus is composed

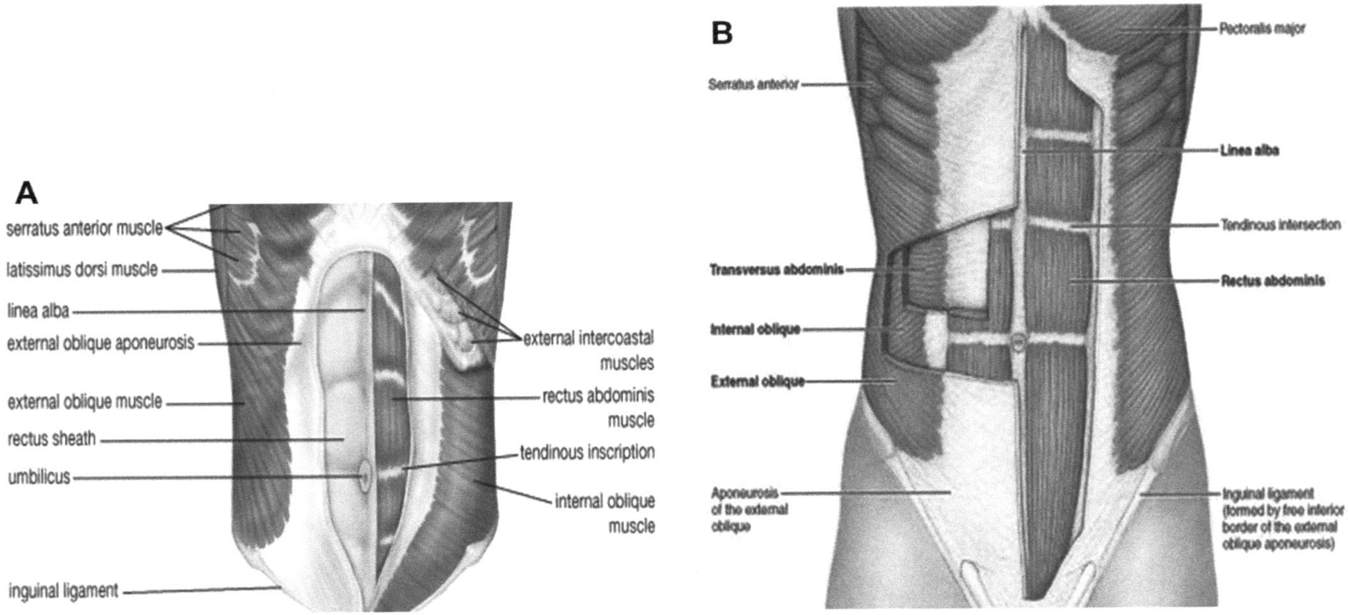

Fig. 2. Abdominal wall musculature (*A*) Superficial layers (*B*) Deep layers.

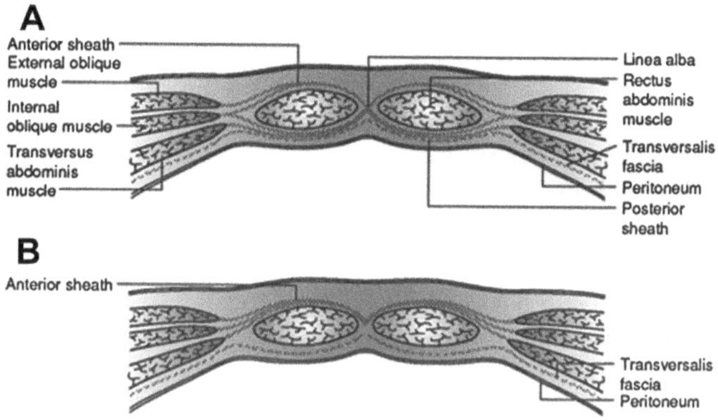

Fig. 3. Composition of rectus sheath above (*A*) and below (*B*) the umbilicus.

of the aponeurosis of the external abdominal oblique and the anterior lamina of the internal abdominal oblique. The transversalis aponeurosis does not participate in the formation of the anterior sheath at this level. The posterior sheath of the rectus muscle superior to the umbilicus is contributed to by the internal abdominal oblique and the transversus abdominis aponeurosis. The external abdominal oblique does not participate in the formation of the posterior portion of the rectus sheath. At a highly variable site inferior to the umbilicus, all the aponeurotic tendons pass anteriorly to form the anterior rectus sheath. The fibers of the posterior sheath are seen to attenuate gradually. This transfer of connective tissue away from the posterior rectus sheath causes the arcuate line of Douglas to form on the posterior surface of the muscle. The tissue covering the deep surface of the rectus muscle inferior to the arcuate line is primarily the transversalis fascia [6]. This anatomic layer is most significant to the surgeon performing a retrorectus hernia repair.

The innervation of the anterior abdominal wall muscles is multiple. The lower intercostal and upper lumbar nerves (T7–T12, L1, L2) contribute most of the innervation to the lateral muscles and the rectus abdominis. The nerves pass anteriorly in a plane between the internal oblique and the transversus abdominis, eventually piercing the lateral aspect of the rectus sheath to innervate the muscle. The external oblique muscle receives branches of the intercostal nerves, which penetrate the internal oblique. The blood supply of the lateral muscles of the anterior wall is primarily from the lower 3 or 4 intercostal arteries, the deep circumflex iliac artery, and the lumbar arteries. The rectus abdominis has a complicated blood supply derived from the superior epigastric artery (a terminal branch of the internal mammary artery), the inferior epigastric artery (a branch of the external iliac artery), and the lower intercostal arteries. The latter arteries enter the sides of the muscle after traveling between the oblique muscles. The superior and inferior epigastric arteries enter the rectus sheath and anastomose near the umbilicus.

DEFINITION OF GIANT VENTRAL HERNIA

There is no consistent or standardized definition of what represents a giant ventral hernia. In the past, ventral hernias have been categorized as large based on the transverse diameter of the defect. However, the critical importance of the definition of a giant ventral hernia is to determine inoperability, so that surgeons can avoid the potentially fatal scenario of being in the operating room with an open abdomen and no options to return the viscera to the abdominal cavity with skin coverage without causing intra-abdominal hypertension. The area of the hernial orifice in relationship to intra-abdominal and hernia sac volumes is more important in determining the severity and complexity of the hernia. Unique to the consideration of giant ventral hernia is the concept of loss of domain. These huge hernias with enormous hernia sacs tend to retain most of the abdominal viscera for prolonged periods. Lack of viscera in the abdominal cavity causes a decrease in abdominal wall muscle elasticity, abdominal wall muscular atrophy, and reduced volume because of disuse.

Decreased intra-abdominal pressure alters the ventilatory equilibrium in these patients, and diaphragmatic descent is often seen. Impaired venous and lymphatic return from long-standing prolapse of the intestines causes edematous thickened bowel, which is difficult to reduce back. In these conditions, forceful replacement of the viscera in the abdominal cavity may prove life-threatening because of development of abdominal compartment syndrome. To objectively quantitate the loss of domain, investigators have tried to calculate the volume of the giant hernia sacs and its ratio with the abdominal cavity volume using multidetector computed tomography scanning. However, these methods need to be validated before widespread application [7].

CAUSE

There are multiple factors that play a role in the development of incisional hernias. Technical flaws at the index operation, including slippage of knots, breakage of sutures, tearing of fascia by sutures, rough handling of tissues, closure of the abdomen under tension, and poor choice of suture material, result in incisional hernias [8]. In addition, several host factors play a role, listed in Box 1 [9,10]. An association between a patient's comorbidities and the incidence of incisional hernia is well known. Genetic factors also play a role. An increased incidence of ventral hernia is noted in certain connective tissue disorders, for example, osteogenesis imperfecta, Marfan syndrome, and Ehlers-Danlos syndrome. Collagen imbalance (type 1–type 3), abnormal matrix metalloproteinase expression, and low growth factor levels are some molecular defects that may be linked to the cause of ventral hernia. A simple incisional hernia may continue to enlarge into a huge complex hernia, reaching a point at which it contains almost all of the abdominal visceral contents. The computed tomographic image shown in Fig. 1 highlights this. Previous unsuccessful attempts at repair of an incisional hernia weaken the abdominal musculature and result in a higher risk of recurrence [11]. Huge ventral hernias may develop after

Box 1: Host factors associated with incisional hernia

Male sex
Old age
Morbid obesity
Abdominal distension
Cigarette smoking
Pulmonary disease
Mechanical ventilation
Type 2 diabetes mellitus
Oral anticoagulants
Malnourishment
Hypoalbuminemia
Anemia/transfusion
Malignancy
Jaundice
Corticosteroid therapy
Chemotherapy
Radiotherapy
Renal failure

extensive resection of the abdominal wall for tumors or massive trauma to the abdominal wall. Intra-abdominal catastrophe requiring serial abdominal washouts and closure achieved by secondary intention or with the aid of split-thickness skin grafts can also result in massive abdominal wall defects.

CLASSIFICATION

To make meaningful decisions about the appropriate management of an incisional hernia, the hernia has to be classified. A classification system developed by experts from the European Hernia Society is shown in Table 1 [6]. Important factors from which ventral hernias are classified are location of hernia, size of defect, reducibility, symptoms, presence or absence of obstruction, and recurrent nature of the hernia. Table 2 shows the Zollinger classification of ventral hernias, which is based on the cause of hernia. Ventral hernias have also been graded depending on the wound status and host factors [12]. Grade 1 (low risk) patients have no previous history of wound infection or comorbidities. Grade 2 patients have comorbidities that predispose to infection but no evidence of ongoing wound infection. These comorbidities include age, smoking history, steroid use, malnutrition, and diabetes mellitus. Grade 3 patients' wounds are contaminated and grade patients 4 have active infection. We recommend customizing the hernia repair based on the grade of hernia.

Table 1
Classification system for incisional hernias

Parameter	Categories
Location	Vertical
	Midline, above or below umbilicus
	Midline, including umbilicus
	Paramedian
	Transverse
	Above or below umbilicus
	Crosses midline
	Oblique
	Above or below umbilicus
	Combined
Size (cm)[a]	<5
	5–10
	>10
Recurrence	Primary
	Multiply recurrent
	Stratification for type of previous repair
Reducibility	Yes
	Obstruction
	No obstruction
	No
	Obstruction
	No obstruction
Symptoms	Asymptomatic
	Symptomatic

[a]Difficult to measure consistently.

CLINICAL PRESENTATION

Most incisional hernias, particularly when reducible, are asymptomatic or cause minimal symptoms, with pain or discomfort when lifting heavy objects, coughing, or standing for long periods. On the other hand, patients with huge ventral hernias (as shown in a clinical image in Fig. 4) can be incapacitated by their hernia because of the presence of a huge pannus, which, in addition to being unsightly, is painful, restricts mobility, commonly causes back problems, and affects respiratory mechanics, with dramatic effects on the functional status and quality of life. These hernias are almost never reducible, not because of the size of the abdominal wall defect but because there has been loss of domain. Some patients may present with a bowel obstruction because the neck of the large hernia sac is very narrow or when there is a Swiss cheese fascial defect pattern. Unique to giant incisional hernias is the patient who has a bowel obstruction caused by factors exclusively within the sac, such as a volvulus or adhesions to the unprotected extra-abdominal bowel caused by inflammation. In this situation, patients can go onto abscess formation or even gangrene and not seem as toxic as patients with more classic intra-abdominal bowel obstructions, presumably because the process becomes relatively isolated from the abdominal cavity proper.

Table 2
Zollinger classification system for ventral abdominal wall hernias

Type	Examples
Congenital	Omphalocele
	Gastroschisis
	Umbilical (infant)
Acquired	Midline
	Diastasis recti
	Epigastric
	Umbilical (adult, acquired, paraumbilical)
	Median
	Supravesical (anterior, posterior, lateral)
	Paramedian
	Spigelian
	Interparietal
Incisional	Midline
	Paramedian
	Transverse
	Special operative sites
Traumatic	Penetrating, autopenetrating[a]
	Blunt
	Focal, minimal injury
	Moderate injury
	Extensive force or shear
	Destructive

[a]Penetration from host tissue such as bone.

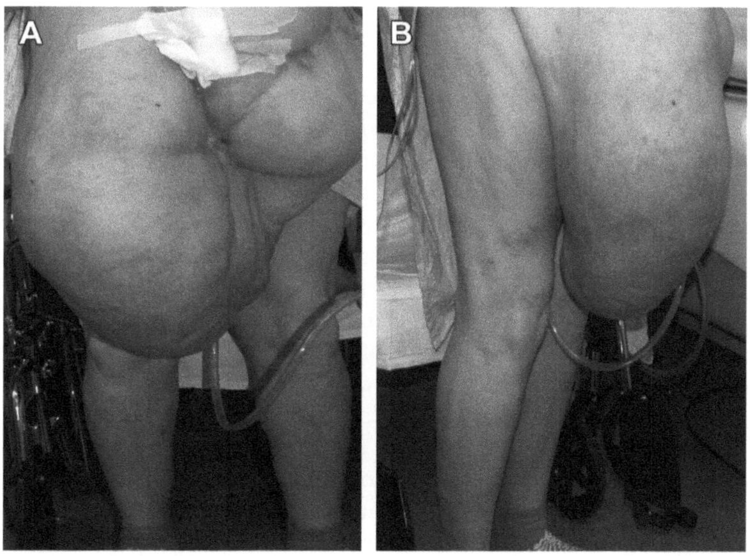

Fig. 4. (*A, B*) Clinical image of a patient with giant ventral hernia with significant loss of domain.

PREOPERATIVE WORKUP

Morbid obesity is a rule rather than exception in patients with giant incisional hernias. Therefore, a comprehensive abdominal wall reconstruction program should include a bariatric arm. A body mass index (BMI) of less than 30 is ideal before repairing the hernia. Incapacitating symptoms or signs of impending bowel obstruction commonly make a prolonged waiting period for weight loss impossible. Because compliance is so poor, bariatric surgery has to be a consideration, but most third-party payers require a minimum of 1 year of supervised weight loss before approving this. Nevertheless, patients need to be thoroughly counseled that the chance of a successful hernia repair is inversely proportional to their BMI and that weight reduction should be the first step.

Before scheduling the patient for surgery, it is vital that any abdominal wall infection (ie, ulceration, open wounds, sinuses, enterocutaneous fistulas, and so forth) must be controlled. This control may entail performing multiple drainage procedures, removal of previous infected prostheses, serial debridements, appropriate wound care, and antibiotics. Because of the large pannus, intertriginous skin problems especially caused by yeast, *Staphylococcus* species and *Corynebacterium* are common and should be treated topically. The complication rate for ventral hernia repair in general is greatly increased in the presence of both clean-contaminated and contaminated cases [13].

All patients with huge ventral hernia must have a computed tomography scan of the abdomen and pelvis to assess the status of the abdominal wall musculature, the defect size, volume of the hernia sac, and also to exclude incidental unsuspected conditions. Some authorities prefer ultrasonography for estimation of the size of the defect [14].

Cardiovascular assessment

Repair of huge ventral hernias is an extensive operation, with a significant operative mortality because of cardiorespiratory complications and pulmonary embolism. The patient experiences a prolonged anesthetic and massive fluid shifts because of third spacing, which continues in the postoperative period. Surgeons are often faced with patients who, despite significant operative risk because of the magnitude of the hernia as well as associated comorbidities, are insistent on having the hernia repaired because their quality of life is so poor that they would rather die than have to continue to live the way they are. Patients should be informed about the potential need for postoperative ventilation, renal failure from intra-abdominal hypertension, and morbidity from wound-related complications. Because most of these operations are performed electively, the cardiopulmonary status of the patient can be thoroughly assessed and medically optimized. Almost all patients should at the minimum undergo pulmonary function studies and stress testing for dynamic cardiac function. Appropriate deep venous thrombosis (DVT) prophylaxis is critical and may even require the placement of a vena cava filter in certain high-risk patients.

PROSTHETIC MATERIAL

A discussion about the repair of a giant incisional hernia is not complete without addressing prosthetic materials. This situation is because prosthesis of some type is always used, except in extenuating circumstances (eg, extensive infection or contamination, allergies, patient refuses foreign material). Use of prosthesis provides a scaffold for ingrowth of fibrous tissue and strengthens the weak abdominal wall. This situation significantly reduces the recurrence rate after incisional hernia repair [15]. Studies have shown that primary suture repair of ventral hernia is associated with a recurrence rate as high as 25% to 55% [3,14]. In a randomized, controlled study from the Netherlands, even small incisional hernias (defects less than 10 cm^2) had a recurrence rate of 67% when primary suture repair was used [16]. In a systematic review published on incisional hernia repairs, recurrence rates ranged from 31% to 63% for direct suture repairs and from 0% to 32% (mostly less than 10%) for prosthetic repairs [17].

In recent years, numerous prosthetic materials have been introduced into the market, making it confusing to decide which should be used. To simplify this situation, the materials can be divided into several classes (ie, noncomposite heavyweight plastic, noncomposite heavyweight membrane, noncomposite lightweight plastic, composite prosthesis, coated prosthesis, absorbable, and biologic). Representative lists of products in each of these categories can be found in Boxes 2 and 3. So how does one decide? Most authorities agree that a synthetic material is preferred over a biologic in the absence of infection or contamination. The choices are between polypropylene (PPL), polyester (PE) or expanded polytetrafluoroethylene (ePTFE). PPL and PE have similar properties and can be used interchangeably. North American surgeons tend to prefer PPL, because they believe that it performs better when considering infection (ie, it less likely to get infected and less likely to have to be explanted when infected), whereas in Europe, PE is more popular, because surgeons there believe that PE has better handling characteristics. ePTFE is commonly referred to as mesh, but it acts more like a membrane. By definition, a mesh has grossly visible interstices (macropores), which allow ingrowth of scar tissue, whereas the pores in ePTFE cannot be seen except microscopically (micropores) and are so small that ingrowth is minimal; therefore, when implanted, the material is encapsulated rather than incorporated, as with a true mesh. The micropores in ePTFE are not so small that they can prevent bacterial penetration and this fact along with the lack of incorporation is believed to be the reason why it is more susceptible to infection and is almost never salvageable when it becomes infected. On the other hand, there is a good side to this lack of incorporation. When placed in contact with intra-abdominal viscera, it does not have a tendency to erode, and fistula formation is almost unheard of. ePTFE is therefore the gold standard material during abdominal wall reconstruction if the prosthesis cannot be isolated from the abdominal cavity and is in contact with the viscera. PPL and PE meshes are contraindicated in this circumstance, because of an unacceptably high incidence or erosion and fistula formation.

Box 2: Commercially available synthetic prostheses for an abdominal wall hernia repair

Noncomposite Heavyweight Plastic Meshes

- Prolene (Ethicon) PPL
- Marlex (Bard) PPL
- SurgiPro (Covidien) PPL
- Parietex (Covidien) PE
- Mersilene (Ethicon) PE

Noncomposite Heavyweight Membranes

- Gore-Tex (W L Gore) polyfluorotetraethylene (ePTFE)
- MotifMesh (Proxy Biomedical)
- Dual Mesh (W L Gore) ePTFE, one side roughened
- Dulex (Bard/Davol) ePTFE, one side roughened

Noncomposite Lightweight Plastic Meshes

- Ultrapro (Ethicon) PP + poliglecaprone-25
- Vipro II (Ethicon) PP + polyglactic acid
- ProLite (Atrium) PPL

Composite Prosthesis (ePTFE + Plastic Mesh)

- ePTFE + heavyweight plastic mesh
    - Composix EX (Bard/Davol) ePTFE + heavyweight PPL
    - Bard Kugel Hernia Patch (Bard/Davol)
    - Ventralex (Bard/Davol)
- ePTFE + lightweight plastic mesh
    - Composix LP (Bard/Davol) ePTFE + lightweight PPL

Coated Prosthesis

- PPL mesh + coating
    - Glucamesh (Brennen) complex carbohydrate, oat β glucan (50 g/m^2)
    - Sepramesh (Genzyme) carboxymethylcellulose-sodium hyaluronate-polyethylene glycol (102 g/m^2)
    - Proceed (Ethicon) polydioxanone-oxidized regenerated cellulose (45 g/m^2)
    - C-Qur (Atrium) omega-3 fatty acid (50 g/m^2)
    - TiMesh (GfE) PP + titanium coat
- PE mesh + coating
    - Parietex composite (Covidien/Sofradim) collagen-polyethylene glycol-glycerol (75 g/m^2)

Absorbable Synthetic

- Polyglactin mesh (Vicryl)
- Polyglycolic acid (Dexon)

Box 3: Commercially available biological prostheses for an abdominal wall hernia repair with approximate price per square centimeter

Human Dermis

- Alloderm (Lifecell) ($26.08)
- Allomax (Bard/Davol) ($26.00)
- Flexhd (MTF)

Porcine Dermis

- Permacol (TSL) (/$8.33)
- Collamend (Bard/Davol) ($16.00)
- Strattice (Lifecell)
- Xenmatrix (Brennan Medical)
- Surgimendtm (TEI Biosciences)

Porcine Small Intestine Submucosa

- Surgisis (Cook) ($3.40)
- Fortagen (Organogenesis)

Fetal Bovine Dermis

- Surgimend (TEI Biosciences) (/$22.00)

Bovine Pericardium

- Tutopatch (Tutogen Medical)
- Veritas (Synovis) ($8.60)

The coated meshes were developed as an alternative to ePTFE when contact with intra-abdominal viscera cannot be avoided. Representative examples along with their specific coating are listed in Box 2. The coating is designed to prevent erosion into viscera. The coating is usually applied only to 1 side of PPL or Polypropylene (PL), with that side facing the viscera and the uncoated side facing the abdominal wall, where ingrowth is desirable. Neither ePTFE nor the coated meshes completely prevent adhesions, as shown by the findings when patients who have had them implanted are reexplored for some reason. It remains to be seen if the coated prosthesis affords the same protection on long-term follow-up as ePTFE, with its long track record of safety.

Lightweight, large-pore prosthetics have become popular in recent years, because they seem to be associated with less chronic discomfort and better abdominal wall mechanics. It is not clear whether the lightweight (eg, less than 35 g/m^2) or the larger pores or both are responsible for this popularity. Regardless, there have been reports of burst mesh with the lightweight material, and therefore, they should be used with caution when considering giant hernias [18].

Another new class of prostheses is the biologics. They are called biologics because they are derived from living tissue (ie, human, porcine, or fetal bovine skin, porcine small intestine submucosa, and bovine pericardium), as shown in Box 3. These donor tissues are processed to remove hair, cells, and cell components as well as other antigens present in the matrix, leaving only the highly organized collagen architecture and surrounding extracellular matrix. In general, these tissues possess the physical and mechanical characteristics of a clinically acceptable synthetic prosthesis, in that they initially have sufficient mechanical strength to withstand the physiologic and anatomic stresses of the abdominal wall and present a biological scaffold to support tissue regeneration. It has been theorized that they might be more physiologic and therefore result in less chronic pain and better recovery than the synthetics, although this theory remains unproved. It seems that they can be safely placed in contact with intra-abdominal viscera and are believed by many authorities to perform better than a synthetic mesh in a contaminated wound. Their major drawback is expense when compared with a synthetic.

OPERATIVE APPROACHES

The basic principles that guide the repair of a giant ventral hernia are modified from those used for simple incisional hernias. However, they almost always include the use of some type of prosthesis, if any chance of success is to be achieved. Rarely, a pure tissue repair can be accomplished using component separation techniques (as discussed later), which are reserved for specific contraindications to a prosthesis such as allergy or the patient's personal preference. Most giant ventral hernias are located in the midline and therefore, for simplicity, the descriptions given later assume this location. The basic principles discussed must be adapted for off-midline or lateral abdominal wall hernias.

Prosthetic material can be positioned in 3 different anatomic planes, as depicted in Fig. 5. An overlay may be placed on top of a simple suture repair, but most authorities believe that it offers minimal advantage over the primary repair and has the same excessive recurrence rates as without a prosthesis [6]. Proponents of the overlay technique mitigate the tension associated with the primary closure by incising the anterior fascia several centimeters lateral to the defect of the hernia, rotating it medially in continuity with the posterior fascia, in effect lengthening the posterior fascia enough to allow for primary closure, isolating the intra-abdominal viscera from the fascia. In the classic procedure described by Chervel, a large synthetic prosthesis widely overlapping the unclosed anterior fascial defect is then placed (Fig. 6) [19].

In the inlay procedure, the prosthesis is circumferentially sutured to the edges of the fascial defect; this was the standard of care for most of the latter half of the twentieth century. It was attractive because it was tension free and easy to perform. Long-term follow-up studies have shown this operation not to be durable, with frequent recurrent herniation at the mesh-tissue interface. It is now considered unacceptable in most instances. However, there

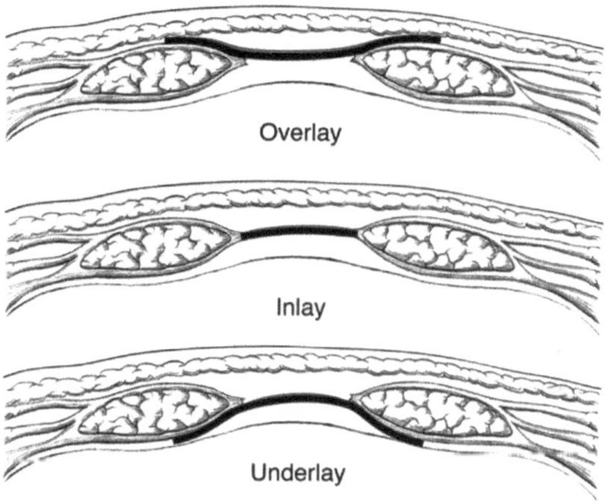

Fig. 5. Various positions for placement of prosthesis during ventral hernia repair.

are situations in which the hernia defect is so large that abdominal wall closure cannot be obtained any other way, even with sophisticated adjuvant strategies such as component separation. It therefore needs to be a part of the armamentarium of the complex abdominal wall reconstruction surgeon. When a hernia defect is bridged, the abdominal viscera must be protected to prevent erosion and subsequent fistula formation. A peritoneal flap constructed from the hernia sac or omentum is sometimes technically possible to isolate the viscera from the abdominal wall. When contact with intra-abdominal organs cannot be avoided, ePTFE or a composite prosthesis is indicated. The coated prosthesis and the biologics also are applicable in this situation but do not have a track record to ensure that erosion into the abdominal viscera does not occur [20].

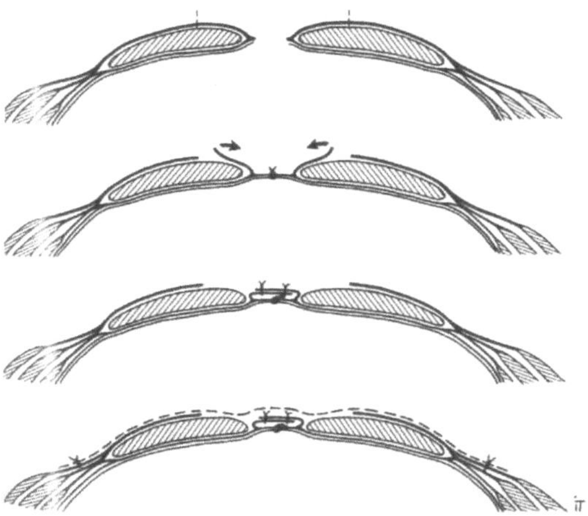

Fig. 6. Chervel technique of ventral hernia repair with the use of overlay mesh.

In addition to the high recurrence rate associated with the inlay mesh repair, even when there is no true recurrence of hernia, many patients perceive that the hernia bulge has come back because of lack of muscular covering overlying the prosthesis, which stretches over time. Therefore, the current gold standard open repair for a midline incisional hernia is primary repair of the posterior rectus sheath followed by reapproximation of the rectus muscles after a prosthesis has been placed behind them. This operation was initially described for treatment of large and multiply recurrent hernias requiring abdominal wall reconstruction but is now being used even for smaller hernias [21]. Minor modifications of the basic procedure have been published by Rives, Stoppa, Velamenta, and others [22,23]. The term Rives-Stoppa technique is commonly used to refer to the procedure in the literature, but retromuscular prosthetic repair is more descriptive and is preferred [24,25]. The operation is characterized by placement of a large prosthesis in the space between the rectus muscle and the posterior fascia or the transversalis fascia, depending on which part of the abdomen is being repaired (ie, there is no posterior fascia below the arcuate line). It involves creating extensive flaps by dissecting the skin and subcutaneous tissue off the external fascia, well lateral to the hernia defect on either side. This strategy often allows the musculoaponeurotic components of the abdominal wall to be advanced to the point at which the posterior and anterior fascial layers can be closed primarily. Once the flaps have been created, the fascia is opened at the edges of the defect, thereby affording entry into the plane between the posterior surface of the deepest muscle and the underlying peritoneum and posterior fascia. A combination of blunt and electrocautery dissection works best for creating a large space to accommodate a sizable prosthesis extending at least 5 cm beyond the defect [26]. The posterior rectus sheaths are approximated to each other primarily if possible. If the posterior sheath cannot be approximated because of tension, then the use of ePTFE or dual-layer prosthesis should be considered instead of the standard mesh. The prosthesis is then placed in the space deep to the muscle and secured in this position with sutures placed via a suture passer at the periphery of the retromuscular pocket (Fig. 7). The sutures pull the prosthesis laterally and firmly affix it to the abdominal wall; they are then tied in the subcutaneous tissue above the fascia. Some surgeons prefer to avoid using these full-thickness sutures because of concern over the possibility of wound pain resulting from neuromuscular entrapment and use sutures or staples to secure the mesh to posterior fascia as far laterally as possible. The retromuscular mesh repair is the most common approach for repair of large incisional hernias.

A laparoscopic repair has now become an accepted technique for ventral hernias, with acceptable short-term and long-term outcomes. However, it has found little place in the repair of huge ventral hernias, because of the wide separation of muscular elements of the abdominal wall. Prosthetic material that is used to bridge a huge gap even when wide overlap can be obtained invariably balloons through the original defect with time, making the patient feel that the hernia has returned. Further contraindicating laparoscopy is the commonly associated

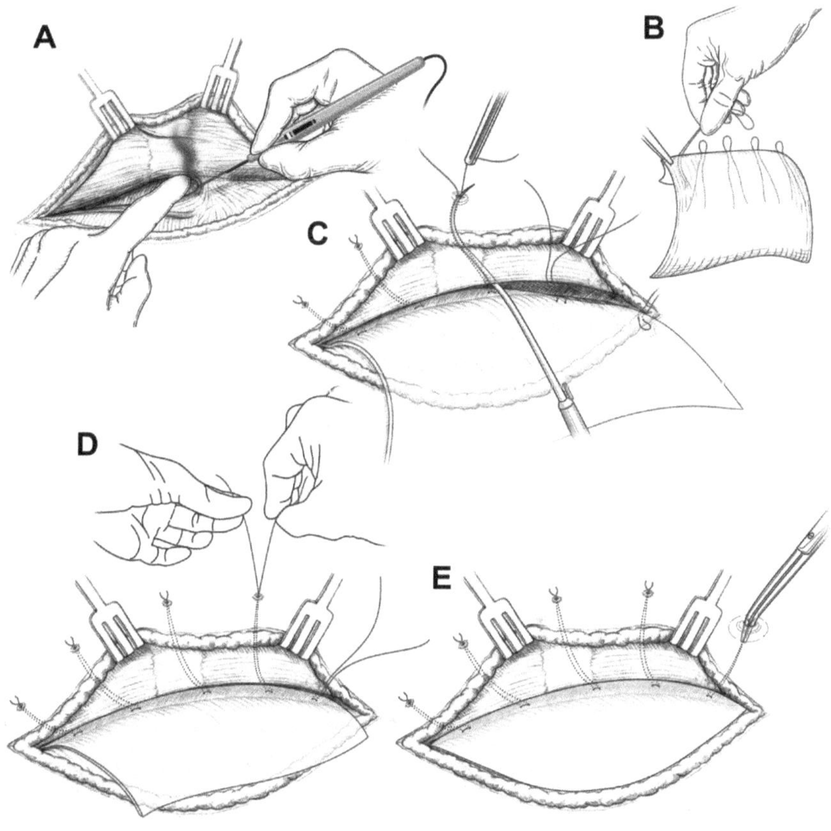

Fig. 7. The technique for placing a prosthesis behind the rectus muscle as described by Flament. (*A*) Creation of the retromuscular space. (*B*) Preparing the prosthesis with sutures with long tails circumferentially. (*C*) A suture passer being used to pass the suture at the periphery of the retromuscular pocket into the subcutaneous plane. (*D*) Sutures tied down in the subcutaneous space, securing the prosthesis to the lateral side of the rectus envelope. (*E*) Final appearance of mesh over the posterior rectus sheath but behind the rectus muscle.

extensive intra-abdominal adhesions caused by multiple previous operations. Laparoscopy can occasionally be helpful as an adjuvant to aid in initial adhesiolysis and to confirm complete fascial closure without incorporation of intra-abdominal viscera at the conclusion of an open procedure. The concepts of minimal invasion for giant ventral hernias have also been applied in the form of endoscopic component separation, which is described in a separate section later.

COMPONENT SEPARATION TECHNIQUE

Closure of rectus sheath commonly fails with giant hernias, with significant loss of domain, because the fascial edges are widely separated from each other. Under such circumstances, there is a role for component separation of the abdominal wall, which allows medialization of the rectus muscles to achieve approximation of the abdominal musculature in the midline.

Component separation was first popularized by Ramirez and colleagues in the 1990s [27]. Several modifications of the operation have been published since then [28–30]. Originally, it was proposed as a tissue repair for incisional hernias with contaminated wounds to avoid the use of a prosthesis. However, this technique is being commonly used synchronously with a sublay prosthesis for repair of huge defects of the abdominal wall [24].

The technique involves making a long midline incision through the scar to expose the hernia. The hernial sac is dissected to the fascial edge. Flaps are fashioned by dissecting the skin and subcutaneous fat off the underlying anterior sheath of the rectus abdominis and the aponeurosis of the external oblique muscle. The aponeurosis of the external oblique muscle is then transected longitudinally, just lateral to the lateral edge of the rectus sheath (Figs. 8 and 9). It is important to extend this incision in the external oblique aponeurosis onto the chest wall at least 5 to 7 cm cranial to the costal margin. The external oblique muscle is separated from the internal oblique muscle as far laterally as possible. This step is safe because the neurovascular bundle (comprising the intercostal nerves and vessels) lies deep to the internal oblique muscle. The result is that the internal oblique muscle and the rectus abdominis muscle slide medially for 7 to 10 cm, so that the edges of the rectus sheath defect can be brought together without undue tension and sutured primarily in the midline [28]. If primary closure is still not possible without undue tension, an additional 2 to 4 cm can be gained by separating the posterior rectus sheath from the rectus abdominis. For very large hernias, transection of the transverse abdominis muscle may give extra gain [31]. Care must be taken not to damage the neurovascular bundle, which runs between the internal oblique muscle and the transversus abdominis to enter the rectus sheath posterolaterally.

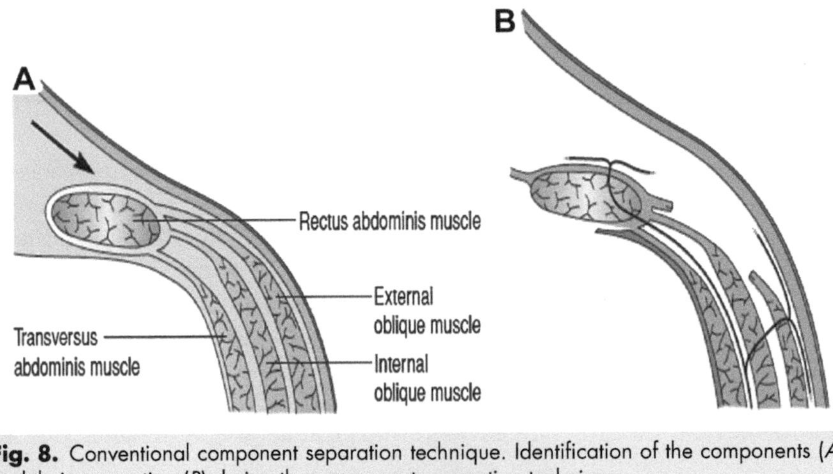

Fig. 8. Conventional component separation technique. Identification of the components (*A*) and their separation (*B*) during the component separation technique.

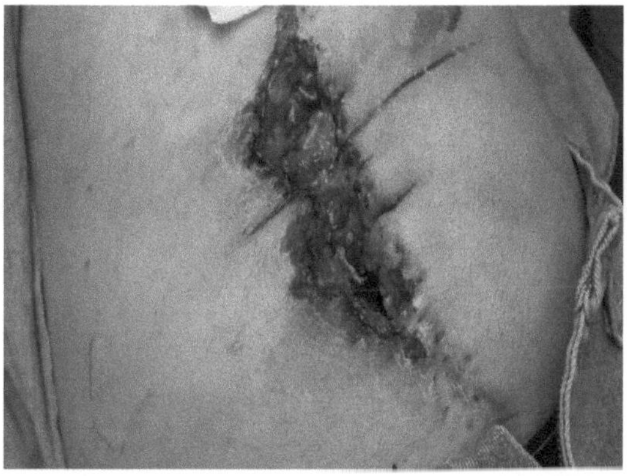

Fig. 9. Clinical picture of a patient who developed ischemia and skin necrosis of the right skin flap after component separation for a giant ventral hernia (note that the left skin flap is viable).

Several investigators have published good outcomes of component separation technique for huge ventral hernias [28,29,32–37]. The rate of recurrence after component separation has been reported to range from 10% to 30% after a 2-year follow-up [38]. Most recurrent hernias after this technique are small and require no further treatment. We believe that to prevent long-term recurrence of hernia, there is a complementary role of mesh alongside the component separation technique, as has been shown by other investigators as well [2,30,39]. A study comparing only component separation versus component separation with overlay of biologics reported a significantly lower recurrence rate in the latter (13% vs 0%) [39]. de Vries Reilingh and colleagues [2] compared component separation technique with prosthetic repair in a randomized controlled trial for patients with giant midline abdominal wall hernias. Recurrence rates were 60% after prosthetic repair versus 53% after component separation during a follow-up of 36 months (statistically no difference). The component separation technique is frequently complicated by wound healing disturbances. Certain modifications of the classic Ramirez technique for component separation have been described to save the blood supply via the periumbilical epigastric perforators to prevent wound breakdown [28,40].

ENDOSCOPIC COMPONENT SEPARATION

Endoscopic component separation was developed to address the well-known wound-related complications of open component separation caused by the large undermining of skin flaps with disruption of the blood supply to the abdominal wall such as seromas, abscesses, or flap necrosis. The technique involves making a 2-cm to 4-cm incision just below the costal margin in the anterior axillary line [41]. This incision must be lateral to the attachment of external oblique aponeurosis to the rectus sheath. Some investigators make this skin incision from within the peritoneal cavity after palpating the lateral border of the rectus sheath [42]. In either case, the space between the external and internal oblique muscle is bluntly dissected out to make space for the dissector balloon (Covidien, Mansfield, MA). Under camera guidance, the dissector balloon is inflated. The balloon bluntly dissects the space between the external oblique and internal oblique muscles lateral to the linea semilunaris and is aided further by carbon dioxide insufflation. The external aponeurosis, which is seen separate from the deeper internal oblique, is then divided from the costal margin to the pubic symphysis using Endo Shears (Covidien, Mansfield, MA).

OTHER SURGICAL OPTIONS

Wide separation of the medial edge of rectus muscle along with an atrophic abdominal wall musculature with huge ventral hernias is sometimes a recipe for failure of abdominal wall reconstruction, even with the combined application of bilateral component separation and the retromuscular prosthesis. Often, the volume of hernia sac exceeds the volume in the abdominal cavity. Closure of the abdominal wall under such circumstances has a high risk of intra-abdominal hypertension and abdominal compartment syndrome [43]. For such complex cases; it is always wise to plan backup options.

MEDIALIZATION

A recent study of a small series of patients (n = 8) proposed a medialization procedure that consists of temporary closure of the abdominal wall with ePTFE followed by scheduled serial visits to the operating room to tighten the prosthesis by excising a strip in the middle and then suturing the edges together [44]. Definitive closure of the abdominal wall was achieved using component separation after a mean 6 serial visits to the operating room in this study.

ROLE OF PROGRESSIVE PNEUMOPERITONEUM PRECEDING VENTRAL HERNIA REPAIR

The use of preoperative progressive pneumoperitoneum (PPP) for repair of huge incisional hernias was first described by Goni Moreno in 1940 [45]. PPP stretches the abdominal cavity by increasing the length of the abdominal muscles and the diaphragm [46–48]. Room air (or CO_2) is injected intraperitoneally daily via a needle or an implantable catheter with or without a subcutaneous port, to tolerance (ie, development of shoulder pain, difficulty breathing, or development of subcutaneous emphysema). Patients or family members are taught to administer this injection so that the procedure can be performed as an outpatient. Some surgeons prefer to use pressure monitoring, keeping less than 15 mm Hg, but this complicates the technique because of the need for in-hospital monitoring. In addition to increasing the capacity of the abdominal cavity, pneumoperitoneum may also cause adhesiolysis and improve diaphragmatic function.

PPP has been more commonly applied in Europe with good results for large ventral hernias [49,50]. In a recent study, safety and feasibility of this approach were shown in 16 patients [51]. Nonetheless, 7 of these 16 patients still required ileocectomy or lateral relaxing incision on the rectus sheath to achieve abdominal wall closure. In another small series of 9 patients, pneumoperitoneum was sufficient to reduce the visceral contents, permitting a retrorectus repair in 80% patients [52]. Of 9 patients, 1 patient with diabetes mellitus developed an abdominal wall abscess requiring drainage in the postoperative period. Many surgeons in North America are skeptical about the approach, questioning how one ensures that the air injected stays in the peritoneal cavity and does not leak into the hernia sac, enlarging it further. Also of concern is the possibility of infection and the cost, especially if in-hospital monitoring is needed.

ROLE OF FLAPS AND GRAFTS

The use of flaps and dermal grafts for abdominal wall reconstruction is usually reserved for patients in whom the conventional component separation repair with a retromuscular prosthesis is not feasible. Most experience has been with fascia lata, which has been shown to retain its shape and tensile strength for an extended period [53]. Harvesting is easy and donor-site morbidity is low (13%–17%). A longitudinal incision on the lateral thigh is used to dissect the fascia from the fascia lata muscle. Girotto and colleagues [34] used free fascia lata grafts along with component separation to repair very large, contaminated abdominal wall defects in 78 patients. Wound infection occurred in 32 patients, with recurrence in 29% of the patients after a follow-up of 6 months. Full-thickness skin has been used to bridge fascial defects for incisional hernia repair. Autodermal grafts are easily available because of the redundant skin overlying the hernia, and its harvesting does not increase morbidity. After the harvest, the subcutaneous layer is removed and the graft is placed with the dermis toward the peritoneal contents. A wound complication rate of 20% has been reported without any complications from overgrowth of adnexal skin structures [14].

Pedicled or free vascularized flaps are used as the last resort, because these are complex procedures and leave large donor-site defects, causing additional morbidity. The tensor fasciae latae (TFL) pedicle flap is most commonly used for lower abdominal wall hernias, because it combines well-vascularized tissue with a strong fascia that can resist intra-abdominal pressure. Williams and colleagues [54] reconstructed abdominal wall defects in 9 patients with a pedicled TFL flap; in 5 patients, there was a contaminated or infected environment. Three flaps needed revision because of flap necrosis. Donor-site morbidity was 50%. There were no recurrences after a mean follow-up of 21 months. Harpf and colleagues [55] used this flap in 4 patients. After a follow-up of more than 11 months, none of the patients had a reherniation. Other flap options for the lower abdomen include a rectus femoris flap, a gracilis, or a vastus lateralis flap. The rectus femoris myocutaneous flap is a long but narrow flap that can be used to repair defects in the lower abdomen. It is pedicled on the lateral circumflex femoral artery. Caulfield and colleagues [56] reconstructed 13 abdominal hernias with this flap. Only 2 had major complications: hematoma and loss of a split skin graft at the donor site. There were no recurrences after a follow-up of 3 to 18 months. A significant loss of muscle strength during knee flexion was noted after flap harvest. For the upper abdomen, the workhorse is the latissimus dorsi flap.

Free flaps represent the next level in extraordinary strategies for abdominal wall reconstruction. Upper abdominal defects may be repaired using a free vascularized TFL flap. The results using this free flap have been described in 4 retrospective case series containing a total of 20 patients [38]. Partial flap necrosis was seen in 5 of 20 patients. A free latissimus dorsi flap for abdominal wall defects has also been used [57]. Anterolateral thigh and rectus femoris have all been described in the literature. Abdominal wall transplantation represents the extreme when considering free flaps and has been reported [58].

TISSUE EXPANSION

Tissue expanders can be used in cases in which either skin or the myofascial elements of the abdominal wall are deficient [59]. They are implanted subcutaneously or subfascially, depending on the tissue needed. The expanders are then gradually inflated until the desired amount of extra tissue is obtained. The limitation of the technique is the delay in definitive repair while the expansion is ongoing and the considerable amount of pain that patients complain of. The intra-abdominal placement of tissue expanders has also been described to address the issue of loss of domain, but this is primarily confined to the pediatric literature [60].

RESECTION OF INTRA-ABDOMINAL VISCERA

There are situations when, despite applying all these techniques, even the most experienced surgeon is not able to replace the abdominal contents and close the fascia without causing significant increase of intra-abdominal pressure. In these circumstances, that the last resort of the surgeon is to resect intra-abdominal viscera to reduce the volume needing to be reduced. The options include performing total omentectomy, subtotal colectomy, and removal of retroperitoneal fat. The downside of opening the gastrointestinal tract is the lack of freedom in using all possible prosthesis in such a wound, especially if there is any contamination.

COMPLICATIONS OF GIANT VENTRAL HERNIA REPAIR

In a meta-analysis, the overall complication rate after open ventral hernia repair was 27% (Box 4) [61]. Prosthesis-related infection remains a major problem repair and is one of the most important risk factors for recurrence. The chance of prosthesis infection is increased with preexisting infection, skin ulceration, obesity, incarceration, and enterotomy during repair. Seromas, which can lead to infection, are a common occurrence, as a result of extensive flap dissection and the large prosthesis required for giant incisional hernias. Suction drains are useful but are likely to result in prosthesis infection if left in place too long. Topical instillation of talc, tetracycline, and numerous other agents

Box 4: Complications of giant ventral hernia repair

Postoperative Complications
Bleeding
Postoperative ileus
Myocardial infarction
Deep venous thrombosis
Pulmonary thromboembolism
Enterocutaneous fistula

Complications Caused by Loss of Domain
Abdominal compartment syndrome
Renal failure
Need for prolonged ventilation

Wound-Related Complications
Seroma
Ischemia of the skin flaps
Skin necrosis
Skin ulceration
Wound infection
Prosthesis infection
Dehiscence (superficial or deep)

Long-Term Complications
Recurrence

has been tried to prevent or decrease seroma formation, but none has been shown to be consistently effective.

Lowe and colleagues [35] retrospectively looked at the complications after reconstruction of abdominal wall defects with component separation. The commonest complications seen were postoperative ileus (27%), cardiorespiratory complications (46% cumulative), wound ischemia (20%), wound infection (40%), and enterocutaneous fistula (43%). Other investigators have also reported wound complication rate as high as 30% to 50% [2,28,35,62]. In a systematic review of studies looking at the outcomes of component separation, wound complications were seen in 85 of the cumulative 354 patients (23.8%, confidence intervals 18.3 to 29.8%) [38]. Wound infection was the most common complication found in 18.9%, seroma in 2.4% hematoma in 2.4%, and skin necrosis in 1.5%. High rates of wound-related complications after component separation are caused by extremely large wound surfaces, which are formed by mobilization of the skin and subcutaneous fascia from abdominal wall muscles. The other explanation is division of perforator vessels while raising these flaps, which causes ischemia, skin necrosis, and infection. Perforators are vital for the abdominal wall, because blood supply by the intercostals, superficial circumflex iliac and external pudendal vessels is often already compromised from previous incisions.

SUMMARY

Repair of huge ventral hernias is technically challenging for the surgeon and a major operation for the patient and should be performed by experienced surgeons in centers that are used to caring for patients who are commonly massively obese with significant comorbidities. Preoperative medical optimization of patients is an important part in the overall management of these large hernias. Conventional component separation with retromuscular mesh repair is the workhorse operation, which successfully deals with many giant ventral hernias, but multiple alternative strategies must be available to address situations in which myofascial elements are completely deficient or there is significant loss of domain The complexity of this surgery is reflected by recurrence rates ranging from 10% to 30% and wound complication rates as high as 40% to 50% in experienced centers.

References

[1] Rutkow IM. Epidemiologic, economic, and sociologic aspects of hernia surgery in the United States in the 1990s. Surg Clin North Am 1998;78(6):941–51, v–vi.
[2] de Vries Reilingh TS, van Goor H, Charbon JA, et al. Repair of giant midline abdominal wall hernias: "components separation technique" versus prosthetic repair: interim analysis of a randomized controlled trial. World J Surg 2007;31(4):756–63.
[3] Luijendijk RW, Hop WC, van den Tol MP, et al. A comparison of suture repair with mesh repair for incisional hernia. N Engl J Med 2000;343(6):392–8.
[4] Carlson MA, Ludwig KA, Condon RE. Ventral hernia and other complications of 1,000 midline incisions. South Med J 1995;88(4):450–3.
[5] Richard AT, Quinn TH, Fitzgibbons RJ. Abdominal wall hernias. In: Mulholland MW, editor. Greenfield's surgery: scientific principles and practice. 5th edition. Philadelphia: Lippincott Williams & Wilkins; 2010. p. 1159–98.
[6] Korenkov M, Paul A, Sauerland S, et al. Classification and surgical treatment of incisional hernia. Results of an experts' meeting. Langenbecks Arch Surg 2001;386(1):65–73.
[7] Agnew SP, Small W Jr, Wang E, et al. Prospective measurements of intra-abdominal volume and pulmonary function after repair of massive ventral hernias with the components separation technique. Ann Surg 2010;251(5):981–8.
[8] Sanders RJ, DiClementi D. Principles of abdominal wound closure. II. Prevention of wound dehiscence. Arch Surg 1977;112(10):1188–91.
[9] Chan G, Chan CK. A review of incisional hernia repairs: preoperative weight loss and selective use of the mesh repair. Hernia 2005;9(1):37–41.
[10] Millikan KW. Incisional hernia repair. Surg Clin North Am 2003;83(5):1223–34.
[11] Flum DR, Horvath K, Koepsell T. Have outcomes of incisional hernia repair improved with time? A population-based analysis. Ann Surg 2003;237(1):129–35.
[12] Ventral Hernia Working Group, Breuing K, Butler CE, Ferzoco S, et al. Incisional ventral hernias: review of the literature and recommendations regarding the grading and technique of repair. Surgery 2010;148(3):544–58.

[13] Choi JJ, Palaniappa NC, Dallas KB, et al. Use of mesh during ventral hernia repair in clean-contaminated and contaminated cases: outcomes of 33,832 cases. Ann Surg 2012;255(1):176–80.
[14] Korenkov M, Sauerland S, Arndt M, et al. Randomized clinical trial of suture repair, polypropylene mesh or autodermal hernioplasty for incisional hernia. Br J Surg 2002;89(1):50–6.
[15] Paajanen H, Hermunen H. Long-term pain and recurrence after repair of ventral incisional hernias by open mesh: clinical and MRI study. Langenbecks Arch Surg 2004;389(5): 366–70.
[16] Burger JW, Luijendijk RW, Hop WC, et al. Long-term follow-up of a randomized controlled trial of suture versus mesh repair of incisional hernia. Ann Surg 2004;240(4):578–83 [discussion: 583–5].
[17] Cassar K, Munro A. Surgical treatment of incisional hernia. Br J Surg 2002;89(5):534–45.
[18] Schippers E. Central mesh rupture–myth or real concern?. In: Schumpelick V, Fitzgibbons R, editors. Recurrent hernia: prevention and treatment. Berlin: Springer-Verlag; 2007. p. 371–6.
[19] Licheri S, Erdas E, Pisano G, et al. Chevrel technique for midline incisional hernia: still an effective procedure. Hernia 2008;12(2):121–6.
[20] Fitzgibbons RJ, Richards A, Quinn TH. Open repair of abdominal wall hernia. In: ACS surgery: principles and practice. 6th edition. Hamilton (Ontario): Decker; 2007.
[21] Flament JB, Palot JP, Burde A. Treatment of major incisional hernias. Probl Gen Surg 1995;12:151.
[22] Temudom T, Siadati M, Sarr MG. Repair of complex giant or recurrent ventral hernias by using tension-free intraparietal prosthetic mesh (Stoppa technique): lessons learned from our initial experience (fifty patients). Surgery 1996;120(4):738–43 [discussion: 743–4].
[23] Wantz GE. Incisional hernioplasty with mersilene. Surg Gynecol Obstet 1991;172(2): 129–37.
[24] Cox TC, Pearl JP, Ritter EM. Rives-Stoppa incisional hernia repair combined with laparoscopic separation of abdominal wall components: a novel approach to complex abdominal wall closure. Hernia 2010;14(6):561–7.
[25] Yaghoobi Notash A, Yaghoobi Notash A Jr, Seied Farshi J, et al. Outcomes of the Rives-Stoppa technique in incisional hernia repair: ten years of experience. Hernia 2007;11(1):25–9.
[26] Klinge U, Conze J, Krones CJ, et al. Incisional hernia: open techniques. World J Surg 2005;29(8):1066–72.
[27] Ramirez OM, Ruas E, Dellon AL. "Components separation" method for closure of abdominal-wall defects: an anatomic and clinical study. Plast Reconstr Surg 1990;86(3): 519–26.
[28] de Vries Reilingh TS, van Goor H, Rosman C, et al. "Components separation technique" for the repair of large abdominal wall hernias. J Am Coll Surg 2003;196(1):32–7.
[29] Ennis LS, Young JS, Gampper TJ, et al. The "open-book" variation of component separation for repair of massive midline abdominal wall hernia. Am Surg 2003;69(9):733–42 [discussion: 742–3].
[30] Kolker AR, Brown DJ, Redstone JS, et al. Multilayer reconstruction of abdominal wall defects with acellular dermal allograft (AlloDerm) and component separation. Ann Plast Surg 2005;55(1):36–41 [discussion: 41–2].
[31] Ewart CJ, Lankford AB, Gamboa MG. Successful closure of abdominal wall hernias using the components separation technique. Ann Plast Surg 2003;50(3):269–73 [discussion: 273–4].
[32] DiBello JN Jr, Moore JH Jr. Sliding myofascial flap of the rectus abdominus muscles for the closure of recurrent ventral hernias. Plast Reconstr Surg 1996;98(3):464–9.
[33] Cohen M, Morales R Jr, Fildes J, et al. Staged reconstruction after gunshot wounds to the abdomen. Plast Reconstr Surg 2001;108(1):83–92.

[34] Girotto JA, Chiaramonte M, Menon NG, et al. Recalcitrant abdominal wall hernias: long-term superiority of autologous tissue repair. Plast Reconstr Surg 2003;112(1):106–14.
[35] Lowe JB 3rd, Lowe JB, Baty JD, et al. Risks associated with "components separation" for closure of complex abdominal wall defects. Plast Reconstr Surg 2003;111(3):1276–83 [quiz: 1284–5]; [discussion: 1286–8].
[36] Shestak KC, Edington HJ, Johnson RR. The separation of anatomic components technique for the reconstruction of massive midline abdominal wall defects: anatomy, surgical technique, applications, and limitations revisited. Plast Reconstr Surg 2000;105(2):731–8 [quiz: 739].
[37] van Geffen HJ, Simmermacher RK, van Vroonhoven TJ, et al. Surgical treatment of large contaminated abdominal wall defects. J Am Coll Surg 2005;201(2):206–12.
[38] de Vries Reilingh TS, Bodegom ME, van Goor H, et al. Autologous tissue repair of large abdominal wall defects. Br J Surg 2007;94(7):791–803.
[39] Espinosa-de-los-Monteros A, de la Torre JI, Marrero I, et al. Utilization of human cadaveric acellular dermis for abdominal hernia reconstruction. Ann Plast Surg 2007;58(3):264–7.
[40] Maas SM, van Engeland M, Leeksma NG, et al. A modification of the "components separation" technique for closure of abdominal wall defects in the presence of an enterostomy. J Am Coll Surg 1999;189(1):138–40.
[41] Rosen MJ, Jin J, McGee MF, et al. Laparoscopic component separation in the single-stage treatment of infected abdominal wall prosthetic removal. Hernia 2007;11(5):435–40.
[42] Maas SM, de Vries RS, van Goor H, et al. Endoscopically assisted "components separation technique" for the repair of complicated ventral hernias. J Am Coll Surg 2002;194(3):388–90.
[43] Munegato G, Brandolese R. Respiratory physiopathology in surgical repair for large incisional hernias of the abdominal wall. J Am Coll Surg 2001;192(3):298–304.
[44] Lipman J, Medalie D, Rosen MJ. Staged repair of massive incisional hernias with loss of abdominal domain: a novel approach. Am J Surg 2008;195(1):84–8.
[45] Moreno IG. Chronic eventrations and large hernias; preoperative treatment by progressive pneumoperitomeum; original procedure. Surgery 1947;22(6):945–53.
[46] Buddee FW, Coupland GA, Reeve TS. Large abdominal wall herniae: an easy method of repair without prosthetic material, with the induction of pneumoperitoneum. Aust N Z J Surg 1975;45(3):265–70.
[47] Caldironi MW, Romano M, Bozza F, et al. Progressive pneumoperitoneum in the management of giant incisional hernias: a study of 41 patients. Br J Surg 1990;77(3):306–7.
[48] Coelho JC, Brenner AS, Freitas AT, et al. Progressive preoperative pneumoperitoneum in the repair of large abdominal hernias. Eur J Surg 1993;159(6–7):339–41.
[49] Raynor RW, Del Guercio LR. The place for pneumoperitoneum in the repair of massive hernia. World J Surg 1989;13(5):581–5.
[50] Toniato A, Pagetta C, Bernante P, et al. Incisional hernia treatment with progressive pneumoperitoneum and retromuscular prosthetic hernioplasty. Langenbecks Arch Surg 2002;387(5–6):246–8.
[51] Mayagoitia JC, Suarez D, Arenas JC, et al. Preoperative progressive pneumoperitoneum in patients with abdominal-wall hernias. Hernia 2006;10(3):213–7.
[52] Dumont F, Fuks D, Verhaeghe P, et al. Progressive pneumoperitoneum increases the length of abdominal muscles. Hernia 2009;13(2):183–7.
[53] Peacock EE Jr. Subcutaneous extraperitoneal repair of ventral hernias: a biological basis for fascial transplantation. Ann Surg 1975;181(5):722–7.
[54] Williams JK, Carlson GW, deChalain T, et al. Role of tensor fasciae latae in abdominal wall reconstruction. Plast Reconstr Surg 1998;101(3):713–8.
[55] Harpf C, Ninkovic M, Kronberger P, et al. Dynamic and functional abdominal wall stabilization, reconstruction of extensive abdominal wall defects. Chirurg 1997;68(5):488–92 [in German].

[56] Caulfield WH, Curtsinger L, Powell G, et al. Donor leg morbidity after pedicled rectus femoris muscle flap transfer for abdominal wall and pelvic reconstruction. Ann Plast Surg 1994;32(4):377–82.
[57] Houston GC, Drew GS, Vazquez B, et al. The extended latissimus dorsi flap in repair of anterior abdominal wall defects. Plast Reconstr Surg 1988;81(6):917–24.
[58] Cipriani R, Contedini F, Santoli M, et al. Abdominal wall transplantation with microsurgical technique. Am J Transplant 2007;7(5):1304–7.
[59] Van Geffen HJ, Simmermacher RK. Incisional hernia repair: abdominoplasty, tissue expansion, and methods of augmentation. World J Surg 2005;29(8):1080–5.
[60] Clifton MS, Heiss KF, Keating JJ, et al. Use of tissue expanders in the repair of complex abdominal wall defects. J Pediatr Surg 2011;46(2):372–7.
[61] Goodney PP, Birkmeyer CM, Birkmeyer JD. Short-term outcomes of laparoscopic and open ventral hernia repair: a meta-analysis. Arch Surg 2002;137(10):1161–5.
[62] Harth KC, Rosen MJ. Endoscopic versus open component separation in complex abdominal wall reconstruction. Am J Surg 2010;199(3):342–6 [discussion: 346 7].

Advances in Surgery 47 (2013) 29–43
ADVANCES IN SURGERY

Laparoscopic Colon Resection

Is It Being Utilized?

Sean Joseph Langenfeld, MD, Jon S. Thompson, MD*, Dmitry Oleynikov, MD

Department of Surgery, University of Nebraska Medical Center, 983280 Nebraska Medical Center, Omaha, NE 68198-3280, USA

Keywords

• Laparoscopy • Colectomy • Laparoscopic colectomy • Trends • Utilization • Colon cancer • Learning curve

Key points

- Laparoscopic colectomy is safe and effective in the treatment of benign and malignant diseases, and offers several short-term and long-term benefits over the open approach.
- The use of laparoscopy for colon resections was initially low, but newer studies show a use rate of 40% to 50% with a conversion rate of 10% to 20%.
- Disparities in laparoscopic colectomy still exist and are based on multiple patient, surgeon, and hospital factors.
- Roadblocks to use include a steep learning curve, a possible lack of adequate operative volume, and variable hospital support.
- The future includes an increased role of laparoscopy in rectal surgery, and an increased role for emerging technologies such as robotics and natural orifice surgery.

Laparoscopic colon resection was first described in 1991 [1,2]. At the time, the investigators cited the enthusiasm and widespread adoption of laparoscopy to treat gallbladder and appendiceal disease as an impetus for exploring its usefulness in colon surgery. Over the next 10 years, numerous other publications further explored the use of laparoscopy to treat benign and malignant diseases of the colon. However, open colectomy remained the

Disclosures: The authors have no relevant financial disclosures.

*Corresponding author. *E-mail address*: jthompso@unmc.edu

0065-3411/13/$ – see front matter
http://dx.doi.org/10.1016/j.yasu.2013.02.003

dominant approach, and concerns about the safety and efficacy of laparoscopic colectomy arose.

Since that time, multiple well-designed randomized controlled trials (RCTs) have shown laparoscopic colectomy to be safe and effective. Despite this situation, early studies suggested that the use of laparoscopy remained low. Variability in the definition of laparoscopic colectomy as well as a lack of appropriate procedure codes limited the accuracy of these studies, and the true level of use remained largely unknown.

With more standardized definitions and the presence of dedicated procedure codes, the use of laparoscopy for colonic disease can now be accurately predicted, and nationwide trends can be assessed. This article explores the safety and efficacy of laparoscopic colectomy, provides an accurate estimate of its current use, and identifies epidemiologic factors affecting implementation. In addition, potential roadblocks to use are explored, current areas of controversy are discussed, and opinion on the future of minimally invasive colon surgery is provided.

COMPLEX VERSUS SIMPLE LAPAROSCOPY

Cholecystectomy is an example of changing trends in the use of laparoscopy. After laparoscopic cholecystectomy was proven to be safe and effective, there was an increase in its use in both urban and rural hospital settings [3]. A study of the Nationwide Inpatient Sample (NIS) showed an increase in elective laparoscopic cholecystectomies from 3.5% in 1989 to 73.7% in 1992. The same study showed an increase in the use of laparoscopy for urgent cholecystectomy from 4.9% in 1990 to 54.6% in 1992. The investigators interpreted these data to represent a short learning curve of approximately 1 year, after which surgeons became more comfortable applying a laparoscopic approach to urgent cases.

Just a few years after laparoscopic cholecystectomy was introduced, it had become the standard of care. Although enthusiasm for laparoscopic colon resections was high in select circles, this procedure did not experience the same increase in use that was shown for cholecystectomy (Fig. 1). Many believed laparoscopic cholecystectomy to be a technically more simple operation with an easier learning curve. Operative steps were more limited and operative times were shorter for cholecystectomy. Retraction was easier for cholecystectomy, and there was less need for an experienced assistant such as a resident or surgical partner. Although colectomy required working in multiple quadrants, cholecystectomy was limited to a single quadrant with less need for changes in the camera and angles.

In addition to the perception that laparoscopic colectomy was technically more difficulty, there was also concern that a laparoscopic approach to colon cancer would compromise oncologic principles and possibly lead to an inferior oncologic outcome. A fear existed that laparoscopic colectomy would result in smaller specimen sizes and would hinder high ligation of blood vessels and adequate nodal sampling. There were also multiple studies that reported tumor

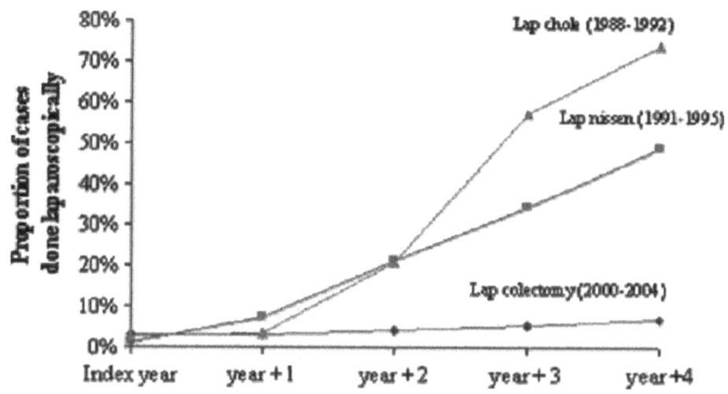

Fig. 1. Trend in proportion of cases performed laparoscopically over a similar 5-year to 7-year period, in which the index year is the year that the proportion of cases performed laparoscopically was greater than 3%. (*From* Kemp JA, Finlayson SR. Nationwide trends in laparoscopic colectomy from 2000 to 2004. Surg Endosc 2008;22:1183; with permission.)

recurrence at the laparoscopic port sites [4,5], one of which reported tumor recurrence in 3 of 14 patients [6]. Other studies showed incisional recurrence after laparoscopy to be equivalent to open colectomy at approximately 1% [7,8], but large prospective studies were lacking.

THE FIRST STEP: PROVING OUTCOMES OF LAPAROSCOPIC SURGERY ARE EQUIVALENT TO OPEN SURGERY

Many of the early questions regarding the safety and efficacy of laparoscopic colectomy were answered in the early 2000s. Several well-designed RCTs were conducted comparing open and laparoscopic colectomy for cancer.

The COST (Clinical Outcomes of Surgical Therapy) trial was initiated in 1994 and published in 2004 [9]. This trial was a large collaborative effort involving multiple centers across North America, which became a landmark study addressing laparoscopic colectomy for colon cancer. This prospective RCT involved 872 patients, with a median follow-up of 4.4 years. It showed laparoscopic colectomy to be noninferior to open colectomy in regards to recurrence rate, time to recurrence, and overall survival. This study also found no significant difference in complication rate or 30-day mortality between the 2 groups. In addition, patients in the laparoscopic colectomy group had a significantly shorter median hospital stay and a shorter duration of narcotic use.

The COLOR (Colon Cancer Laparoscopic or Open Resection) trial was a multicenter European RCT initially published in 2005, with long-term follow-up reported in 2009 [10,11]. It looked at 1076 patients with colon cancer and showed laparoscopic colectomy to be equivalent to the open approach in terms of specimen length and number of lymph nodes harvested. It also showed equivalent 3-year survival between the 2 groups. The laparoscopic group had a quicker recovery of bowel function with decreased narcotic use and decreased length of stay.

The MRC CLASICC trial (UK Medical Research Council trial of conventional vs laparoscopic-assisted surgery) was initially published in 2005 [12]. This was a multicenter UK trial similar in design to the COST trial. It involved 794 patients with colon or rectal cancer randomized to either open or laparoscopic resection. The initial publication had a short median follow-up, but subsequent 3-year and 5-year follow-up results were published [13,14]. This trial once again showed equivalent recurrence rates, disease-free survival, and overall survival for open and laparoscopic colectomies for colon cancer. It also reported a port-site recurrence rate of 2.4% in the laparoscopic group.

An important aspect of the MRC CLASICC trial was that it included patients with rectal cancer, whereas these patients were excluded from the COST and COLOR trials. Patients undergoing laparoscopic low anterior resection for rectal cancer had a nonsignificant trend toward an increased positive circumferential resection margin compared with open surgery (12.4% vs 6.3%, $P = .19$). In addition, there was a high conversion rate to open surgery of 34%. This situation led to an initial conclusion that routine laparoscopic low anterior resection for rectal cancer could not be justified. However, 3-year and 5-year follow-up studies showed that there was no difference in local recurrence, disease-free survival, or overall survival between the open and laparoscopic groups.

A subsequent Cochrane review assessing the long-term outcomes of laparoscopic colectomy for colon cancer was performed [15]. This review reported 33 RCTs, 12 of which had long-term follow-up. This review concluded that recurrence rates and long-term outcomes are equivalent between laparoscopic and open surgery for colon cancer.

In addition to oncologic equivalence, another Cochrane review of 25 RCTs looked at short-term outcomes after surgery and determined that incisional hernia rates and reoperation rates were equivalent between open and laparoscopic colectomy. Rates of deep vein thrombosis and cardiopulmonary complications were also similar [16].

OTHER BENEFITS OF LAPAROSCOPY

The COST trial reported that patients who underwent laparoscopic colectomy had a shorter median hospital stay and a shorter duration of narcotic use than the open colectomy group. In addition, this study showed a modest but significant improvement in quality-of-life scores [17].

Other benefits of laparoscopy have been described at length. The previously mentioned Cochrane review of short-term outcomes after surgery evaluated pooled data from 25 RCTs in an attempt to summarize these benefits [15]. Compared with open surgery, laparoscopic colectomy showed decreased pain intensity, decreased postoperative ileus, improved pulmonary function, decreased length of stay, decreased surgical site infections, and decreased total morbidity. Duepree and colleagues [18] in 2003 looked at their single-center experience retrospectively and found that compared with open surgery, laparoscopic bowel resection was associated with lower incidences of incisional hernia

(12.9% vs 2.4%) and small bowel obstruction requiring hospitalization and conservative management (6.1% vs 1.9%).

ASSESSMENTS OF NATIONWIDE TRENDS IN USE

Once laparoscopic colectomy was proved to be safe and effective with several short-term advantages over open surgery, the next step was to encourage widespread implementation. However, early reports on use had disappointing results.

Kemp and Finlayson used the NIS to look at trends in use of laparoscopic colectomy before the publication of the COST trial [19]. These investigators reported that the proportion of elective colectomies being performed laparoscopically increased from 3% in 2000 to 6.5% in 2004. For 2004, they calculated that 8.2% of colectomies for benign disease were laparoscopic, whereas the rate in cancer surgery was 4.3%. At that time, there were not distinct codes for laparoscopic colectomy within the *International Classification of Diseases, Ninth Revision, Clinical Modification* (ICD-9-CM). Instead, the investigators identified cases using procedure modifier codes for laparoscopy (54.21) or laparoscopic lysis of adhesions (54.51).

Steele and colleagues [20] in 2008 used the NIS to look specifically at laparoscopic colectomy for cancer and found that from 2003 to 2004, 3.3% of colectomies within the NIS were performed laparoscopically. Robinson and colleagues [21] in 2011 used the same database to look at 2005 to 2007, hoping to find a trend for any changes in use after the publication of the COST trial. These investigators found an increase in use for colon cancer from 4.7% in 2005% to 6.7% in 2007. For benign disease, a modest increase was found from 25.2% in 2005 to 27.4% in 2007. Once again, these trials used the ICD-9-CM modifier code for laparoscopy (54.21) to identify these patients.

Rea and colleagues [22] in 2011 used a similar approach to the NIS, using ICD-9-CM modifier codes for laparoscopy (54.21) and conversion to an open operation (v64.4), once again trying to identify trends before and after publication of the COST trial. These investigators found that comparing 2001 to 2003 with 2005 to 2007, use of laparoscopy increased from 6.2% to 11.8% for benign disease and from 2.3% to 8.9% for colon cancer. This study added to existing knowledge because it helped to define the conversion rate from laparoscopy to open surgery, which for the 2005 to 2007 was 34.2% for benign disease and 35.6% for malignant disease.

The lack of a specific code for laparoscopic colectomy severely limited these studies because modifier codes for billing were believed to be inconsistently applied to cases. Criticism of this approach was that use was inaccurate and underestimated. In a later study, the SCOAP (Surgical Care and Outcomes Assessment Program) collaborative commented that 2 studies using the same database in the same year (NIS 2007) reported 2 different estimates of laparoscopic colectomy for benign disease (Rea and colleagues = 13.2% vs Robinson and colleagues = 27.4%) [23], thus showing the inaccuracy of this approach.

Taking a different approach, Kiran and colleagues [24] (2010) used the National Surgical Quality Improvement Program (NSQIP) database from 2006 to 2007 to evaluate outcomes after colorectal surgery. Because this database used current procedural terminology codes to collect data, specific codes were available for laparoscopic procedures. In this study, the rate of laparoscopy for colorectal surgery was 31.1%. Within this group, 45.2% of partial colectomies were performed laparoscopically. This study did not comment on different use rates based on benign or malignant diagnoses. In addition, the rate of conversion to an open operation could not be determined. The contrast in use rates between studies within the same period raised concerns that coding error was significantly affecting the accuracy of these studies.

Schoetz took another approach toward determining use in 2006. He looked specifically at colon and rectal surgery fellowship case logs submitted to the American Board of Colon and Rectal Surgery [25]. He found a more impressive increase in use than other studies in the same time period. From 1994 to 2005, use of laparoscopy for colectomy increased from 5.6% to 41.1% for colon cancer, and 6.5% to 44.7% for diverticulitis. Although this study roughly estimated use of laparoscopic colectomy among specialists in colon and rectal surgery, it possibly overestimated use, because case logs represented the fellows' cumulative experience rather than a single surgeon's practice. Because open cases were considered more routine at the time, trainees would have gravitated toward the available laparoscopic cases to increase their exposure to a newer technique.

Probably the most accurate estimation of laparoscopic colectomy use came from the SCOAP collaborative in 2012 [23]. This was a retrospective cohort study of an in-hospital registry (SCOAP) used by 48 hospitals in the states of Washington and Oregon [26]. These investigators identified 9705 patients who underwent a colorectal operation from 2005 to 2010 and went through individual operative reports to determine the details of the case, thus reducing the possibility of coding errors. During that period, 38% of elective colorectal operations used a laparoscopic approach, with a conversion rate of 17.8%. Trends from 2005 to 2010 showed an increase in laparoscopy from 23.3% to 41.6%, and a decrease in conversion rate from 23.5% to 18.1% (Table 1). Because this cohort was limited to the northwest, the study was subject to regional bias, and therefore the results could not necessarily be applied to the rest of the country.

In October 2008, specific ICD-9-CM codes for laparoscopic colectomy became available. Two major studies have used the newly available codes to more accurately assess trends in use. Our institution published a study in September 2012 using the University Health System Consortium (UHC) to identify use rates among academic medical centers and their affiliated hospitals (Table 2) [27]. From October 2008 to December 2011, 85,712 patients were identified who underwent colon resection. The overall rate of laparoscopic colectomy for this period was 42.2%, significantly higher than previous database estimations. The overall conversion rate was 15.8%. There was an increase in use of approximately 7% from 2008 to 2011 (Fig. 2).

Table 1
Use of laparoscopy in elective colorectal operation from 2005 to 2010, overall (n = 9705) and for cancer indications (n = 3568)

	Total number of cases (number of hospitals)	Open cases		Laparoscopic cases		Laparoscopic converted to open cases	
		n	%	n	%	n	%
Overall							
2005	146 (8)	112	76.7	34	23.3	8	23.5
2006	794 (13)	566	71.3	228	28.7	36	15.8
2007	1227 (17)	792	64.5	435	35.5	83	19.1
2008	1808 (27)	1119	61.9	689	38.1	108	15.7
2009	2647 (40)	1631	61.6	1016	38.4	187	18.4
2010	3083 (48)	1800	58.4	1283	41.6	233	18.2
Overall	9704	6020	62	3685	38	655	18
Cancer							
2005	44 (4)	31	70.5	13	29.5	3	23.1
2006	353 (12)	261	73.9	92	26.1	18	19.6
2007	491 (17)	348	70.9	143	29.1	37	25.9
2008	624 (26)	405	64.9	219	35.1	32	14.6
2009	946 (39)	607	64.2	339	35.8	69	20.4
2010	1110 (45)	684	61.6	426	38.4	73	17.1
Overall	3568	2336	65.5	1232	35	232	19

Data from SCOAP Collaborative. Adoption of laparoscopy for elective colorectal resection: a report from the Surgical Care Outcomes Assessment Program. J Am Coll Surg 2012;214:912.

Fox and colleagues [28] in 2012 used the new ICD-9-CM codes to revisit the NIS from 2008 to 2009, specifically looking at laparoscopic colectomy for cancer. For all adults undergoing an elective colectomy for cancer, there was a 44.8% rate of laparoscopy use with a conversion rate of 12.2%.

FACTORS AFFECTING USE

Studies have shown several patient factors to affect the likelihood of having a laparoscopic approach to colon surgery. Patients undergoing laparoscopic colectomy tended to be younger, with fewer comorbidities [19–23,25,27,28], have a higher median household income [20], and were more likely to have private insurance versus Medicare, Medicaid, or self-pay [28]. Some studies showed race to be a factor, with whites more likely to undergo laparoscopic surgery than Hispanics or African Americans [19,27,28]. In most studies, gender was not a significant factor [21,22].

Patient body habitus also played a role in these studies. Obesity, defined as a body mass index greater than 30 (calculated as weight in kilograms divided by the square of height in meters), has been shown to increase operative time, increase length of stay, and increase the rate of conversion to open surgery [29,30]. The effect of obesity on use rates varied between studies and is of unclear significance [22,23]. Despite these findings, laparoscopic colectomy has

Table 2
Comparison of demographic characteristics for patients undergoing laparoscopic or open colectomy

Demographics (n = 85,712)	Laparoscopic (%) (n = 36,228)	Open (%) (n = 49,484)	*P* value
Age (y)			
18–30	8.1	6.7	<.001
31–50	23.9	21.6	<.001
51–64	34.5	33.1	<.001
65+	35.6	40.7	<.001
Sex (%)			
Female	52.6	52.7	.8775
Male	47.3	47.2	.8775
Race (%)			
White	75.6	72.9	<.001
African American	10.8	15.1	<.001
Other	13.5	11.9	<.001
Ethnicity (%)			
Hispanic	3.7	4.7	<.001
Non-Hispanic	96.2	95.2	<.001
Admission Severity of Illness (%)			
Minor/moderate	86.7	59	<.001
Major	12.1	29.4	<.001
Extreme	1.2	11.4	<.001
Admission Type (%)			
Elective	82.6	50.4	<.001
Urgent	17.4	49.6	<.001
Diagnosis (%)			
Diverticulitis	22.1	17.8	<.001
Crohn's disease	8.8	6.3	<.001
Infection	0.24	3.53	<.001
Malignancy	30.1	25.8	<.001
Benign neoplasm	14.5	4.2	<.001
Ulcerative colitis	5.6	4.1	<.001
Obstruction	2	6.2	<.001
Colectomy complications	2.6	8.9	<.001
Gastrointestinal hemorrhage	0.1	0.5	<.001
Trauma	0.1	2.3	<.001
Other	13.7	20.6	<.001

Data from Simorov A, Shaligram A, Shostrom V, et al. Laparoscopic colon resection trends in utilization and rate of conversion to open procedure: a national database review of academic medical centers. Ann Surg 2012;256:464.

been shown to be safe in obese patients without an increased risk of postoperative morbidity or mortality [31].

In addition to patient factors, there were several hospital factors as well. Use was higher in urban hospitals compared with rural hospitals [19,20,28], which may have represented a difference in access to technology, equipment, and surgical specialists. Hospitals with higher volumes of colorectal surgery also had

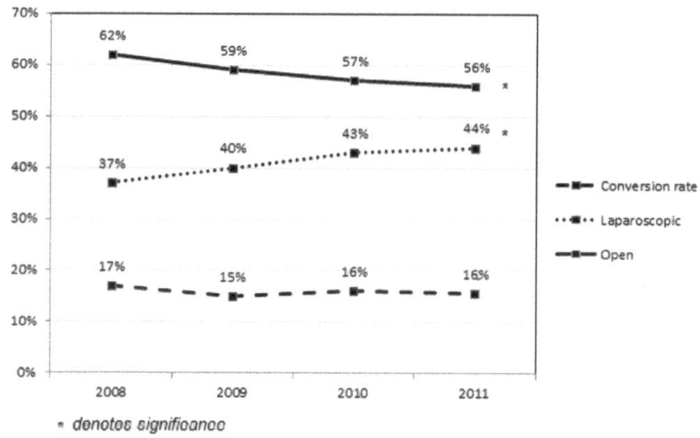

Fig. 2. Trends of colon resections from 2008 to 2011 by approach: laparoscopic, open, and conversion rate to an open procedure. (*From* Simorov A, Shaligram A, Shostrom V, et al. Laparoscopic colon resection trends in utilization and rate of conversion to open procedure: a national database review of academic medical centers. Ann Surg 2012;256:463; with permission.)

higher use of laparoscopy [28]. Some studies showed hospital size and number of beds to be a minor factor [19,23,27,28], whereas another showed no significant difference [21]. The effect of the teaching status of a hospital was unclear, because some studies showed teaching hospitals to have an increased rate of laparoscopic colectomy [19,20,28], whereas others showed no difference [23,27].

Use of laparoscopy was regional as well. Early studies showed that hospitals in the south and southeast regions were less likely to use laparoscopy than the west or northeast regions, with slower increases in use rates [19–21,27] The SCOAP collaborative reported that laparoscopy was heavily used in the northwest as well [23]. Like most things in the midwest, use has been average, with reliable and moderate increases slowly over time [19–21,27].

As discussed previously, the underlying diagnosis affected use rates, with use of laparoscopy being higher for benign disease than for cancer [19,22,23,25,27]. Within surgeries performed for colon cancer, patients with localized, node-negative cancer were more likely to undergo a laparoscopic surgery than those with node-positive disease or known metastases [20–22,28].

As expected, the urgency of the patient's admission also affected use, with emergent colectomies having a lower use rate than elective colectomies [12]. Severity of illness (SOI) was also a significant factor, and patients with major or extreme SOI were less likely to undergo laparoscopic surgery than those with minor or moderate SOI [27].

The type and site of colectomy also affected the use of laparoscopy, because some areas of the colon were considered more technically challenging to remove in a laparoscopic fashion. Steele and colleagues [20] excluded patients who underwent transverse colectomies or total colectomies from their study because they "may be less likely to be offered a laparoscopic approach," showing the varying levels of difficulty among different colectomies. Two separate studies of the UHC showed transverse colectomy to have the lowest rate of laparoscopic use (10%) [32] and the highest rate of conversion to open colectomy (20.8%) [27]. Total colectomy has shown nonsignificant trends toward lower use [28], which was variable between different studies. On the other side of the spectrum, ileocolectomy, cecectomy, and right hemicolectomy have shown consistently higher rates of use, with a conversion rate of 15% to 16% [23,24,27,28,32].

CURRENT ROADBLOCKS TO THE WIDESPREAD ADOPTION OF LAPAROSCOPIC COLECTOMY

Laparoscopic colectomy is now known to be safe and effective with several short-term and long-term benefits to the patient, but there are several factors preventing its widespread adoption. One potential roadblock to use is the presence of a more extensive learning curve compared with simple laparoscopy. Several studies have attempted to define the learning curve and estimate its length. These studies showed that operative times and conversion rates decreased with experience, whereas the complication rates did not significantly change [33–35]. The COST, CLASICC, and COLOR trials required participants to have performed at least 20 laparoscopic colectomies as one of the quality measures. Other studies have estimated the learning curve to be between 50 and 60 laparoscopic colectomies [36,37]. Despite these estimates, the number of cases required to obtain proficiency is still unknown.

Because a significant learning curve exists, surgeons may not receive adequate training during residency. Graduating residents have seen an increase in the average number of laparoscopic colectomies performed, from 2 in 1999 to 13 in 2008 [38]. Despite this increase, the numbers are still less than the 20-case minimum required to participate in the COST trial, and the level of resident participation within these cases is difficult to assess. Attending surgeons who are themselves early in the learning curve may not feel comfortable allowing residents to perform a substantial portion of these cases.

The presence of surgical fellows may also limit resident experience. Of senior residents in 1 survey, 61% stated that the presence of a fellow of minimally invasive surgery negatively affected their experience with complex laparoscopy [39].

After graduation from residency, another potential roadblock is a lack of adequate volume of colectomies to develop and maintain laparoscopic expertise. Most colectomies are performed by general surgeons, with only 11.5% performed by board-certified colon and rectal surgeons [40]. However, general surgeons perform an average of only 11.16 partial colectomies per year, with 14 colectomies placing a general surgeon in the 70th percentile and 23 colectomies placing them in the 90th percentile [41]. If the average surgeon is performing less than 12 colectomies per year, it could take a long time to become proficient in an advanced technique.

Roadblocks also exist among fellowship-trained surgeons. Steele and colleagues [42] in 2011 performed a survey study of colon and rectal surgery fellowship graduates to determine impediments to performing laparoscopic surgery. The survey reported that use of laparoscopy for colon and rectal surgery was equivalent between academic and private practice surgeons. However, the private practice group was more likely to perceive a lack of hospital equipment and a lack of adequate support as roadblocks to laparoscopic use. In addition, a larger percentage of private practice surgeons reported a surgical partner as an assistant on laparoscopic cases (43% vs 8%, $P<.001$). This study highlights potential environmental factors limiting use despite adequate training and experience.

CONTROVERSIES

Because the main reason for this review is to determine how much laparoscopy is being used in colon surgery, the definition of laparoscopy is important. As was previously discussed, early studies assessing use did not have access to specific ICD-9-CM codes for laparoscopic colectomies, and had to use back-door approaches to define a case as laparoscopic. Now that specific codes exist, database interpretation is more accurate, but the qualities of a surgery that label it as laparoscopic are still at the discretion of the surgeons and coders. The approach, operative steps, and technique of a laparoscopic colectomy are not standardized, especially because many surgeons taught themselves laparoscopy with very little formal training.

The definition of laparoscopic-assisted is therefore a moving target. Major vessels may be ligated laparoscopically, or the surgeon may choose to ligate them in an open fashion once the specimen is exteriorized. Some anastomoses are performed intracorporally, whereas others are routinely performed in an extracorporeal fashion. The incision length varies based on the size of the specimen and the preference of the operating surgeon.

Another uncertainty is how to define a conversion, and what percentage of the procedure must be performed laparoscopically to avoid the label of a conversion to open. Hand-assisted laparoscopic approaches complicate this definition. Whereas some consider a hand-assisted approach to be a conversion, others use it primarily, and believe it should be considered part of a laparoscopic procedure.

An important factor to consider is whether or not laparoscopic and open surgery are truly equivalent in most surgeons' hands. The COST trial had strict criteria for surgeons included in the study and consisted primarily of experts. Early in the learning curve, a surgeon may not be able to offer an oncologically equivalent resection using a laparoscopic approach, and perhaps should gain initial experience in patients with favorable anatomy and benign disease.

THE FUTURE OF LAPAROSCOPIC COLECTOMY

It is possible that as a surgical community we have reached our peak with laparoscopy, and the increases in use will slow down or cease. However, this scenario is unlikely. Attending comfort in performing and teaching laparoscopy has increased significantly over the last 20 years. With surgical residents being exposed to an increasing number of complex laparoscopic surgeries, one can assume that they will be more likely to use laparoscopy in practice, and will be more aggressive in attempting complex surgeries using a laparoscopic approach.

If the trend does continue to increase over time, it is unclear if it represents a more widespread adoption of laparoscopy or increasing surgeon subspecialization and increased access to specialty care. Perhaps the percentage of colectomies performed by specialists will increase, whereas the use among general surgeons will have a more modest increase.

There will always be a role for open colectomy. Some cases are still difficult to perform laparoscopically. Although it has not been specifically studied, multiple previous surgeries and the presence of adhesions will continue to necessitate the occasional open surgical approach. Emergency colectomies will also likely have a slower progression toward laparoscopy, because equipment and clinical expertise may not be available for these cases, and the patient's physiology may not allow a more time-consuming approach.

Disease process will also likely continue to affect use rates. Except for gallbladder cancer, most cholecystectomies are performed in the same standard fashion. Colectomies, on the other hand, vary based on a need for high ligation of the mesenteric arteries, mobilization of the splenic flexure, adequate surgical margins, and several other important factors.

As mentioned earlier, laparoscopic surgery for rectal cancer is a different topic and requires a separate review of equal or greater length. Laparoscopic surgery in the pelvis is difficult, and its complexity may hinder its widespread adoption even more than that seen with colectomy.

Robotic surgery, natural orifice surgery, and single-incision laparoscopic surgery are adjuncts to laparoscopy that were not discussed in this review. Their role in the future of minimally invasive surgery remains unclear, but they offer potential technical and cosmetic advantages that may increase their role in colon resections as time goes on. It will be interesting to monitor their increasing rates of use in the future.

As minimally invasive colectomy becomes more prevalent, the surgeon must not view a conversion to open surgery as a treatment failure, but rather as an appropriate step in certain complex cases to ensure the safety and adequacy of a case. The possibility and rationale for a conversion to open surgery should remain a routine portion of informed consent. As resident experience with laparoscopy increases, the surgical educator must ensure that residents continue to maintain their skills in open surgery so that they are prepared for complex situations in which laparoscopy is not appropriate.

SUMMARY

Since its inception, the use of laparoscopy for colon surgery has slowly increased, albeit at a slower rate than for cholecystectomy. Initial concerns about the safety and efficacy of laparoscopy have been addressed, and it is now known to have several potential short-term and long-term benefits for the patient. Early studies likely underestimated use of laparoscopy because of coding error. Currently, 40% to 50% of colectomies in the United States are performed laparoscopically, with a 10% to 20% rate of conversion to an open operation. The definitions of laparoscopy and conversion to open remain at the discretion of the surgeons and their coders. Disparities still exist among use based on several patient, hospital, and surgeon factors. In the future, we will likely see a continuing increase in use as the new generation of surgeons enters practice, and there will be an increasing role for laparoscopy in rectal surgery. The benefit and extent of robotic surgery, natural orifice surgery, and single-incision surgery for minimally invasive colectomies are yet to be defined.

References

[1] Jacobs M, Verdeja JC, Goldstein HS. Minimally invasive colon resection (laparoscopic colectomy). Surg Laparosc Endosc 1991;1(3):144–50.
[2] Fowler DL, White SA. Laparoscopy-assisted sigmoid resection. Surg Laparosc Endosc 1991;1(3):183–8.
[3] Kemp JA, Zuckerman RS, Finlayson SR. Trends in adoption of laparoscopic cholecystectomy in rural versus urban hospitals. J Am Coll Surg 2008;206(1):28–32.
[4] Alexander R, Jaques B, Mitchell K. Laparoscopic-assisted colectomy and wound recurrence. Lancet 1993;341:249–50.
[5] Johnstone PA, Rohde DC, Swartz SE, et al. Port site recurrences after laparoscopic and thoracoscopic procedures in malignancy. J Clin Oncol 1996;14:1950–6.
[6] Berends FJ, Kazemier G, Bonjer HJ, et al. Subcutaneous metastases after laparoscopic colectomy. Lancet 1994;344:58.
[7] Vukasin P, Ortega AE, Greene FL, et al. Wound recurrence following laparoscopic colon cancer resection. Dis Colon Rectum 1996;39:s20–3.
[8] Kwok SP, Lau WY, Carey PD, et al. Prospective evaluation of laparoscopic-assisted large bowel excision for cancer. Ann Surg 1996;223:170–6.
[9] Clinical Outcomes of Surgical Therapy Study Group. A comparison of laparoscopically assisted and open colectomy for colon cancer. N Engl J Med 2004;350:2050–9.
[10] COLOR Study Group. Laparoscopic surgery versus open surgery for colon cancer: short-term outcomes of a randomized trial. Lancet Oncol 2005;6:477–84.
[11] COLOR Study Group. Survival after laparoscopic surgery versus open surgery for colon cancer: long-term outcome of a randomised clinical trial. Lancet Oncol 2009;10:44–52.
[12] Guillou PJ, Quirke P, Thorpe H, et al. Short-term endpoints of conventional versus laparoscopic-assisted surgery in patients with colorectal cancer (MRC CLASICC trial): multicentre, randomized controlled trial. Lancet 2005;365:1718–26.
[13] Jayne DG, Guillou PJ, Thorpe H, et al. Randomized trial of laparoscopic-assisted resection of colorectal carcinoma: 3-year results of the UK MRC CLASICC Trial Group. J Clin Oncol 2007;25:3061–8.
[14] Jayne DG, Thorpe HC, Copeland J, et al. Five-year follow-up of the Medical Research Council CLASICC trial of laparoscopically assisted versus open surgery for colorectal cancer. Br J Surg 2010;97:1638–45.
[15] Kuhry E, Schwenk W, Gaupset R, et al. Long-term outcome of laparoscopic surgery for colorectal cancer: a Cochrane systematic review of randomized controlled trials. Cancer Treat Rev 2008;34(6):498–504.
[16] Schwenk W, Haase O, Neudecker J, et al. Short term benefits for laparoscopic colorectal resection. Cochrane Database Syst Rev 2005;(3):CD003145.

[17] Weeks JC, Nelson H, Gelber S. Short term quality-of-life outcomes following laparoscopic-assisted colectomy vs. open colectomy for colon cancer: a randomized trial. JAMA 2002;287(3):321–8.
[18] Duepree HJ, Senagore AJ, Delaney CP, et al. Does means of access affect the incidence of small bowel obstruction and ventral hernia after bowel resection? Laparoscopy versus laparotomy. J Am Coll Surg 2003;197:177–81.
[19] Kemp JA, Finlayson SR. Nationwide trends in laparoscopic colectomy from 2000 to 2004. Surg Endosc 2008;22:1181–7.
[20] Steele SR, Brown TA, Rush RM, et al. Laparoscopic vs open colectomy for colon cancer: results from a large nationwide population-based analysis. J Gastrointest Surg 2008;12: 583–91.
[21] Robinson CN, Chen GJ, Balentine CJ, et al. Minimally invasive surgery is underutilized for colon cancer. Ann Surg Oncol 2011;18:1412–8.
[22] Rea JD, Cone MM, Diggs BS, et al. Utilization of laparoscopic colectomy in the United States before and after the clinical outcomes of surgical therapy study group trial. Ann Surg 2011;254:281–8.
[23] SCOAP Collaborative. Adoption of laparoscopy for elective colorectal resection: a report from the Surgical Care Outcomes Assessment Program. J Am Coll Surg 2012;214: 909–18.
[24] Kiran RP, El-Gazzaz GH, Vogel JD, et al. Laparoscopic approach significantly reduces surgical site infections after colorectal surgery: data from National Surgical Quality Improvement Program. J Am Coll Surg 2010;211:232–8.
[25] Schoetz DJ. Evolving practice patterns in colon and rectal surgery. J Am Coll Surg 2006;203:322–7.
[26] Flum DR, Fisher N, Thompson J, et al. Washington state's approach to variability in surgical processes/outcomes: Surgical Clinical Outcomes Assessment Program. Surgery 2005;138: 821–8.
[27] Simorov A, Shaligram A, Shostrom V, et al. Laparoscopic colon resection trends in utilization and rate of conversion to open procedure: a national database review of academic medical centers. Ann Surg 2012;256:462–8.
[28] Fox J, Gross CP, Longo W, et al. Laparoscopic colectomy for the treatment of cancer has been widely adopted in the United States. Dis Colon Rectum 2012;55:501–8.
[29] Mustain WC, Davenport DL, Hourigan JS, et al. Obesity and laparoscopic colectomy: outcomes from the ACS-NSQIP database. Dis Colon Rectum 2012;55:429–35.
[30] Makino T, Shukla PJ, Rubino F, et al. The impact of obesity on perioperative outcomes after laparoscopic colorectal resection. Ann Surg 2012;255:228–36.
[31] Poulsen M, Ovesen H. Is laparoscopic colorectal cancer surgery in obese patients associated with an increased risk? Short-term results from a single center study of 425 patients. J Gastrointest Surg 2012;16:1554–8.
[32] Carmichael JC, Masoomi H, Mills S, et al. Utilization of laparoscopy in colorectal surgery for cancer at academic medical centers: does site of surgery affect rate of laparoscopy? Am Surg 2011;77:1300–4.
[33] Ozturk E, da Luz Moreira A, Vogel JD. Hand-assisted laparoscopic colectomy: the learning curve is for operative speed, not for quality. Colorectal Dis 2010;12:e304–9.
[34] Kang JC, Jao SW, Chung MH, et al. The learning curve for hand-assisted laparoscopic colectomy: a single surgeon's experience. Surg Endosc 2007;21:234–7.
[35] Waters JA, Chihara R, Moreno J, et al. Laparoscopic colectomy: does the learning curve extend beyond colorectal surgery fellowship? JSLS 2010;4:325–31.
[36] Tekkis PP, Senagore AJ, Delaney CP. Evaluation of the learning curve in laparoscopic colorectal surgery: comparison of right-sided and left-sided resections. Ann Surg 2005;242: 83–91.
[37] Wishner JD, Baker JW, Hoffman GC, et al. Laparoscopic-assisted colectomy. The learning curve. Surg Endosc 1995;9:1179–83.

[38] Alkhouri F, Martin JT, Contessa J. The impact of laparoscopy on the volume of open cases in general surgery training. J Surg Educ 2010;67:316–9.
[39] Brown NM, Helmer SD, Yates CL. The revised ACGME laparoscopic operative requirements: how have they impacted resident education? Surg Endosc 2012;26:1737–43.
[40] Etzioni DA, Cannom RR, Madoff RD. Colorectal procedures: what proportion is performed by American Board of Colon and Rectal Surgery-certified surgeons? Dis Colon Rectum 2010;53:713–20.
[41] Hyman N. How much colorectal surgery do general surgeons do? J Am Coll Surg 2002;194:37–9.
[42] Steele SR, Stein SL, Bordeianou LG, et al. The impact of practice environment on laparoscopic colectomy utilization following colorectal residency: a survey of the ASCRS Young Surgeons. Colorectal Dis 2012;14:374–81.

Advances in Surgery 47 (2013) 45–57

ADVANCES IN SURGERY

Safety of Surgical Resident Training

Usama Ahmed Ali, MD[a], Jon D. Vogel, MD[b,*]

[a]Department of Colorectal Surgery, Digestive Disease Institution, Cleveland Clinic, 9500 Euclid Avenue, JJ4N, Cleveland, OH 44195, USA; [b]Department of Colorectal Surgery, Digestive Disease Institution, Cleveland Clinic, 9500 Euclid Avenue, Desk A30, Cleveland, OH 44195, USA

Keywords

• Surgical training • Surgery • Training • Safety • Resident • Surgical outcome

Key points

- The current structure of resident participation in surgical procedures is safe, with no negative impact on mortality or major complications.
- For laparoscopic surgery, training and simulation are advisable to ameliorate potential negative effects of learning curves.
- The influence of duty-hour restriction on patient safety remains controversial.
- With the introduction of structured work shifts for residents, a focused effort to educate residents on adequate and effective communication and hand-offs is an important part of ensuring patient safety.
- Adequate training under stressful conditions can help improve resident performance in emergencies on the floor and in the Emergency Department.

INTRODUCTION

Residency training in the United States was first formalized and developed by Dr William Osler and Dr William Steward Halsted, at The Johns Hopkins Hospital, in the late nineteenth century [1]. The goal was to ensure that future physicians and surgeons mastered the necessary skills to become independent practitioners in the field. By the end of the twentieth century, residency had become an indispensable part of medical practice, with more than 80% of all surgical procedures conducted in teaching hospitals with resident participation [2,3]. Resident training and participation are thus an integral part of patient care and are of paramount importance for the sustainability of our health care system. This fact inevitably raises the question of whether participation of

Disclosure: No conflicting interest exists for all authors.

*Corresponding author. *E-mail address*: vogelj@ccf.org

0065-3411/13/$ – see front matter
http://dx.doi.org/10.1016/j.yasu.2013.02.009

surgical residents in health care has an impact on outcome, especially in terms of safety. Several studies have attempted to study this topic, with large variation in research questions, methods, study setting, and outcome measures. In this article these studies are reviewed, and their potential implication for practice and research discussed.

SAFETY OF RESIDENT PARTICIPATION IN SURGICAL PROCEDURES

Several studies have attempted to assess the impact of resident involvement in surgical procedures on postoperative morbidity and mortality. Table 1 provides an overview of the most important studies in this regard. A recent study by Kiran and colleagues [4] provided the first direct matched comparison to assess the impact of resident involvement on a large scale. This study compared resident participation with no resident participation in surgeries performed on 60,711 patients from the American College of Surgeons National Surgical Quality Improvement Program (ACS-NSQIP). The ACS-NSQIP database is the first validated national, outcome-based, risk-adjusted, performance-controlled platform for the measurement and subsequent improvement of medical health care delivery [2,3,5–9]. The ACS-NSQIP database collects a variety of preoperative, intraoperative, and 30-day postoperative data in patients undergoing surgical procedures [7,10–12]. Variables are collected in many national hospitals in a uniform and controlled manner, offering an opportunity to directly evaluate the effects of various factors on surgical safety, including resident involvement, while optimally correcting for potential confounders [2,3,5–8]. In their study, Kiran and colleagues [4] found that there was no difference in rate of mortality and major complications between the 2 groups. A slight increase in mild surgical complications was seen in the residents group, which was mainly driven by an increase in the rate of superficial wound infection (3.0% vs 2.2%, $P<.001$). No difference was seen in other individual complications, such as deep surgical-site infection or reoperation rate. In addition, operative time was longer when residents were involved (mean [SD] 122 [80] vs 97 [67] minutes, $P<.001$). Although a clear explanation of the difference in wound infection rate was not available, the investigators argued that the longer operative time observed in the residency group may have played a role. Of note, subgroup analyses in the same study comparing surgeries with residents of different postgraduate year (PGY) levels (PGY 1–2, PGY 3–5, and PGY $\geq$6) with matched groups without resident involvement provided results that were consistent with the main findings of the study. Superficial wound infection and operative time were significantly higher when residents were involved, whereas severe complications and mortality showed no difference. This result further strengthened the reliability of these findings. Other strengths of the study are the use of the NSQIP data, which are considered particularly reliable, and the use of extensive matching to reduce the influence of potential confounding variables on outcomes.

The main conclusion of the study was that the current form of resident involvement can be considered safe and responsible. In particular, mortality

Table 1
Overview of studies on impact of resident participation on safety of surgical procedures

Study	N	Type of analysis	Comparison	Patient selection	Mortality	Morbidity
Kiran et al [4], 2012	60,711	Matched comparison	Resident vs no resident	All surgeries in the ACS-NSQP database	No difference	No difference in major complications Slightly higher rate of SSI
Raval et al [13], 2011	607,683	Regression	Resident vs no resident	All general and vascular surgeries in the ACS-NSQP database	No difference	Increased morbidity
Tseng et al [14], 2011	37,907	Regression	Resident vs no resident	Seven general surgical procedures from the ACS-NSQP database	Slightly decreased mortality	Increased morbidity
Karatas et al [15], 2008	811	Direct comparison	Resident vs no resident	Otologic surgeries	NA	No difference
Fischer et al [16], 2006	164	Cohort	Resident vs national best-practice benchmark	Pancreaticoduodenectomy	No difference[a]	No difference[a]
Offner et al [17], 2003	1071	Historic comparison and Regression	Resident vs no resident	Level I trauma patients	No difference	No difference in complications Shorter time in ER and shorter hospital stay in resident group
Khuri et al [2], 2001	690,811	Regression	Teaching vs nonteaching hospitals	All noncardiac surgery from the VA-NSQIP database	No difference	Increased morbidity

Abbreviations: ACS-NSQIP, American College of Surgeons National Surgical Quality Improvement Program; ER, emergency room; NA, no data available; SSI, superficial surgical infection; VA-NSQIP, Veteran Affaire National Surgical Quality Improvement Program.

[a]Based on conclusion of investigators. No formal comparison performed (ie, no *P* value provided).

and major morbidity were similar when residents participated in surgical operations. The investigators advised surgeons to be more aware of the potential association of longer operative time and higher rates of wound infection. Where possible, surgeons should prevent prolongation of operative time beyond what is needed for patient care and essential resident training, although the investigators acknowledged the difficulty of implementing this in practice.

Two recent studies using the same ACS-NSQIP database to examine the impact of resident involvement on surgical outcome found slightly different results (see Table 1) [13,14]. These studies did not compare surgeries with and without resident involvement, but rather used regression analysis to correct for potential differences between these groups. Raval and colleagues [13] included all general surgical and vascular procedures from 2006 to 2009 for a total sample of 607,683 surgical cases. Tseng and colleagues [14] included a total of 37,907 patients undergoing a selected number of general surgical procedures from 2005 to 2007. The results of both studies were similar. Resident participation in surgical procedures was associated with slightly higher morbidity rates but slightly decreased mortality rates. Tseng and colleagues [14] were not able to provide a clear explanation of these seemingly conflicting results, despite performance of various post hoc analyses in an attempt to do so. Raval and colleagues [13] also conducted several post hoc analyses, with interesting results. When an analysis was performed accounting for hospital-level variation, the difference in morbidity was minimized and mortality no longer reached significance. None of the studies examined individual complications to further specify the cause of the increased morbidity. Both studies concluded that patients and other stakeholders can be reassured that resident involvement in surgical care is safe, because the differences observed were small.

In a different approach, Khuri and colleagues [2] studied the differences in outcome between teaching and nonteaching hospitals, using the Veterans Affairs National Surgical Quality Improvement Program (VA-NSQIP) to obtain data from 690,811 noncardiac operations performed in 128 hospitals. Based on logistic regression, the study examined the relationship between teaching and nonteaching hospitals and 30-day postoperative mortality and morbidity. It was found that in teaching hospitals the residents were the primary surgeons in more than 90% of the operations. As expected, the patient populations in teaching hospitals had a higher prevalence of risk factors, underwent more complex operations, and had longer operation times. Therefore, unadjusted mortality and morbidity rates were higher in teaching hospitals. After correction for differences in patient severity, no difference was observed in mortality between teaching and nonteaching hospitals. However, differences in morbidity persisted. The investigators explained this by the poor performance of the regression-risk adjustment, as evidenced by the low c-index associated with these models in their analysis [2].

This finding might offer an explanation for the differences observed in the 2 studies by Raval and colleagues [13] and Tseng and colleagues [14] discussed earlier. The limitation of regression analysis in not fully correcting for confounders may be related to the difference in case mix between teaching (ie, with residents) and nonteaching (ie, without residents) hospitals. It can be expected that there is a group of patients that is almost exclusively treated in either of these settings. For example, patients who need simple procedures and do not have many comorbidities are more likely to be treated in a nonteaching hospital, whereas patients with complex surgeries or with many comorbidities are almost exclusively treated in teaching hospitals. Because no adequate controls are available for these patients, regression will not be able to fully correct for such differences. When matching is used, patients without appropriate controls are excluded, effectively avoiding this problem.

Certain studies have also investigated the impact of resident involvement in specific types of surgery. Karatas and colleagues [15] examined the effect of resident participation in otologic procedures in 811 patients, and observed no difference in complications or success rates after surgery. Similarly, Fischer and colleagues found no difference in morbidity or mortality when comparing outcomes of Whipple procedures performed by residents vs the national best-practice benchmark [16]. Offner and colleagues [17] reported on the impact of resident involvement in the management of level I trauma patients. Of interest, they found that resident participation does not affect outcome in terms of morbidity or mortality, but did significantly improve the efficiency of trauma care delivery, as evidenced by shorter time in the emergency room and shorter hospital stay. The results of these studies are summarized in Table 1.

Several studies also investigated the impact of varying levels of supervision on resident performance and safety [18–20]. None of these studies identified a difference in outcome for varying levels of resident supervision, or between operations performed by residents alone or by residents and attending surgeons. However, this does not mean that supervision is not important. An important limitation of these studies is that supervision is often selected based on the assessment of the attending. Therefore, the conclusion of these results is that physicians seem to appropriately select the level of supervision needed based on a resident's competence and skills, without compromising patient outcome.

In summary, the majority of current studies support the notion that resident participation in surgical procedures is safe. None of the studies showed an increase in mortality. Some studies showed a small increase in complication rate when residents were involved. The best available evidence shows that this is probably caused by a small increase in mild surgical complications such as superficial wound infection, and may be related to the longer operative time when residents are involved.

SAFETY OF RESIDENT PARTICIPATION IN LAPAROSCOPIC SURGERY

Laparoscopic surgery has now become the standard technique for many common operative procedures such as cholecystectomy and appendectomy.

The use of laparoscopy for other, more complex operations is on the increase, meaning that residents are expected to participate in these types of surgeries at an early stage of their training. Because learning curves are more pronounced in laparoscopic surgery, the safety of resident participation in this type of surgery warrants a more focused discussion. Methods and findings of studies addressing safety of resident involvement in laparoscopic cholecystectomy and appendectomy are summarized in Table 2.

Several studies addressed the safety of resident participation in laparoscopic cholecystectomy, but all had important methodological limitations, making it difficult to draw a reliable conclusion. A recent large study compared the outcome of laparoscopic cholecystectomy performed by residents and attending surgeons [21]. Mortality was similar in both groups, but the resident group showed lower morbidity and shorter hospital stay. Unfortunately, the baseline characteristics of both groups were not equal. The rate of urgent surgery, body mass index, and American Society of Anesthesiologists (ASA) classification were higher in the attending group. A matched study by Bencini and colleagues [22] showed no difference in mortality and morbidity after laparoscopic cholecystectomy procedures performed by residents versus experienced staff surgeons. Again, the matching was not extensive and differences existed in important confounding variables. In this case the ASA classification was higher in the group operated on by experienced surgeons, effectively favoring the resident group. In addition, fewer patients in the resident group required additional concomitant procedures (3% vs 7%, respectively; $P = .009$). Kauvar and colleagues [23] compared outcomes after laparoscopic cholecystectomy performed by junior residents (PGY 1–3) and senior residents (PGY >3), and observed a higher rate of overall postoperative complications in the junior resident group (5.6% vs 0.78%, $P < .05$) [23]. The investigators explained that their residents, up to that point, learned to perform laparoscopic cholecystectomy solely through observation in the operating room, and did not participate in simulation training or other teaching methods specifically aimed at laparoscopic skills. The investigators suggested that these educational techniques might improve outcome, and concluded that the results of their study may help surgical educators maximize both resident learning and operative efficiency and safety.

Two recent studies addressed the safety of resident participation in laparoscopic appendectomy. Again, results were somewhat conflicting. Mahmoud and colleagues [18] performed a randomized controlled trial comparing outcomes of laparoscopic appendectomy performed by either junior residents under supervision of a senior resident (residents only group) or junior residents under supervision of an attending surgeon (resident and attending group). The trial showed no difference between both groups regarding complications and mortality. It was concluded that senior surgical residents can act safely as teaching assistants for junior residents. This trial was limited by the fact that residents performed the operations in both groups, making a direct evaluation of the role of residents impossible. Lin and colleagues [24], on the other hand,

Table 2
Overview of studies on impact of resident participation on safety of selected laparoscopic surgical procedures

Study	N	Type of analysis	Comparison	Patient selection	Mortality	Morbidity
Fahrner et al [21], 2012	1747	Direct comparison	Resident vs no resident	Laparoscopic cholecystectomy	No difference	Fewer complications in residents group[a]
Bencini et al [22], 2008	342	Matched	Resident vs staff surgeons	Laparoscopic cholecystectomy	No difference	No difference[b]
Kauvar et al [23], 2006	315	Regression	Junior vs senior residents	Laparoscopic cholecystectomy	NA	Higher complications in junior residents group
Mahmoud et al [18], 2012	120	Randomized controlled trial	Residents only vs residents and attending	Laparoscopic appendectomy	NA	No difference
Lin et al [24], 2010	306	Direct comparison	First 20 vs subsequent 20 surgeries for each resident	Laparoscopic appendectomy	No difference	Higher complications in less experienced residents

Abbreviation: NA, no data available.
[a]Nonresident group included patients with higher American Society of Anesthesiologists (ASA) classification.
[b]Nonresident group included patients with more urgent surgeries, higher body mass index, and higher ASA classification.

compared the outcome of laparoscopic appendectomy for 6 residents during their first 20 surgeries versus their subsequent 20 procedures. Higher complication rates were observed for residents during their first 20 procedures. Residents in this study attended a certified laparoscopic surgery workshop, and used simulation to practice laparoscopic surgery. Residents also assisted in several procedures, and were evaluated and found to be proficient and safe by a consulting surgeon before operating independently. The investigators concluded that operative duration and complication rate were significantly reduced with increasing experience of residents, and that stringent supervision is required in the initial phase of the learning curve.

In summary, studies regarding this topic have important limitations, but do demonstrate that mortality is similar in the groups that were studied while the impact of resident participation on morbidity was variable. Better designed studies correcting for potential confounders and aiming to directly evaluate the role of resident participation are needed, especially in the case of laparoscopic cholecystectomy and appendectomy, because these are often the first types of laparoscopic surgeries that residents embark on. It does seem that with improved supervision and specific teaching approaches directed toward laparoscopic skills, the safety of early resident participation in laparoscopic surgery can be improved. The benefit of such training programs has been shown in several studies that included other surgical approaches such as colectomies and gastric bypass surgery [25–28].

RESIDENT WORK RESTRICTION AND SAFETY

In a recent article, Van Eaton and colleagues [29] identified 3 key current challenges for surgical resident training. The first of these was a new restriction of duty hours proposed in 2011. The aim of these restrictions can be easily deduced from the name of the committee formed for this purpose: "Optimizing Graduate Medical Trainee Hours and Work Schedules to Improve Patient Safety" [29]. The proposed changes do not alter the maximum permitted work hours per week (remaining at 80 hours), but do put some restrictions on durations of shifts, on-call frequency, minimum time off between scheduled shifts, and the maximum frequency of in-hospital night shifts. The most notable change may be the 5-hour protected sleep period between 10 PM and 8 AM during a 30-hour duty period. The recommendation of a 48-hour off-duty period after 3 or 4 consecutive nights may prove to be challenging for many programs, because they are currently relying on night-shift teams to comply with the 2003 restriction of on duty hours.

There has been great controversy about whether the previous 2003 restriction of work hours has improved patient safety. A large number of studies have shown a decrease in mortality rate after implementation of these restrictions [30–32]. However, similar decreases have been observed in nonteaching hospitals over the same period [30]. This finding has raised doubts about the relationship between the restriction of working hours and the decrease in mortality. In addition, most studies were retrospective in nature, limiting the studies' ability to reliably identify causal relationships. The effect of restriction of work hours on morbidity and medical errors also remains unclear. Some studies show higher rates of complications and errors before the implementation of the 80-hour work schedule, whereas other reports show an increase in such events after the implementation of these restrictions [30]. A recent meta-analysis found no difference between pooled complications in both periods (odds ratio [OR] 1.03, 95% confidence interval [CI] 0.67–1.57) [33]. This finding has led a recent review to conclude that as a result of methodological concerns and the lack of hard evidence linking fatigue and underperformance in medical practice, it is unclear whether the goals of the reductions in work hours have been achieved [30].

In general, the sentiments of both surgical residents and program directors seem to be against any further restriction of work hours. Both seem to think that further reduction of work hours will not improve patient safety [34,35]. In addition, they raise the concern that further reductions may jeopardize adequate surgical training, affect the quality of the learning environment, and further complicate program administration, all of which ultimately could negatively affect patient outcomes [35,36].

Although controversy regarding this topic is likely to continue, careful evaluation of the actual impact of any further restriction seems warranted. Such assessment includes better studies to evaluate the relationship between restriction of working hours and safety. Pilot studies in which work-hour restrictions are implemented in a limited number of hospitals or departments, and the outcomes compared with those of adequate controls, may be the best next step.

CONTINUATION OF CARE AND HAND-OFFS

One of the consequences of the modern organization of health care is the increased number of caregivers for each patient. This situation is related to the growing size of health care institutions and the recent restriction of work hours necessitating frequent switches between caregivers. Hand-off refers to the process of communication that takes place when a primary caregiver transfers this responsibility to another person [37]. Hand-offs are critical in patient care, as they constitute opportunities for important information to become lost or be misunderstood. Several studies have investigated the effect of switching of primary caregivers on outcomes of care. A case-control study at an urban tertiary center showed that potential preventable adverse events were strongly associated with cross-coverage by a physician from another team (OR 6.1; 95% CI 1.4–26.7) [38]. Other studies have also shown that cross-coverage and gaps in communication can lead to ordering more (duplicate) tests and longer hospital stays [39,40]. Moreover, an analysis of litigation cases showed that teamwork breakdowns were a leading contributing factor for litigation (70% of all litigation cases) [41]. Hand-off problems were one of the most prevalent types of teamwork problem, and were found to be disproportionately more common among errors that involved trainees [41]. This issue is, therefore, of great importance in ensuring the safety of resident participation in care.

To be able to prevent these deleterious effects of poor communication, there needs to be a more deliberate and focused effort to educate residents on adequate and effective hand-offs [37]. Several examples of such efforts have been described, and have been shown to improve the outcome of care. A recent study showed that simply agreeing on a set of policies aimed at increasing effective and consistent resident-attending communication can substantially reduce potentially harmful communication breakdowns [42]. These policies were agreed on internally and were reinforced by simple measures, such as a pocket information card for residents and periodic reminders. After implementation of these measures, the proportion of critical events not conveyed to an attending surgeon decreased from 33% to 2% [42]. These results were corroborated by another study, which showed that simplifying and standardizing the hand-off instrument results in substantial increases in accuracy, completeness, and number of tasks transferred during hand-off at a surgical department [43]. Others have described the use of computerized systems to aid in ensuring complete and effective communication. Van Eaton and colleagues [44] describe a centralized, Web-based computerized rounding and sign-out system in a surgical department, developed specifically as a consequence of the recent restriction on residents' work hours. This system was shown to significantly reduce the number of patients missed during rounds, and increase the quality of reporting and the continuity of care. It also was able to save residents up to 3 hours per week, facilitating meeting the 80-hour work week.

Regardless of the approach used, implementing some form of structure for hand-offs seems an obvious necessity in surgical practice in the twenty-first century. Recently, a checklist containing 10 essential points for an efficient and safe hand-off has been formulated by the surgical services at the Johns Hopkins Hospital [45]. This list might provide an appropriate guideline for the formulation of such systems in other services.

IMPACT OF STRESS ON PERFORMANCE OF RESIDENTS

An important part of surgical training is preparing residents to deal with emergencies. Knowledge and skills in such stressful situations might not be sufficient if residents cannot cope with the associated stress. Studies have shown that residents tend to perform less effectively when faced with a stressful situation. One study compared surgical and trauma residents with experts in 12 basic emergencies [46]. The study found that in simple clinical scenarios, residents had significant deficits in cognitive performance when compared with experts in the areas of secondary evaluation, follow-up of the presenting problem, and total performance [46]. The investigators suggested the need for the development of educational systems to enhance performance of residents under such stressful conditions. A second study compared performance of residents in simulated trauma scenarios under low and high stress conditions [47], and found that performance scores and postscenario recall were significantly lower in the high-stress situation. The investigators concluded that these findings highlight a potential threat to patient safety that needed to be addressed.

There is no doubt that experience is an important factor for developing competence in stressful situations. However, adequate teaching and training have been shown to improve residents' skills and performance. A study investigated the effect of a single 8-hour period of intensive simulation resuscitation training, and found that this significantly improved self-assessed theoretical knowledge and procedural skill competence for residents [48]. Another study showed that simulation training can reduce levels of anxiety, and improve clinical performance and nontechnical skills [49]. Implementation of adequate training under stressful conditions is therefore an important part of ensuring the safety of resident participation.

SUMMARY

The current structure of residency training allows for safe participation of residents in the care of surgical patients. In part, this is likely due to the ability of attending-level surgeons and educators to adequately select and provide the supervision needed for different levels of residents. Nonetheless, efforts have to be made to ensure the optimal safety of patients in several settings of modern health care. For laparoscopic surgery, training and simulation are highly advisable in preparing residents to perform well in the early stage of their learning curves. Attention has to be given to safe and complete hand-offs, especially with the increased focus on restricting work hours and the increased number of changing shifts. Measures to ensure optimal preparation of surgical residents to perform well in stressful situations should also be taken, because such situations are an intrinsic part of this specialty. It is only by focusing on all these aspects that we can ensure the safety for our patients and provide the best possible training for the next generation of surgeons.

References

[1] Rankin JS. William Stewart Halsted: a lecture by Dr Peter D Olch. Ann Surg 2006;243: 418–25.
[2] Khuri SF, Najjar SF, Daley J, et al. Comparison of surgical outcomes between teaching and nonteaching hospitals in the Department of Veterans Affairs. Ann Surg 2001;234: 370–82.
[3] Khuri SF, Henderson WG, Daley J, et al. Successful implementation of the Department of Veterans Affairs' national surgical quality improvement program in the private sector: the Patient Safety in Surgery study. Ann Surg 2008;248:329–36.
[4] Kiran RP, Ahmed AU, Coffey JC, et al. Impact of resident participation in surgical operations on postoperative outcomes: national surgical quality improvement program. Ann Surg 2012;256:469–75.
[5] Daley J, Forbes MG, Young GJ, et al. Validating risk-adjusted surgical outcomes: site visit assessment of process and structure. National VA Surgical Risk Study. J Am Coll Surg 1997;185:341–51.
[6] Fink AS, Campbell DA Jr, Mentzer RM Jr, et al. The National Surgical Quality Improvement Program in non-veterans administration hospitals: initial demonstration of feasibility. Ann Surg 2002;236:344–53.
[7] Fink AS. Adjusted or unadjusted outcomes. Am J Surg 2009;198:S28–35.
[8] Khuri SF, Daley J, Henderson W, et al. The Department of Veterans Affairs' NSQIP: the first national, validated, outcome-based, risk-adjusted, and peer-controlled program for the

measurement and enhancement of the quality of surgical care. National VA Surgical Quality Improvement Program. Ann Surg 1998;228:491–507.
[9] Nathan H, Raut CP, Thornton K, et al. Predictors of survival after resection of retroperitoneal sarcoma: a population-based analysis and critical appraisal of the AJCC staging system. Ann Surg 2009;250:970–6.
[10] Davenport DL, O'Keeffe SD, Minion DJ, et al. Thirty-day NSQIP database outcomes of open versus endoluminal repair of ruptured abdominal aortic aneurysms. J Vasc Surg 2010;51: 305–9.
[11] Fink AS, Hutter MM, Campbell DC Jr, et al. Comparison of risk-adjusted 30-day postoperative mortality and morbidity in department of veterans affairs hospitals and selected university medical centers: general surgical operations in women. J Am Coll Surg 2007;204: 1127–36.
[12] Visser BC, Keegan H, Martin M, et al. Death after colectomy: it's later than we think. Arch Surg 2009;144:1021–7.
[13] Raval MV, Wang X, Cohen ME, et al. The influence of resident involvement on surgical outcomes. J Am Coll Surg 2011;212:889–98.
[14] Tseng WH, Jin L, Canter RJ, et al. Surgical resident involvement is safe for common elective general surgery procedures. J Am Coll Surg 2011;213:19–26.
[15] Karatas E, Durucu C, Baglam T, et al. Outcomes of otologic surgeries with special interest in learning curves of residents in a tertiary referral setting. Ann Otol Rhinol Laryngol 2008;117:103–5.
[16] Fischer CP, Hong JC. Early perioperative outcomes and pancreaticoduodenectomy in a general surgery residency training program. J Gastrointest Surg 2006;10(4):478–82.
[17] Offner PJ, Hawkes A, Madayag R, et al. General surgery residents improve efficiency but not outcome of trauma care. J Trauma 2003;55:14–9.
[18] Mahmoud A, Ward C, Padmesh H, et al. Safety and feasibility of the teaching assistant role of senior surgical residents: a prospective randomized study. J Surg Educ 2012;69(2): 249–52.
[19] Itani KM, DePalma RG, Schifftner T, et al. Surgical resident supervision in the operating room and outcomes of care in Veterans Affairs hospitals. Am J Surg 2005;190:725–31.
[20] Kazaure HS, Roman SA, Sosa JA. The resident as surgeon: an analysis of ACS-NSQIP. J Surg Res 2012;178(1):126–32.
[21] Fahrner R, Turina M, Neuhaus V, et al. Laparoscopic cholecystectomy as a teaching operation: comparison of outcome between residents and attending surgeons in 1,747 patients. Langenbecks Arch Surg 2012;397:103–10.
[22] Bencini L, Bernini M, Martini F, et al. Safety of laparoscopic cholecystectomy performed by surgical residents. Chir Ital 2008;60:819–24.
[23] Kauvar DS, Braswell A, Brown BD, et al. Influence of resident and attending surgeon seniority on operative performance in laparoscopic cholecystectomy. J Surg Res 2006;132:159–63.
[24] Lin YY, Shabbir A, So JB. Laparoscopic appendectomy by residents: evaluating outcomes and learning curve. Surg Endosc 2010;24:125–30.
[25] Fried GM, Feldman LS, Vassiliou MC, et al. Proving the value of simulation in laparoscopic surgery. Ann Surg 2004;240:518–25.
[26] Iordens GI, Klaassen RA, van Lieshout EM, et al. How to train surgical residents to perform laparoscopic Roux-en-Y gastric bypass safely. World J Surg 2012;36:2003–10.
[27] Lin E, Szomstein S, Addasi T, et al. Model for teaching laparoscopic colectomy to surgical residents. Am J Surg 2003;186:45–8.
[28] Hashimoto DA, Gomez ED, Danzer E, et al. Intraoperative resident education for robotic laparoscopic gastric banding surgery: a pilot study on the safety of stepwise education. J Am Coll Surg 2012;214:990–6.
[29] Van Eaton EG, Tarpley JL, Solorzano CC, et al. Resident education in 2011: three key challenges on the road ahead. Surgery 2011;149:465–73.

[30] Baldwin K, Namdari S, Donegan D, et al. Early effects of resident work-hour restrictions on patient safety: a systematic review and plea for improved studies. J Bone Joint Surg Am 2011;93:e5.
[31] Fletcher KE, Reed DA, Arora VM. Patient safety, resident education and resident well-being following implementation of the 2003 ACGME duty hour rules. J Gen Intern Med 2011;26: 907–19.
[32] Privette AR, Shackford SR, Osler T, et al. Implementation of resident work hour restrictions is associated with a reduction in mortality and provider-related complications on the surgical service: a concurrent analysis of 14,610 patients. Ann Surg 2009;250:316–21.
[33] Jamal MH, Doi SA, Rousseau M, et al. Systematic review and meta-analysis of the effect of North American working hours restrictions on mortality and morbidity in surgical patients. Br J Surg 2012;99:336–44.
[34] Borman KR, Jones AT, Shea JA. Duty hours, quality of care, and patient safety: general surgery resident perceptions. J Am Coll Surg 2012;215:70–7.
[35] Shea JA, Willett LL, Borman KR, et al. Anticipated consequences of the 2011 duty hours standards: views of internal medicine and surgery program directors. Acad Med 2012;87: 895–903.
[36] De Martino RR, Brewster LP, Kokkosis AA, et al. The perspective of the vascular surgery trainee on new ACGME regulations, fatigue, resident training, and patient safety. Vasc Endovascular Surg 2011;45:697–702.
[37] Babu MA, Nahed BV, Heary RF. Investigating the scope of resident patient care handoffs within neurosurgery. PLoS One 2012;7:e41810.
[38] Petersen LA, Brennan TA, O'Neil AC, et al. Does housestaff discontinuity of care increase the risk for preventable adverse events? Ann Intern Med 1994;121:866–72.
[39] Stewart BA, Fernandes S, Rodriguez-Huertas E, et al. A preliminary look at duplicate testing associated with lack of electronic health record interoperability for transferred patients. J Am Med Inform Assoc 2010;17:341–4.
[40] Lofgren RP, Gottlieb D, Williams RA, et al. Post-call transfer of resident responsibility: its effect on patient care. J Gen Intern Med 1990;5:501–5.
[41] Singh H, Thomas EJ, Petersen LA, et al. Medical errors involving trainees: a study of closed malpractice claims from 5 insurers. Arch Intern Med 2007;167:2030–6.
[42] Arriaga AF, Elbardissi AW, Regenbogen SE, et al. A policy-based intervention for the reduction of communication breakdowns in inpatient surgical care: results from a Harvard surgical safety collaborative. Ann Surg 2011;253:849–54.
[43] Wayne JD, Tyagi R, Reinhardt G, et al. Simple standardized patient handoff system that increases accuracy and completeness. J Surg Educ 2008;65:476–85.
[44] Van Eaton EG, Horvath KD, Lober WB, et al. A randomized, controlled trial evaluating the impact of a computerized rounding and sign-out system on continuity of care and resident work hours. J Am Coll Surg 2005;200:538–45.
[45] Kemp CD, Bath JM, Berger J, et al. The top 10 list for a safe and effective sign-out. Arch Surg 2008;143:1008–10.
[46] Young JS, Dubose JE, Hedrick TL, et al. The use of "war games" to evaluate performance of students and residents in basic clinical scenarios: a disturbing analysis. J Trauma 2007;63: 556–64.
[47] Harvey A, Bandiera G, Nathens AB, et al. Impact of stress on resident performance in simulated trauma scenarios. J Trauma 2012;72(2):497–503.
[48] Langhan TS, Rigby IJ, Walker IW, et al. Simulation-based training in critical resuscitation procedures improves residents' competence. CJEM 2009;11:535–9.
[49] Muller MP, Hansel M, Fichtner A, et al. Excellence in performance and stress reduction during two different full scale simulator training courses: a pilot study. Resuscitation 2009;80:919–24.

Advances in Surgery 47 (2013) 59–79

ADVANCES IN SURGERY

Current Management of the Zollinger-Ellison Syndrome

Geoffrey W. Krampitz, MD, Jeffrey A. Norton, MD*

Stanford University School of Medicine, Department of Surgery, 300 Pasteur Drive, H3591, Stanford, CA 94305-5655, USA

Keywords

• Zollinger-Ellison • Gastrinoma • Gastrin • Ulcer
• Gastroesophageal reflux disease • Diarrhea • Octreotide

Key points

- Zollinger-Ellison Syndrome (ZES) should be considered in patients with upper gastrointestinal tract symptoms (gastroesophageal reflux disease, peptic ulcer disease) with or without secretory diarrhea, or in those with peptic ulcer disease and primary hyperparathyroidism or family history suspicious for multiple endocrine neoplasia type 1 (MEN1).
- The initial workup should include a measurement of serum gastrin, serum calcium, gastric pH, and/or basal acid output when off antacid medications.
- Gastric acid hypersecretion should be controlled with proton-pump inhibitors.
- Localization studies including positron emission tomography, somatostatin receptor scintigraphy, computed tomography, magnetic resonance imaging, and endoscopic ultrasonography should be performed initially to evaluate for metastases and identify surgically resectable disease.
- In patients with MEN1, surgical correction of hyperparathyroidism (3½-gland parathyroidectomy) should precede surgical resection of the primary tumor, as patients have multiple tumors and are seldom cured; however, surgical resection is recommended for pancreatic neuroendocrine tumors larger than 2.5 cm because of malignant potential.
- All patients with localized sporadic gastrinoma should undergo surgical exploration for tumor resection, regardless of the results of imaging studies.

Disclosures: None.

*Corresponding author. *E-mail address*: janorton@stanford.edu

0065-3411/13/$ – see front matter
http://dx.doi.org/10.1016/j.yasu.2013.02.004

INTRODUCTION

Zollinger-Ellison Syndrome (ZES) is caused by gastrinoma, which is the second most common functional pancreatic neuroendocrine tumor (PNET). Gastrin hypersecretion from gastrinoma leads to increased production of gastric acid and severe peptic ulcer disease. In their landmark description, Robert Zollinger and Edwin Ellison correlated the triad of pancreatic tumors, hypersecretion of gastric acid, and unusual peptic ulcer disease in a series of patients at Ohio State University in 1955 [1]. Zollinger and Ellison correctly attributed the patients' intractable peptic ulcer disease to their pancreatic tumors that we now know were gastrinomas.

Gastrinoma has a yearly incidence of approximately 1 to 3 cases per million people in the United States [2]. ZES is the underlying cause in approximately 0.1% to 1% of patients with peptic ulcer disease [3]. Patients with ZES commonly present with signs and symptoms of peptic ulcer disease, gastroesophageal reflux disease (GERD), and secretory diarrhea. Because of the widespread availability of accurate immunoassays to measure serum concentrations of gastrin, gastrinoma is increasingly diagnosed and treated at an early stage of disease. Nevertheless, the mean time from symptoms to diagnosis is up to 8 years in many studies, underscoring the need for increased awareness of ZES [4]. In 80% of cases ZES occurs sporadically; however, approximately 20% of patients have the familial form associated with multiple endocrine neoplasia type 1 (MEN1). Fifty percent of patients with MEN1 have ZES, making gastrinoma the most common functional neuroendocrine tumor in MEN1. As a result, MEN1 must always be excluded during the workup of ZES. A significant family history of ulcers and peptic ulceration occurring at a young age are clues to familial gastrinoma. In addition, peptic ulcers in association with hyperparathyroidism and/or nephrolithiasis, pituitary tumors, benign thyroid tumors, benign and malignant adrenocortical tumors, lipomas, and cutaneous angiofibromas all may indicate MEN1.

CHARACTERISTICS

Size and location

Approximately 80% of gastrinomas are found within the gastrinoma triangle. The gastrinoma triangle is the anatomic area bounded by the junction of the cystic and common bile ducts superiorly, the junction of the second and third portions of the duodenum laterally, and the neck of the pancreas medially [5]. Gastrinomas are 3 times more likely to occur in the duodenum than in the pancreas, with the highest proportion in the first portion of the duodenum, becoming progressively less common toward the distal duodenum (Fig. 1) [6]. Duodenal gastrinomas (mean size 0.95 cm) are often smaller than pancreatic tumors (mean size 2.1 cm) [7]. In MEN1, both pancreatic and duodenal gastrinomas are multiple. Primary gastrinomas have been reported in several ectopic anatomic sites including the jejunum, stomach, liver, spleen, mesentery, ovary, heart, and lymph nodes [8]. Gastrinomas have been found in extrapancreatic, extraintestinal lymph nodes with no identifiable primary pancreatic or duodenal

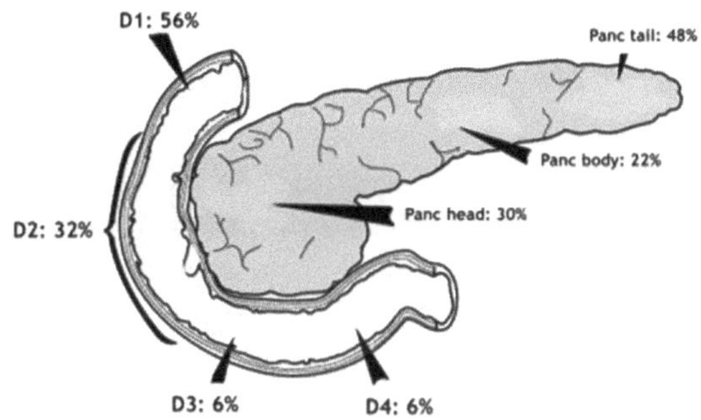

Fig. 1. Distribution of gastrinomas throughout the duodenum and pancreas. Duodenal gastrinomas are concentrated in the proximal duodenum and are progressively less frequent in the distal duodenum. Pancreatic gastrinomas are most commonly found in the tail of the pancreas. D, duodenum; Panc, pancreas. (*From* Cisco RM, Norton JA. Surgery for gastrinoma [review]. Adv Surg 2007;41:168; with permission from Elsevier.)

tumor [9–11]. Whether these represent lymph node primary tumors or metastases from occult pancreatic or intestinal primary tumors is controversial. In one series of 138 patients who underwent exploration for gastrinoma, 10% of patients with sporadic ZES achieved long-term cure after resection of a lymph node only. These patients were followed for a mean of 10 years, suggesting that these tumors represent true lymph node primary gastrinoma (Fig. 2) [9].

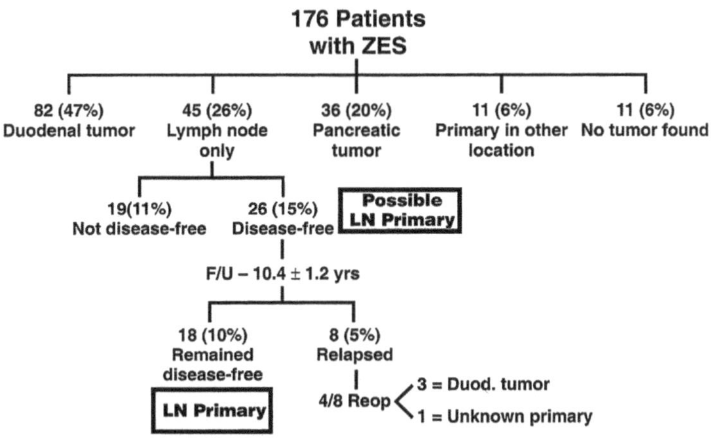

Fig. 2. Distribution of patients with ZES, dependent on surgical results. Of the 176 patients with ZES undergoing exploratory laparotomy, 45 had a lymph node (LN) only removed, and 26 of the 45 patients (15%) were disease-free postresection and had a possible primary lymph node gastrinoma. Duod., duodenal; F/U, follow-up. (*From* Norton JA, Alexander HR, Fraker DL, et al. Possible primary lymph node gastrinoma: occurrence, natural history, and predictive factors: a prospective study. Ann Surg 2003;237(5):652; with permission from Lippincott Williams & Wilkins.)

The discovery that neuroendocrine cells may be found within abdominal lymph nodes offers a possible explanation for the origin of these tumors [12,13].

Metastatic potential and survival

Gastrinomas are slow growing, but approximately 60% to 90% are malignant, with patients having lymph node, liver, or distant metastatic disease at the time of diagnosis. In 25% of cases, the tumor may pursue a particularly aggressive course. Pancreatic gastrinomas have a 50% incidence of liver metastases, compared with 10% for duodenal tumors. In addition, tumors in the distal pancreas are more likely to metastasize to the liver than are tumors arising within the gastrinoma triangle [14]. Overall, however, gastrinomas of the duodenum and pancreas appear to have a similar incidence of metastases. Because liver metastases have a direct effect on survival, pancreatic gastrinomas have a decreased long-term survival in comparison with duodenal primary tumors. Patients without liver metastases have a 95% 20-year survival after surgery, whereas patients with diffuse bilobar liver metastases have a 10-year survival of only 15%. Patients who have a solitary liver metastasis or fewer than 5 discrete metastases in both liver lobes have an intermediate survival (60% at 15 years) [15]. The extent of liver involvement is therefore the most important predictor of survival in gastrinoma (Fig. 3).

Lymph node involvement and survival

Gastrinoma is associated with lymph node involvement in 50% to 80% of patients. Duodenal gastrinomas have a 70% incidence of lymph node metastases,

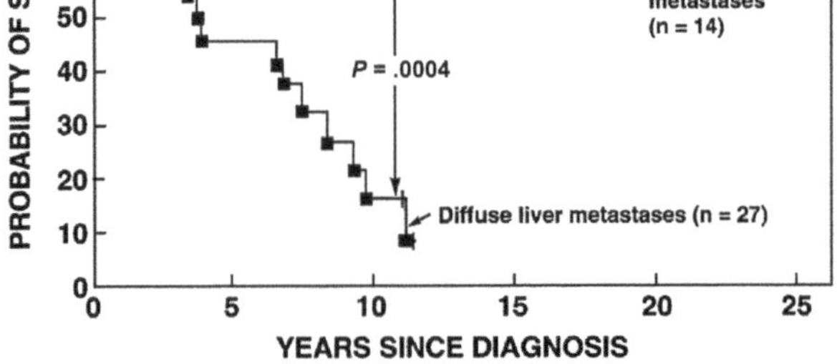

Fig. 3. Effect of the extent of liver tumor on the survival of 212 patients. Disease-related survival is plotted in the form of a Kaplan-Meier distribution. Numbers in parentheses refer to the number of patients in each group. (*From* Norton JA, Jensen RT. Resolved and unresolved controversies in the surgical management of patients with Zollinger-Ellison syndrome. Ann Surg 2004;240(5):766; with permission from Lippincott Williams & Wilkins.)

compared with 40% for pancreatic tumors [14]. In contrast to the well-established effect of liver metastases on survival in patients with PNETs, the effect of lymph node metastases on patient survival is controversial. A recent analysis of the Surveillance, Epidemiology, and End Results database from 1980 to 2004 involving 2350 patients with PNETs, the presence of lymph node involvement without liver metastases did not affect survival [16]. This finding supports a host of other studies [16–32] that also determined that lymph node metastases do not significantly decrease survival in patients with PNETs.

Nevertheless, some studies [33–35] have reported that lymph node involvement can be an important prognostic factor in PNETs. The conclusions of some of these studies are limited because it is not apparent whether the analysis included only lymph node involvement or lymph node and liver metastases. However, a recent study from 2 academic institutions of 326 patients with PNETs, the majority of which were gastrinomas, specifically analyzed the effect of lymph node involvement on survival [36]. Although overall survival was not significantly different between patients with and without lymph node metastases, patients with lymph node metastases had a shorter time to development of metachronous liver metastases than those without lymph node metastases. This difference was related to the number of lymph nodes involved. A subgroup analysis of patients with long-term follow-up demonstrated that significant differences occurred in disease-related survival among patients with no metastases, lymph node metastases only, and liver metastases. Furthermore, the decrease in disease-related survival was related to the number of lymph nodes involved with tumor (Fig. 4). Thus, for patients with gastrinoma, new studies suggest that lymph node involvement may affect disease-related survival, but longer follow-up is required to identify a significant difference.

Diagnosis

The diagnostic evaluation of a patient in whom ZES is suspected begins by obtaining a fasting serum concentration of gastrin. Hypergastrinemia (>100 pg/mL) occurs in all patients with ZES. Therefore, a normal fasting serum gastrin concentration effectively excludes ZES. Proton-pump inhibitors (PPI) may cause a false-positive increase in serum concentration of gastrin. Medicines that inhibit secretion of gastric acid should be withheld for at least 1 week before measurement of the serum gastrin concentration.

Patients with ZES also have hypersecretion of gastric acid. Achlorhydria is a common cause of hypergastrinemia, and secretion of gastric acid is measured to exclude this condition. A basal acid output (BAO) greater than 15 mEq/h (>5 mEq/h in patients who have undergone previous acid-reducing operations) is diagnostic of ZES. However, many hospitals are unable to measure acid output, and the measurement of gastric pH is simpler and more widely available. A gastric pH of 2 or less is consistent with ZES.

Finally, the secretin test is also positive in most patients with ZES. An increase of greater than 200 pg/mL in the fasting serum level of gastrin at 2 to 15 minutes following intravenous secretin administration is diagnostic of

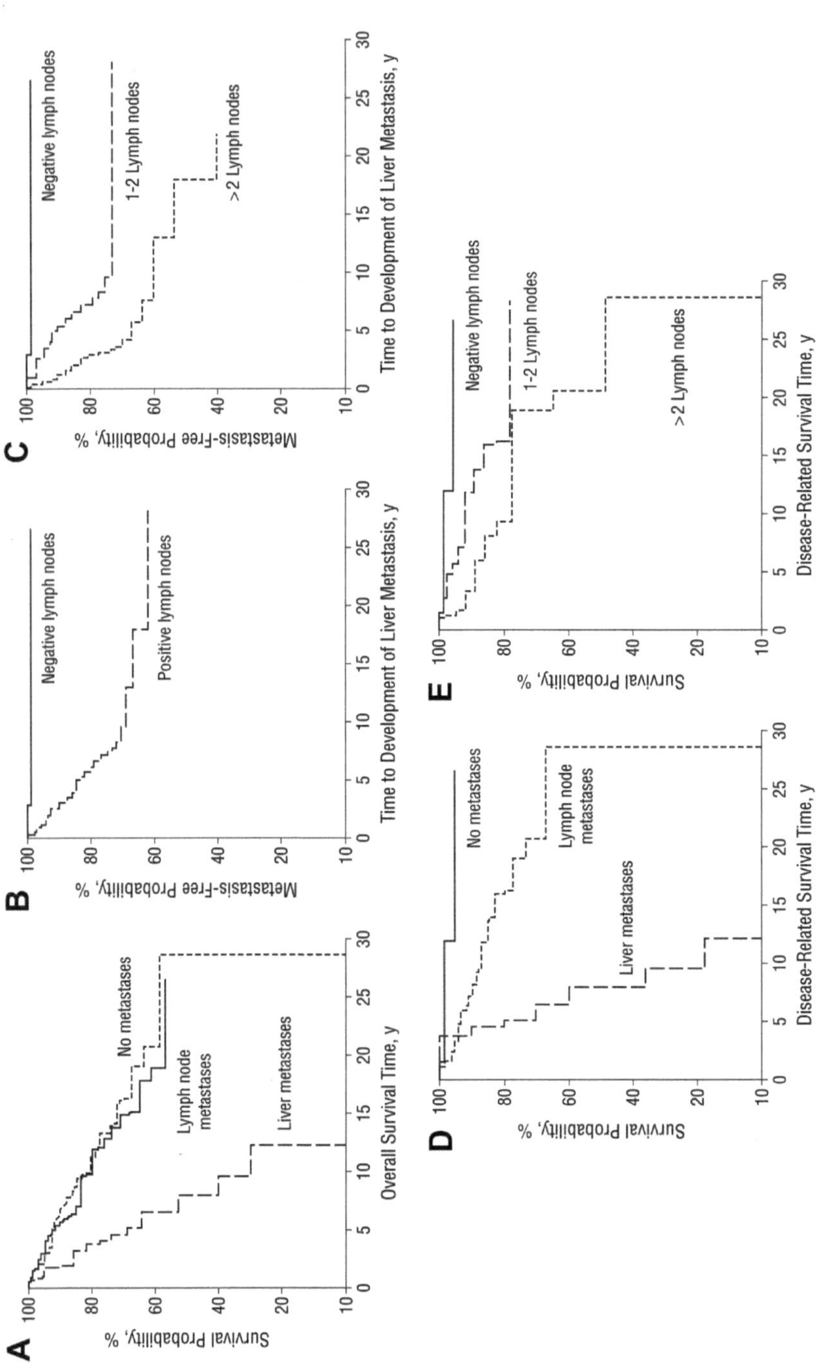
A
Survival Probability, %
Overall Survival Time, y
No metastases
Lymph node metastases
Liver metastases
B
Metastasis-Free Probability, %
Time to Development of Liver Metastasis, y
Negative lymph nodes
Positive lymph nodes
C
Metastasis-Free Probability, %
Time to Development of Liver Metastasis, y
Negative lymph nodes
1-2 Lymph nodes
>2 Lymph nodes
D
Survival Probability, %
Disease-Related Survival Time, y
No metastases
Lymph node metastases
Liver metastases
E
Survival Probability, %
Disease-Related Survival Time, y
Negative lymph nodes
1-2 Lymph nodes
>2 Lymph nodes

ZES. However, approximately 15% of patients with gastrinoma may have a negative secretin test. The laboratory tests for the diagnosis of ZES are summarized in Table 1.

All patients undergoing an initial workup for ZES should be screened for MEN1. ZES is the initial clinical manifestation in 40% of patients with MEN1, and the onset of ZES symptoms may precede the diagnosis of primary hyperparathyroidism [37]. The initial screen should include a serum calcium and parathyroid hormone measurement. If primary hyperparathyroidism is detected, the patient has MEN1. Surgery for the primary hyperparathyroidism (3½-gland parathyroidectomy) is recommended as the initial procedure before any surgery for the gastrinoma [38].

GASTRINOMA LOCALIZATION

Noninvasive localization studies

The diagnosis of ZES can be achieved by clinical symptoms and biochemical analysis. However, locating the primary tumor and identifying any evidence of metastases is critical to developing appropriate treatment strategies. Localization of gastrinomas should begin with noninvasive imaging to assess the extent of tumor spread and exclude unresectable metastatic disease. Invasive modalities can then be used to localize the primary tumor before surgery, because accurate localization of gastrinomas offers the best chance at curative resection. The sensitivities of various tumor localization modalities are summarized in Table 2. Gastrinomas appear as hyperattenuating lesions in the arterial and venous phases on contrast-enhanced computed tomography (CT), a finding that indicates their rich capillary network. Smaller lesions tend to be more homogeneous, and larger lesions are more likely to demonstrate heterogeneous enhancement, a finding attributable to areas of cystic degeneration, necrosis, fibrosis, and calcification [39]. Calcified tumors are larger and are more commonly associated with lymph node metastasis, synchronous liver metastasis, and higher tumor

Fig. 4. Kaplan-Meier plots. (*A*) Overall survival. (*B, C*) Time to development of liver metastases. (*D, E*) Disease-related survival. For National Institutes of Health (NIH) and Stanford University Hospital patients (n = 326), overall survival was not significantly different between patients with lymph node involvement and those without metastases (*A*). As a result, the time to development of liver metastases was analyzed, and a significant difference ($P<.001$) was found between the 2 groups (*B*). This difference in time to development of liver metastases was related to the number of lymph nodes involved ($P<.001$) (*C*). Because of the longer follow-up time for the NIH cohort (n = 216), an analysis of disease-related survival was performed on this subgroup (*D*); significant differences were found among patients with no metastases, lymph node metastases only, and liver metastases ($P<.001$). The extent of lymph node involvement was then examined in a subgroup analysis (*E*) whereby disease-related survival was found to decrease as a function of the number of lymph nodes involved with tumor ($P=.004$). (*From* Krampitz GW, Norton JA, Poultsides GA, et al. Lymph nodes and survival in pancreatic neuroendocrine tumors. Arch Surg 2012;147(9):825; with permission from the American Medical Association.)

Table 1
Diagnosis of gastrinoma

Fasting measurement off acid-reducing medication	Normal range	Gastrinoma range	Sensitivity (%)
Gastrin	<100 pg/mL	>100 pg/mL	99
Basal acid output	2–5 mEq/h	>15 mEq/h (>5 mEq/h in patients who have undergone previous acid-reducing operations)	98
Gastric pH		≤2	
Gastrin after secretin stimulation test	<200 pg/mL increase above baseline	≥200 pg/mL increase above baseline	85

grade [40]. Previous studies found that abdominal CT detects approximately 50% of gastrinomas, and the sensitivity of CT depends greatly on tumor size, tumor location, and the presence of metastases [41]. CT reliably detects gastrinomas larger than 3 cm in diameter, whereas tumors smaller than 1 cm in diameter are rarely detected. Intermediate tumors between 1 and 3 cm are identified in 30% of cases. Primary gastrinomas that arise within the pancreas are identified much more reliably than those in extrapancreatic, extrahepatic locations (80% vs 35%). In addition, CT scanning identified only 50% of liver metastases. New multidetector CT scanners and 3-dimensional imaging software have improved the detection of small lesions by allowing thin collimation, optimizing the timing of data acquisition, and administering contrast material intravenously [42]. Arterial and portal venous phases are complementary, as some lesions may be seen in only one phase but not the other. In addition, custom pancreatic imaging protocols that include a late arterial phase and thin slices have improved the sensitivity of CT. A recent study reviewing the multiphase helical CT scans

Table 2
Sensitivities of tumor localization modalities

	% of tumors localized			
Modality	Overall	Pancreas	Duodenum	Liver metastases
Noninvasive				
Transabdominal ultrasonography	20–30	—	—	14
Abdominal computed tomography	50	80–100	35	50
Abdominal magnetic resonance imaging	25	—	—	83
Somatostatin receptor scintigraphy	71–90	—	50	—
DOTA-TOC PET	97	—	—	—
Invasive				
Endoscopic ultrasonography	85	75–100	28–57	—
Palpation	65	91	60	—
Intraoperative ultrasonography	83	95	58	—
Duodenotomy	—	—	100	—

Abbreviation: DOTA-TOC PET, ^{68}Ga-tetraazacyclododecanetetraacetic acid–tyrosine-3-octreotide positron emission tomography.

of 30 patients with small PNETs (mean size 1.3 cm) found an overall sensitivity of 83% for CT. Moreover, in the 13 cases where pancreatic-phase images were obtained, a sensitivity of 100% was reported [43]. Examples of CT imaging of gastrinoma are shown in Fig. 5A and B.

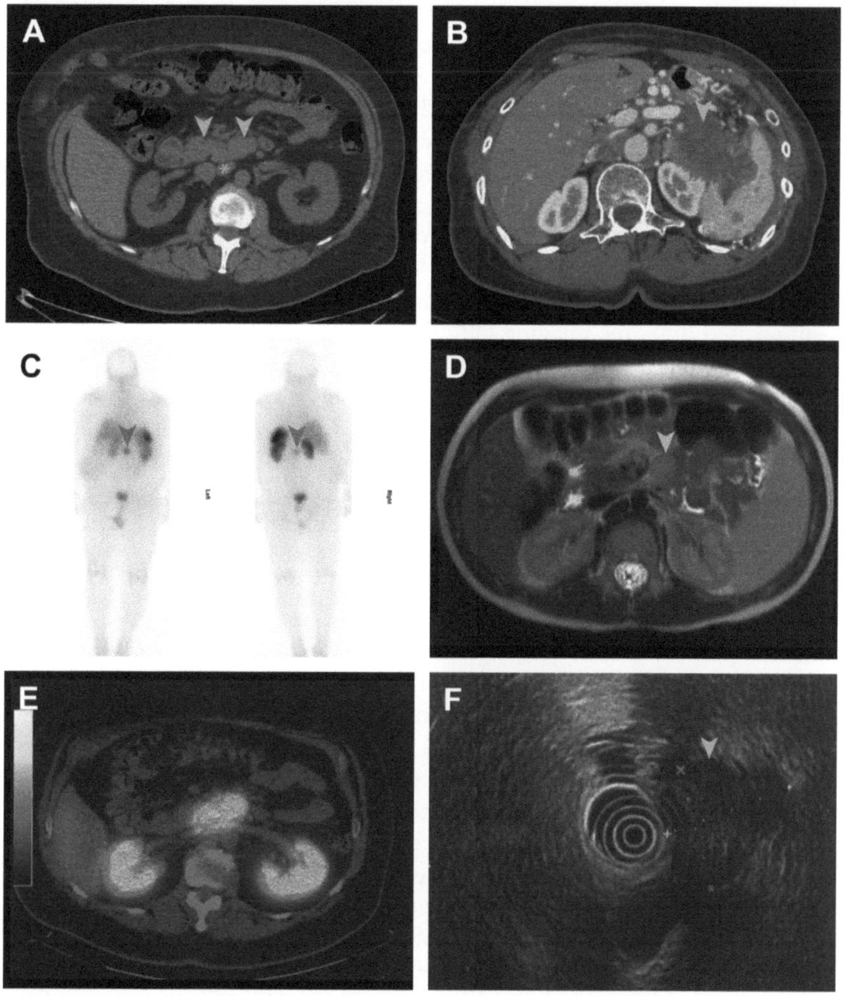

Fig. 5. Imaging modalities for gastrinoma. (*A*) Portal venous-phase CT of low grade tumor (*arrowheads*) and lymph node metastasis (*asterisk*). (*B*) Arterial-phase CT of intermediate-grade gastrinoma invading the spleen and kidney (*arrowhead*). (*C*) Anterior (*left*) and posterior (*right*) octreoscans of the patient from panel *A* 4 hours following administration of ^{111}In-octreodide. The arrowheads denote the gastrinoma. (*D*) T2-weighted MR image of a mesenteric gastrinoma (*arrowhead*). (*E*) ^{68}Ga-Tetraazacyclododecanetetraacetic acid–tyrosine-3-octreotide (DOTA-TOC) positron emission tomography (PET) scan of the patient from panels *A* and *C*. Note that the PET image is more vivid than the octreoscan. (*F*) Endoscopic ultrasonogram of a pancreatic head gastrinoma (*arrowhead*) in a patient with ZES and MEN1.

Magnetic resonance imaging (MRI) is also able to image gastrinomas. Gastrinomas are relatively hypervascular compared with the normal pancreas, and therefore appear hypointense on T1-weighted imaging, both with and without fat saturation, and hyperintense on T2 imaging (see Fig. 5D) [39]. Previous studies found that abdominal MRI had a low sensitivity (25%) in localizing primary gastrinomas, but was particularly useful in detecting hepatic metastases (sensitivity of 83%). Gastrinoma metastases in the liver appear hypointense on T1-weighted imaging and hyperintense on dynamic T2-weighted imaging, with distinct peripheral enhancement. With the use of hepatobiliary agents, including gadoxetic acid and dimeglumine gadobenate, metastases appear hypointense during the hepatocyte-specific phase because they do not contain hepatocytes. Involved peripancreatic lymph nodes also demonstrate prominent enhancement. More recent pancreatic MRI protocols to evaluate for PNETs include both T1-weighted and T2-weighted sequences, either with or without fat suppression, as well as gadolinium contrast material–enhanced T1-weighted fat-suppressed dynamic imaging [39]. One study addressing the utility of MRI in detecting small (<2 cm) PNETs found overall sensitivity of 85%, specificity of 100%, positive predictive value of 100%, and negative predictive value of 73% [44]. Another study comparing biphasic CT and MRI found that both modalities have similar effectiveness in detecting PNETs [45].

Somatostatin receptor scintigraphy (SRS), also called octreoscan, uses Indium (^{111}In)-labeled octreotide, which has a strong avidity for type 2 somatostatin receptors (SSR2) that are highly expressed on gastrinoma cells. During SRS, patients suspected of harboring gastrinoma are administered 6 mCi of ^{111}In-labeled octreotide by intravenous injection. Gamma recorders estimate tracer uptake at particular time points (usually 4 hours, and if necessary 24 and 48 hours) after administration of the radioactive compound. An example of SRS imaging of gastrinoma is shown in Fig. 5C. One prospective study using SRS in 146 gastrinoma patients found sensitivity of 71%, specificity of 86%, positive predictive value of 85%, and negative predictive value of 52% [46]. With a high pretest probability, as in the setting of ZES, SRS has overall sensitivity of approximately 90%, specificity approaching 100%, and positive predictive value near 100% [46,47]. The sensitivity of SRS for gastrinoma exceeds most other imaging modalities combined (including CT and MR) [48]. SRS altered clinical management in half of the patients, reflecting the ability of SRS not only to identify the primary tumor location but also to clarify equivocal results generated by conventional imaging studies [49]. The accuracy of SRS can be further improved by single-photon emission computed tomography (SPECT) [50,51]. SRS/SPECT enables convenient whole-body imaging to detect the presence of gastrinomas throughout the body. Like CT, the sensitivity of SRS correlates directly with the size of tumors. SRS is able to detect 96% of gastrinomas larger than 2.2 cm, but only 30% of tumors smaller than 1.1 cm. SRS has a sensitivity of 64% for intermediate tumors between 1.1 and 2.2 cm in size. Because duodenal gastrinomas are usually subcentimeter in size (Fig. 6), SRS fails to detect about 50% of these tumors [7,52,53]. A

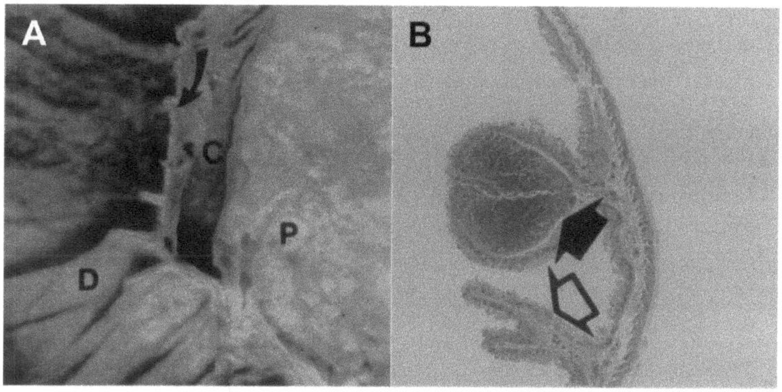

Fig. 6. Subcentimeter-sized gastrinomas in the wall of the duodenum in a patient with ZES and MEN1. (*A*) The bisected duodenum (D), common bile duct (C), and head of the pancreas (P). A small gastrinoma is present in the duodenal mucosa (*arrow*). (*B*) A histologic section of a duodenal gastrinoma (*solid arrow*). The size of the tumor barely exceeds the size of a normal mucosal fold (*open arrow*) (hematoxylin and eosin, original magnification ×10). (*From* Pipeleers-Marichal M, Somers G, Willems G, et al. Gastrinomas in the duodenums of patients with multiple endocrine neoplasia type 1 and the Zollinger-Ellison syndrome. N Engl J Med 1990;322(11):726; with permission from the Massachusetts Medical Society.)

positive SRS study strongly predicts the presence of tumor, but the variable negative predictive value (33%–100%) cautions against excluding a tumor on the basis of a negative study. SRS has a false-positive localization rate of about 12%. Extra-abdominal false-positive localization scans are more common than intra-abdominal false-positive scans, and are attributed to thyroid, breast, or granulomatous lung disease [54]. The most common cause of false-positive intra-abdominal SRS scans is accessory spleens, localization to prior operative sites, and renal parapelvic cysts. Only 2.7% of these false-positive results actually altered management, suggesting the importance of a high awareness of other potential causes for a positive SRS scan.

For most tumors, conventional positron emission tomography (PET) allows for more precise tumor localization than SRS. However, PNETs usually do not demonstrate increased fluorodeoxyglucose (FDG) uptake unless they are poorly differentiated. The poor uptake of FDG by PNETs limits the use of FDG PET in the localization of PNETs. However, a variety of octreotide-conjugated radionuclides have been developed that can be used for imaging PNETs by PET. Octreotide may be conjugated with the chelator tetraazacyclododecanetetraacetic acid (DOTA). DOTA-octreotide may be further modified with the addition of tyrosine to form DOTA-tyrosine-3-octreotide (DOTA-TOC), which demonstrates a very high affinity for SSR2. In addition, sodium iodide may be added to form DOTA-1-NaI-octreotide (DOTA-NOC), which demonstrates a high affinity for subtypes 2, 3, and 5 [55]. Gallium-68 (^{68}Ga) is a generator-produced positron-emitting nuclide that may be used to label DOTA and its analogues, which allows for high-contrast imaging and detection of small liver, lymph node, and bone metastases and primary tumors in patients with PNETs. Fig. 5E shows an example of ^{68}Ga-DOTA-TOC PET imaging in a patient with PNETs. Recent clinical studies have shown that these radioconjugates are effective for both imaging and therapy [55]. A recent study assessing the diagnostic efficacy of ^{68}Ga-DOTA-TOC PET in neuroendocrine tumors found that ^{68}Ga-DOTA-TOC PET had a higher sensitivity than SRS and dedicated CT in detecting primary tumors and metastases [56]. Additional somatostatin analogues with different receptor affinity, as well as other peptides, are currently under investigation, and may improve diagnostic and therapeutic capabilities in the future.

Invasive localization studies

Endoscopic ultrasonography (EUS) is an invasive procedure that combines endoscopy and ultrasound to produce high-quality, detailed, cost-effective images of the walls of the hollow gastrointestinal tract and adjacent organs during surveillance for gastrinoma (see Fig. 5F). EUS has a sensitivity between 80% and 94% for detecting pancreatic gastrinomas, but only 43% to 50% for duodenal tumors [52,57]. There is great variability in the sensitivities for EUS localization of pancreatic (75%–100%) and duodenal (28%–57%) tumors among several studies reviewed. Whether the differences in sensitivities are due to operator dependence, patient populations, or instrumentation is unclear. The authors hypothesize that ultrasonography needs a homogeneous background as seen in the pancreas (and not the duodenum), such that the gastrinoma appears sonolucent and is more clearly delineated. Nevertheless, the low sensitivity of EUS for duodenal tumors, given the high frequency of small duodenal gastrinomas, is a significant limitation [58]. EUS may provide some insight in distinguishing different types of pancreatic lesions; however, the specificity of using morphologic features alone to differentiate pancreatic lesions is only 53% [57]. Furthermore, EUS-guided fine-needle aspiration of the tumor mass may provide a histopathologic diagnosis in approximately 68% of cases before surgery [59].

Intraoperative ultrasonography (IOUS) is very useful for localizing intrapancreatic gastrinoma. IOUS can localize pancreatic tumors as small as 5 mm, and is therefore a powerful adjunct for detecting tumors not identified during preoperative imaging [53,60]. However, IOUS is poor at detecting duodenal gastrinomas [61], and does not substitute for duodenotomy with direct bifingered palpation.

Duodenotomy (opening the duodenum during surgery) is necessary to allow direct inspection and exploration of the duodenal mucosa. Duodenal gastrinomas originate in the submucosa of the duodenum, but they often pucker the mucosa and can be precisely palpated as a small nodule between the thumb and forefinger when the duodenum is opened. A recent prospective study of patients with sporadic ZES has shown a significantly higher cure rate following duodenotomy, both immediately and long term [62]. Duodenotomy was particularly important in the detection of small duodenal tumors, allowing localization of 90% of tumors smaller than 1 cm versus only 50% discovered on preoperative imaging. Duodenotomy is the intraoperative procedure of choice for detection of gastrinoma, and should be performed in all surgical explorations for gastrinoma. Duodenal wall gastrinomas occur in greatest density more proximally in the duodenum. Regional lymph nodes should be systematically sampled, as lymph node metastases may be inapparent at exploration and will be found in 55% of patients with duodenal tumors. Furthermore, imaging-negative patients most commonly have duodenal gastrinomas as the primary site of tumor. Duodenotomy has been essential in finding these small tumors [63]. Gastrinomas can ultimately be found by an experienced surgeon in nearly all patients [63–66].

TREATMENT

Medical management

The introduction of PPIs has made control of symptoms and medical management of gastric-acid hypersecretion routine in all patients with ZES. PPIs provide potent, specific, and durable inhibition of the production of gastric acid [67]. Oral omeprazole and intravenous pantoprazole must be dose adjusted in patients with ZES to normalize BAO levels to less than 15 mEq/h (<5 mEq/h in patients who have reflux esophagitis or who have had prior operations to reduce acid secretion, such as subtotal gastrectomy) [68]. Measuring BAO after initiating drug therapy is necessary because relief of symptoms alone is not a reliable indicator of effective acid control [69,70]. The typical dose of pantoprazole is 80 mg by mouth twice daily. This medication should be taken on an empty stomach. Conversely, if acid hypersecretion is controlled, epigastric discomfort resolves and ulcers heal in virtually all patients [71,72]. Because of the recent advances in the effective medical treatment of ZES, total gastrectomy is no longer indicated in patients with gastrinoma. However, even with symptomatic control and negative imaging studies, patients with sporadic gastrinoma should be referred for surgical exploration because of the high probability of tumor resection and cure [63].

Surgical management

MEN1 and ZES

Hypercalcemia resulting from primary hyperparathyroidism (HPT) can significantly exacerbate the symptoms and elevate serum gastrin levels in patients with ZES. Thus, in ZES and coexistent HPT, neck exploration for resection of parathyroid hyperplasia should be performed before surgery for the gastrinoma. In these patients, subtotal parathyroidectomy (3½ glands with the cervical thymus) can significantly decrease end-organ effects of hypergastrinemia, allowing for better medical control of ZES symptoms, and may even normalize abnormal serum levels of gastrin and abnormal secretin tests [38].

Gastrinomas associated with MEN1 tend to be multiple and small (Fig. 6), usually originate in the duodenum, and frequently develop lymph node metastases; however, these tumors may be more indolent than sporadic tumors and may have a more favorable long-term prognosis [73]. In patients with MEN1 and ZES, surgical resection is seldom curative (0%–10%) but may be effective in preventing or decreasing the development of liver metastases [6]. Tumor size correlates with progression to liver metastasis, which in turn is the strongest predictor of survival. Consequently, in ZES patients with MEN1, surgery is recommended only if there is an identifiable tumor greater than 2.5 cm in size. The operation should include resection of body and tail PNETs, enucleation of palpable pancreatic head tumors, duodenotomy with excision of duodenal tumors, and peripancreatic lymph node sampling [74]. The goal of such an operation is to prevent the development of liver metastases and thus decrease tumor-related mortality, not to cure ZES [6]. However, this approach is controversial because some other investigators have documented cure of ZES patients with MEN1 by performing a Whipple pancreaticoduodenectomy [52]. The authors do not favor this approach because in most of these studies the follow-up is short, patients develop late recurrences, the secretin test and gastrin levels are not routinely performed, and the operative morbidity, mortality, and long-term survival with the surgical approach described above are excellent.

Sporadic gastrinoma

All patients with sporadic gastrinoma who do not have unresectable metastatic disease should undergo exploratory laparotomy for potential cure of ZES [63,75]. A recent study followed 160 ZES patients for a mean of 12 years, and demonstrated that routine surgical removal of gastrinoma increased survival (54 vs 21%) by increasing disease-related survival (23 vs 1%) and decreasing the development of distant disease (rate of metastasis 29% vs 5%) [76]. Surgical exploration and duodenotomy should be performed even in patients without an identifiable tumor on preoperative imaging but with clear biochemical evidence of sporadic ZES, because of the high probability of finding an occult duodenal gastrinoma [76]. A recent study of sporadic ZES patients with negative imaging studies found that duodenal gastrinomas occur in almost every patient (98%); moreover, a substantial subset is cured. Fig. 7 shows the comparison of disease-related and overall survival for the negative and positive imaging patients. All the disease-related deaths occurred in patients who had liver metastases discovered at the time of surgery. A long delay in referring these patients for surgery because of a lack of positive imaging findings likely contributed to the disease progression. Thus, surgery should be routinely undertaken early in sporadic ZES patients, even in those with negative imaging studies [63].

Gastrinomas localized to the duodenum may be locally resected with adequate margins [77]. Resection should allow for nonconstricting closure of the remaining duodenum, and special attention must be paid to avoid injury to the ampulla of Vater, which may be mistaken for a gastrinoma. Regional lymph nodes should be systematically sampled and excised, as lymph node metastases may be unapparent at exploration and will be found in 55% of patients with duodenal tumors. Resection of a single duodenal gastrinoma and regional lymph node dissection resulted in a cure in 60% of patients with sporadic gastrinoma [53]. Multiple duodenal gastrinomas localized to either the upper or lower aspects of the duodenum may undergo partial resection of

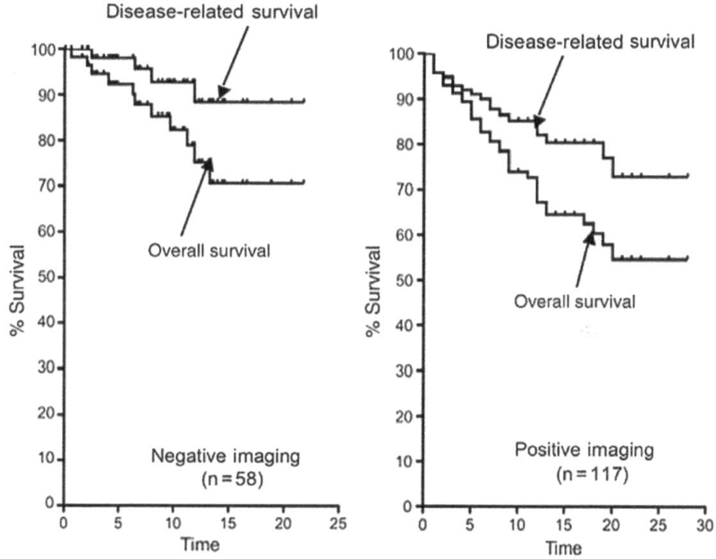

Fig. 7. Survival of patients with image-negative gastrinomas. Kaplan-Meier plot of the disease-related and overall survival for the negative and positive imaging patients. Negative imaging patients had an overall 20-year survival of 71% compared with 58% for the positive imaging patients, and the disease-related survival was 88% compared with 73% ($P = .015$). (*From* Norton JA, Fraker DL, Alexander HR, et al. Value of surgery in patients with negative imaging and sporadic Zollinger-Ellison syndrome. Ann Surg 2012;256(3):514; with permission from Lippincott Williams & Wilkins.)

the duodenum. For patients with large tumors or ampullary involvement, a pylorus-preserving pancreaticoduodenectomy may be indicated [53].

Patients with pancreatic disease should undergo mobilization of the pancreas and palpation with IOUS. For disease in the body and tail of the pancreas, distal pancreatectomy is indicated. Pancreatic head and neck tumors not involving major ductal or vascular structures are enucleated. For bulky large tumors localized to the pancreatic head, a pylorus-preserving pancreaticoduodenectomy may be necessary [78]. The authors have demonstrated that mesenteric vascular resection and reconstruction is not a contraindication to gastrinoma resection. In carefully selected patients with involvement of the superior mesenteric vein and portal vein, the results have been excellent. Thirty percent of patients with vascular resection for PNET were disease-free, and the 10-year survival was 60% [79].

Advanced disease

Because 60% to 90% of gastrinomas are malignant, management of advanced disease is a significant problem. At the time of diagnosis of ZES, 25% to 33% of patients have liver metastases [8] with 5% to 15% limited to 1 lobe of the liver [32,52]. In these patients, resection of both primary and metastatic gastrinoma should be considered [8]. The long-term (10-year) survival of patients with resected liver metastases from gastrinoma is 60%. The cure rate is infrequent, as tumors will recur late. Other cytoreductive strategies, such as transarterial chemoembolization (TACE) and radioembolization, and radiofrequency ablation (RFA) may be performed preoperatively or in lieu of an operation in the case of liver metastases [80]. However, these procedures have not been as effective as surgery. Although surgery remains the primary option for patients for both early-stage and advanced disease, the treatment of patients with metastatic PNET requires a multidisciplinary approach. In PNETs that present at advanced stage, medical treatments play a pivotal role in controlling both symptoms and tumor mass in the majority of patients. Nonsurgical therapeutic approaches include: chemotherapy; biotherapies including somatostatin analogues and interferon; targeted therapies including antiangiogenic therapy, epidermal growth factor inhibition, multireceptor tyrosine kinase inhibition, and mammalian target of rapamycin (mTOR) inhibition, RFA, TACE and radioembolization, and polypeptide radionuclide receptor therapy; and external radiation therapies including radiorobotic surgery [81–84]. Recently, everolimus and sunitinib demonstrated significant antitumor activity in patients with malignant PNETs [82]. RADIANT-3 is a randomized, double-blind, placebo-controlled, multicenter, phase 3 study of everolimus, an oral inhibitor of the mTOR, which showed antitumor activity in patients with advanced PNETs in 2 prior phase 2 studies [85,86]. In RADIANT-3, 410 patients with advanced neuroendocrine tumors with radiologic evidence of disease progression were randomized to receive everolimus or placebo in conjunction with the best supportive therapy [83]. Patients receiving everolimus had significantly prolonged progression-free survival compared with placebo (4.6 vs 11.0 months), representing a 65% reduction in the estimated risk of disease progression or death. Furthermore, patients receiving everolimus had a low rate of adverse events [83]. Similarly, a recent multinational, randomized, double-blind, placebo-controlled, phase 3 trial evaluated the efficacy of sunitinib, an oral inhibitor of platelet-derived growth factor receptors (PDGFRs) α and β, stem-cell factor receptor (c-kit), and vascular endothelial growth factor receptor (VEGFR)-2 and VEGFR-3, which showed antitumor activity in patients with advanced PNETs in prior phase 1 and 2 trials [87,88]. In this trial, a total of 171 patients with advanced PNETs progressing within 1 year were randomized to receive the best supportive care with either sunitinib or placebo. Patients receiving sunitinib had improved progression-free survival (11.4 vs 5.5 months), overall survival, and objective response rate (9.3% vs 0%) in comparison with placebo [84].

Each of these therapies has potential because each has had some success, and should be considered based on the extent of tumor, prior treatments, the general health of the patient, and the resources of the institution.

SUMMARY

In summary, ZES is a syndrome caused by gastrinoma, usually located within the gastrinoma triangle and associated with symptoms of peptic ulcer disease,

GERD, and diarrhea. The diagnosis of ZES is made by measuring fasting levels of serum gastrin, BAO, and the secretin stimulation test. Because of the high association of ZES and MEN1, HPT must be excluded by obtaining a serum calcium and parathyroid hormone level. Treatment of ZES consists of medical control of symptoms with PPIs and evaluation for potentially curative surgical intervention. Noninvasive imaging studies including SRS, CT, and MRI should be performed initially to evaluate for metastases and identify resectable disease. Invasive imaging modalities such as EUS may be performed to further evaluate primary tumors. IOUS, palpation, and duodenotomy are used for intraoperative localization of gastrinomas. In patients with MEN1, surgical resection should be pursued only if there is an identifiable tumor larger than 2 cm and after surgery for the primary hyperparathyroidism (3½-gland parathyroidectomy). All patients with resectable localized sporadic gastrinoma should undergo surgical exploration, even those with biochemical evidence but negative imaging studies. Tumor is most commonly found in the duodenum, and the cure rate is high. In patients with liver metastases, surgery should be considered if all identifiable tumor can be safely removed. A multidisciplinary approach including surgical and nonsurgical therapies should be taken in patients with advanced disease.

References

[1] Zollinger RM, Ellison EH. Primary peptic ulcerations of the jejunum associated with islet cell tumors of the pancreas. Ann Surg 1955;142(4):709–23 [discussion: 724–8].

[2] Grobmyer SR, Hochwald SN. Reoperative surgery for the Zollinger-Ellison syndrome. Adv Surg 2010;44:327–46.

[3] Eriksson B, Oberg K, Skogseid B. Neuroendocrine pancreatic tumors. Clinical findings in a prospective study of 84 patients. Acta Oncol 1989;28(3):373–7.

[4] Gibril F, Jensen RT. Zollinger-Ellison syndrome revisited: diagnosis, biologic markers, associated inherited disorders, and acid hypersecretion. Curr Gastroenterol Rep 2004;6(6): 454–63.

[5] Stabile BE, Morrow DJ, Passaro E Jr. The gastrinoma triangle: operative implications. Am J Surg 1984;147(1):25–31.

[6] Cisco RM, Norton JA. Surgery for gastrinoma. Adv Surg 2007;41:165–76.

[7] Behe M, Gotthardt M, Behr TM. Imaging of gastrinomas by nuclear medicine methods. Wien Klin Wochenschr 2007;119(19–20):593–6.

[8] Gibril F, Jensen RT. Advances in evaluation and management of gastrinoma in patients with Zollinger-Ellison syndrome. Curr Gastroenterol Rep 2005;7(2):114–21.

[9] Norton JA, Alexander HR, Fraker DL, et al. Possible primary lymph node gastrinoma: occurrence, natural history, and predictive factors: a prospective study. Ann Surg 2003;237(5): 650–7 [discussion: 657–9].

[10] Norton JA. Advances in the management of Zollinger-Ellison syndrome. Adv Surg 1994;27: 129–59.

[11] Wolfe MM, Alexander RW, McGuigan JE. Extrapancreatic, extraintestinal gastrinoma: effective treatment by surgery. N Engl J Med 1982;306(25):1533–6.

[12] Perrier ND, Batts KP, Thompson GB, et al. An immunohistochemical survey for neuroendocrine cells in regional pancreatic lymph nodes: a plausible explanation for primary nodal gastrinomas? Mayo Clinic Pancreatic Surgery Group. Surgery 1995;118(6):957–65 [discussion: 965–6].

[13] Herrmann ME, Ciesla MC, Chejfec G, et al. Primary nodal gastrinomas. Arch Pathol Lab Med 2000;124(6):832–5.

[14] Sutliff VE, Doppman JL, Gibril F, et al. Growth of newly diagnosed, untreated metastatic gastrinomas and predictors of growth patterns. J Clin Oncol 1997;15(6):2420–31.
[15] Norton JA. Endocrine tumours of the gastrointestinal tract. Surgical treatment of neuroendocrine metastases. Best Pract Res Clin Gastroenterol 2005;19(4):577–83.
[16] Roland CL, Bian A, Mansour JC, et al. Survival impact of malignant pancreatic neuroendocrine and islet cell neoplasm phenotypes. J Surg Oncol 2012;105(6):595–600.
[17] Stabile BE, Passaro E Jr. Benign and malignant gastrinoma. Am J Surg 1985;149(1):144–50.
[18] Pape UF, Jann H, Muller-Nordhorn J, et al. Prognostic relevance of a novel TNM classification system for upper gastroenteropancreatic neuroendocrine tumors. Cancer 2008;113(2): 256–65.
[19] Nikfarjam M, Warshaw AL, Axelrod L, et al. Improved contemporary surgical management of insulinomas: a 25-year experience at the Massachusetts General Hospital. Ann Surg 2008;247(1):165–72.
[20] Kazanjian KK, Reber HA, Hines OJ. Resection of pancreatic neuroendocrine tumors: results of 70 cases. Arch Surg 2006;141(8):765–9 [discussion: 769–70].
[21] Hochwald SN, Zee S, Conlon KC, et al. Prognostic factors in pancreatic endocrine neoplasms: an analysis of 136 cases with a proposal for low-grade and intermediate-grade groups. J Clin Oncol 2002;20(11):2633–42.
[22] Fendrich V, Langer P, Celik I, et al. An aggressive surgical approach leads to long-term survival in patients with pancreatic endocrine tumors. Ann Surg 2006;244(6):845–51 [discussion: 852–3].
[23] Ellison EC, Sparks J, Verducci JS, et al. 50-year appraisal of gastrinoma: recommendations for staging and treatment. J Am Coll Surg 2006;202(6):897–905.
[24] Ekeblad S, Skogseid B, Dunder K, et al. Prognostic factors and survival in 324 patients with pancreatic endocrine tumor treated at a single institution. Clin Cancer Res 2008;14(23): 7798–803.
[25] DiNorcia J, Lee MK, Reavey PL, et al. One hundred thirty resections for pancreatic neuroendocrine tumor: evaluating the impact of minimally invasive and parenchyma-sparing techniques. J Gastrointest Surg 2010;14(10):1536–46.
[26] Bilimoria KY, Talamonti MS, Tomlinson JS, et al. Prognostic score predicting survival after resection of pancreatic neuroendocrine tumors: analysis of 3851 patients. Ann Surg 2008;247(3):490–500.
[27] Chu QD, Hill HC, Douglass HO Jr, et al. Predictive factors associated with long-term survival in patients with neuroendocrine tumors of the pancreas. Ann Surg Oncol 2002;9(9): 855–62.
[28] Jensen RT, Niederle B, Mitry E, et al. Gastrinoma (duodenal and pancreatic). Neuroendocrinology 2006;84(3):173–82.
[29] Schurr PG, Strate T, Rese K, et al. Aggressive surgery improves long-term survival in neuroendocrine pancreatic tumors: an institutional experience. Ann Surg 2007;245(2):273–81.
[30] Fischer L, Kleeff J, Esposito I, et al. Clinical outcome and long-term survival in 118 consecutive patients with neuroendocrine tumours of the pancreas. Br J Surg 2008;95(5): 627–35.
[31] Weber HC, Venzon DJ, Lin JT, et al. Determinants of metastatic rate and survival in patients with Zollinger-Ellison syndrome: a prospective long-term study. Gastroenterology 1995;108(6): 1637–49.
[32] Yu F, Venzon DJ, Serrano J, et al. Prospective study of the clinical course, prognostic factors, causes of death, and survival in patients with long-standing Zollinger-Ellison syndrome. J Clin Oncol 1999;17(2):615–30.
[33] Tomassetti P, Campana D, Piscitelli L, et al. Endocrine pancreatic tumors: factors correlated with survival. Ann Oncol 2005;16(11):1806–10.
[34] Bettini R, Boninsegna L, Mantovani W, et al. Prognostic factors at diagnosis and value of WHO classification in a mono-institutional series of 180 non-functioning pancreatic endocrine tumours. Ann Oncol 2008;19(5):903–8.

[35] Boninsegna L, Panzuto F, Partelli S, et al. Malignant pancreatic neuroendocrine tumour: lymph node ratio and Ki67 are predictors of recurrence after curative resections. Eur J Cancer 2012;48(11):1608–15.
[36] Krampitz GW, Norton JA, Poultsides GA, et al. Lymph nodes and survival in pancreatic neuroendocrine tumors. Arch Surg 2012;147(9):820–7.
[37] Gibril F, Schumann M, Pace A, et al. Multiple endocrine neoplasia type 1 and Zollinger-Ellison syndrome: a prospective study of 107 cases and comparison with 1009 cases from the literature. Medicine (Baltimore) 2004;83(1):43–83.
[38] Norton JA, Cornelius MJ, Doppman JL, et al. Effect of parathyroidectomy in patients with hyperparathyroidism, Zollinger-Ellison syndrome, and multiple endocrine neoplasia type I: a prospective study. Surgery 1987;102(6):958–66.
[39] Lewis RB, Lattin GE Jr, Paal E. Pancreatic endocrine tumors: radiologic-clinicopathologic correlation. Radiographics 2010;30(6):1445–64.
[40] Poultsides GA, Huang LC, Chen Y, et al. Pancreatic neuroendocrine tumors: radiographic calcifications correlate with grade and metastasis. Ann Surg Oncol 2012;19(7): 2295–303.
[41] Wank SA, Doppman JL, Miller DL, et al. Prospective study of the ability of computed axial tomography to localize gastrinomas in patients with Zollinger-Ellison syndrome. Gastroenterology 1987;92(4):905–12.
[42] Horton KM, Hruban RH, Yeo C, et al. Multi-detector row CT of pancreatic islet cell tumors. Radiographics 2006;26(2):453–64.
[43] Fidler JL, Fletcher JG, Reading CC, et al. Preoperative detection of pancreatic insulinomas on multiphasic helical CT. AJR Am J Roentgenol 2003;181(3):775–80.
[44] Thoeni RF, Mueller-Lisse UG, Chan R, et al. Detection of small, functional islet cell tumors in the pancreas: selection of MR imaging sequences for optimal sensitivity. Radiology 2000;214(2):483–90.
[45] Ichikawa T, Peterson MS, Federle MP, et al. Islet cell tumor of the pancreas: biphasic CT versus MR imaging in tumor detection. Radiology 2000;216(1):163–71.
[46] Alexander HR, Fraker DL, Norton JA, et al. Prospective study of somatostatin receptor scintigraphy and its effect on operative outcome in patients with Zollinger-Ellison syndrome. Ann Surg 1998;228(2):228–38.
[47] Gibril F, Reynolds JC, Doppman JL, et al. Somatostatin receptor scintigraphy: its sensitivity compared with that of other imaging methods in detecting primary and metastatic gastrinomas. A prospective study. Ann Intern Med 1996;125(1):26–34.
[48] Schillaci O, Spanu A, Scopinaro F, et al. Somatostatin receptor scintigraphy in liver metastasis detection from gastroenteropancreatic neuroendocrine tumors. J Nucl Med 2003;44(3):359–68.
[49] Modlin IM, Tang LH. Approaches to the diagnosis of gut neuroendocrine tumors: the last word (today). Gastroenterology 1997;112(2):583–90.
[50] Schillaci O, Corleto VD, Annibale B, et al. Single photon emission computed tomography procedure improves accuracy of somatostatin receptor scintigraphy in gastro-entero pancreatic tumours. Ital J Gastroenterol Hepatol 1999;31(Suppl 2):S186–9.
[51] Krausz Y, Keidar Z, Kogan I, et al. SPECT/CT hybrid imaging with 111 In-pentetreotide in assessment of neuroendocrine tumours. Clin Endocrinol (Oxf) 2003;59(5):565–73.
[52] Norton JA, Jensen RT. Resolved and unresolved controversies in the surgical management of patients with Zollinger-Ellison syndrome. Ann Surg 2004;240(5):757–73.
[53] Imamura M, Komoto I, Ota S. Changing treatment strategy for gastrinoma in patients with Zollinger-Ellison syndrome. World J Surg 2006;30(1):1–11.
[54] Meko JB, Doherty GM, Siegel BA, et al. Evaluation of somatostatin-receptor scintigraphy for detecting neuroendocrine tumors. Surgery 1996;120(6):975–83 [discussion: 983–4].
[55] Rufini V, Calcagni ML, Baum RP. Imaging of neuroendocrine tumors. Semin Nucl Med 2006;36(3):228–47.

[56] Gabriel M, Decristoforo C, Kendler D, et al. ^{68}Ga-DOTA-Tyr3-octreotide PET in neuroendocrine tumors: comparison with somatostatin receptor scintigraphy and CT. J Nucl Med 2007;48(4):508–18.
[57] McLean A. Endoscopic ultrasound in the detection of pancreatic islet cell tumours. Cancer Imaging 2004;4(2):84–91.
[58] Rosch T, Lightdale CJ, Botet JF, et al. Localization of pancreatic endocrine tumors by endoscopic ultrasonography. N Engl J Med 1992;326(26):1721–6.
[59] Imaoka H, Yamao K, Bhatia V, et al. Rare pancreatic neoplasms: the utility of endoscopic ultrasound-guided fine-needle aspiration-a large single center study. J Gastroenterol 2009;44(2):146–53.
[60] Norton JA, Cromack DT, Shawker TH, et al. Intraoperative ultrasonographic localization of islet cell tumors. A prospective comparison to palpation. Ann Surg 1988;207(2):160–8.
[61] Norton JA. Intra-operative procedures to localize endocrine tumours of the pancreas and duodenum. Ital J Gastroenterol Hepatol 1999;31(Suppl 2):S195–7.
[62] von Eyben FE, Grodum E, Gjessing HJ, et al. Metabolic remission with octreotide in patients with insulinoma. J Intern Med 1994;235(3):245–8.
[63] Norton JA, Fraker DL, Alexander HR, et al. Value of surgery in patients with negative imaging and sporadic Zollinger-Ellison syndrome. Ann Surg 2012;256(3):509–17.
[64] Thompson NW, Vinik AI, Eckhauser FE. Microgastrinomas of the duodenum. A cause of failed operations for the Zollinger-Ellison syndrome. Ann Surg 1989;209(4):396–404.
[65] Norton JA, Fraker DL, Alexander HR, et al. Surgery to cure the Zollinger-Ellison syndrome. N Engl J Med 1999;341(9):635–44.
[66] Howard TJ, Zinner MJ, Stabile BE, et al. Gastrinoma excision for cure. A prospective analysis. Ann Surg 1990;211(1):9–14.
[67] Wolfe MM, Sachs G. Acid suppression: optimizing therapy for gastroduodenal ulcer healing, gastroesophageal reflux disease, and stress-related erosive syndrome. Gastroenterology 2000;118(2 Suppl 1):S9–31.
[68] Maton PN, Vinayek R, Frucht H, et al. Long-term efficacy and safety of omeprazole in patients with Zollinger-Ellison syndrome: a prospective study. Gastroenterology 1989;97(4):827–36.
[69] Norton JA. Gastrinoma: advances in localization and treatment. Surg Oncol Clin N Am 1998;7(4):845–61.
[70] Maton PN, Frucht H, Vinayek R, et al. Medical management of patients with Zollinger-Ellison syndrome who have had previous gastric surgery: a prospective study. Gastroenterology 1988;94(2):294–9.
[71] Fox PS, Hofmann JW, Decosse JJ, et al. The influence of total gastrectomy on survival in malignant Zollinger-Ellison tumors. Ann Surg 1974;180(4):558–66.
[72] Zollinger RM, Ellison EC, O'Dorisio TM, et al. Thirty years' experience with gastrinoma. World J Surg 1984;8(4):427–35.
[73] Li ML, Norton JA. Gastrinoma. Curr Treat Options Oncol 2001;2(4):337–46.
[74] Norton JA, Fang TD, Jensen RT. Surgery for gastrinoma and insulinoma in multiple endocrine neoplasia type 1. J Natl Compr Canc Netw 2006;4(2):148–53.
[75] Meko JB, Norton JA. Management of patients with Zollinger-Ellison syndrome. Annu Rev Med 1995;46:395–411.
[76] Norton JA, Fraker DL, Alexander HR, et al. Surgery increases survival in patients with gastrinoma. Ann Surg 2006;244(3):410–9.
[77] Frucht H, Norton JA, London JF, et al. Detection of duodenal gastrinomas by operative endoscopic transillumination. A prospective study. Gastroenterology 1990;99(6):1622–7.
[78] Brandi ML, Gagel RF, Angeli A, et al. Guidelines for diagnosis and therapy of MEN type 1 and type 2. J Clin Endocrinol Metab 2001;86(12):5658–71.
[79] Norton JA, Harris EJ, Chen Y, et al. Pancreatic endocrine tumors with major vascular abutment, involvement, or encasement and indication for resection. Arch Surg 2011;146(6): 724–32.

[80] Ehehalt F, Saeger HD, Schmidt CM, et al. Neuroendocrine tumors of the pancreas. Oncologist 2009;14(5):456–67.
[81] Yalcin S. Advances in the systemic treatment of pancreatic neuroendocrine tumors. Cancer Treat Rev 2011;37(2):127–32.
[82] Jensen RT, Delle Fave G. Promising advances in the treatment of malignant pancreatic endocrine tumors. N Engl J Med 2011;364(6):564–5.
[83] Yao JC, Shah MH, Ito T, et al. Everolimus for advanced pancreatic neuroendocrine tumors. N Engl J Med 2011;364(6):514–23.
[84] Raymond E, Dahan L, Raoul JL, et al. Sunitinib malate for the treatment of pancreatic neuroendocrine tumors. N Engl J Med 2011;364(6):501–13.
[85] Yao JC, Lombard-Bohas C, Baudin E, et al. Daily oral everolimus activity in patients with metastatic pancreatic neuroendocrine tumors after failure of cytotoxic chemotherapy: a phase II trial. J Clin Oncol 2010;28(1):69–76.
[86] Yao JC, Phan AT, Chang DZ, et al. Efficacy of RAD001 (everolimus) and octreotide LAR in advanced low- to intermediate-grade neuroendocrine tumors: results of a phase II study. J Clin Oncol 2008;26(26):4311–8.
[87] Faivre S, Delbaldo C, Vera K, et al. Safety, pharmacokinetic, and antitumor activity of SU11248, a novel oral multitarget tyrosine kinase inhibitor, in patients with cancer. J Clin Oncol 2006;24(1):25–35.
[88] Kulke MH, Lenz HJ, Meropol NJ, et al. Activity of sunitinib in patients with advanced neuroendocrine tumors. J Clin Oncol 2008;26(20):3403–10.

Advances in Surgery 47 (2013) 81–98

ADVANCES IN SURGERY

What Laboratory Tests Are Required for Ambulatory Surgery?

Jaime Benarroch-Gampel, MD, MS, Taylor S. Riall, MD, PhD*

Department of Surgery, The University of Texas Medical Branch, 301 University Boulevard, Galveston, TX 77555, USA

Keywords

• Preoperative testing • Ambulatory surgery • Laboratory testing
• Preoperative evaluation • Low-risk surgery

Key points

- Current indications for preoperative testing represent a synthesis of expert opinion, and are not based on a sufficient number of adequately powered and controlled trials.
- Abnormal preoperative test results are considered in many cases of questionable clinical significance, and have not been shown to predict adverse outcomes.
- Elimination of routine testing and more selective use based on patient history and physical examination has been shown to decrease cost without detriment to patient care.

INTRODUCTION

Ambulatory, or same-day, surgery is being used with increasing frequency because of the significant cost savings and increased convenience for patients and health care providers. At present, more than 60% of surgical procedures in North American are performed in the ambulatory setting [1–5]. Ambulatory surgical procedures are performed in patients with no medical problems or those with stable chronic medical illnesses. The procedures are generally less than 1 to 2 hours in duration, and have minimal blood loss, low complication rates, and minimal expected postoperative care. Examples include inguinal hernia repair, umbilical hernia repair, breast biopsy, partial or total mastectomy,

Disclosures: The authors have nothing to disclose.

*Corresponding author. Department of Surgery, The University of Texas Medical Branch, 301 University Boulevard, JSA 6.312b, Galveston, TX 77555-0542. *E-mail address:* tsriall@utmb.edu

0065-3411/13/$ – see front matter
http://dx.doi.org/10.1016/j.yasu.2013.02.005 Published by Elsevier Inc.

hemorrhoidectomy, and arthroscopy. With improvements in surgical and anesthetic techniques, the patient and procedure selection criteria for ambulatory surgery are rapidly expanding, and more patients with multiple preexisting medical conditions are candidates. As the indications for ambulatory surgery have evolved, evidence-based recommendations regarding preoperative testing have lagged. Clear indications for testing in the ambulatory surgery setting have not been defined.

Preoperative testing may be used as part of the screening process, in addition to physician assessment with a comprehensive history and physical examination, to guide appropriate patient selection and optimize perioperative care. Commonly ordered preoperative tests include chest radiograph (CXR), electrocardiography (ECG), hemoglobin/complete blood count (Hb/CBC), creatinine, electrolytes, liver function tests (LFTs), albumin, and coagulation parameters.

There is a broad spectrum of operative factors and patient characteristics that may prompt preoperative testing. Operative factors that are potential indications for testing include expected blood loss greater than 500 mL, prolonged anesthesia time, and high procedure complexity. This article discusses preoperative testing as it applies to ambulatory surgery, so these operative factors do not apply and are not discussed. Potential indications for preoperative testing in the ambulatory setting include extremes of age, symptoms, personal risk factors for disease (eg, smoking, alcohol, family history), and the presence of specific acute and chronic disease processes. For the purposes of this discussion, "routine" preoperative testing is defined as testing in the absence of specific indications.

PREOPERATIVE LABORATORY TESTING: GOALS, BENEFITS, AND RISKS

The goal of preoperative testing is to detect abnormalities that might adversely affect outcomes. In the case of known chronic medical conditions, preoperative testing can be used to assess the current status of disease. Examples include creatinine, potassium, and bicarbonate levels in patients with chronic kidney disease; HbA_{1c} to assess long-term diabetic control; or ECG in patients with heart disease to assess for interval changes from a known baseline. Preoperative testing in asymptomatic or healthy patients has the potential to detect undiagnosed disease processes that may put patients at increased risk for perioperative complications. However, such screening should be reserved for populations at high risk for a specific condition (eg, ECG screening in asymptomatic patients with multiple cardiac risk factors) to avoid high costs and potentially high false-positive rates when the pretest probability of a specific condition is low.

Preoperative testing allows for correction of suspected or unsuspected abnormalities that might adversely affect anesthetic or surgical outcomes. Findings that place patients at higher risk for specific complications allow for optimization of a patient's preoperative health status and establishment of perioperative plans to prevent, anticipate, and better manage problems, enhancing the quality and outcome of the perioperative experience [6,7]. Preoperative testing may also establish baseline values for tests that will be monitored after surgery.

Finally, in some instances preoperative testing is not based on patient characteristics or clinical indications. Testing may be done based on institutional policy or provider preference, or to provide medical-legal protection [5,8,9].

Despite the potential benefits, preoperative testing in the absence of clear indications can lead to prohibitive cost. It is estimated that up to $18 billion are spent annually for preoperative testing in the United States, in many cases for unnecessary tests that do not alter perioperative management [5,10,11]. Previous studies have shown that preoperative testing in the absence of clear indications leads to abnormal results in 30% to 50% of cases [5,8,12–15]. Because of the low prevalence of disease in the ambulatory population and, therefore, the low pretest probability, these abnormal results are often of questionable clinical significance [5,12–14]. Moreover, harm to patients may come from overtreatment of false-positive results or positive results with little clinical significance [16]. Unnecessary preoperative testing increases pain and inconvenience for the patient, and may lead to additional harm and anxiety from further workup required if abnormal values are reported [17]. Roizen [18] reported that in up to 60% of cases, abnormal results of preoperative laboratory testing are not noted or investigated. In these cases, the legal risk for not following up or acting on an abnormal result may be greater than not ordering a test [7].

CURRENT RECOMMENDATIONS FOR PREOPERATIVE LABORATORY TESTING

Current guidelines for preoperative testing in the United States are based on the 2002 Practice Advisory from the American Society of Anesthesiology (ASA) Task Force on Preanesthesia Evaluation [6]. As acknowledged in their report, current scientific literature is insufficient to create evidence-based guidelines, and their current recommendations represent a synthesis of expert opinion and data from small, nonrandomized, and/or underpowered studies. In Canada, guidelines for preoperative laboratory testing are given by the Canadian Anesthesiologists' Society (CAS) [19] and the Ontario Preoperative Testing Grid (OPTG) [12].

The ASA, CAS, and OPTG advocate against the use of routine preoperative testing. In the ASA practice advisory, they state that preoperative tests without indications lack utility and should be ordered on a selective basis according to information obtained during medical record reviews, patient's interview, and preoperative physical examination. However, the guidelines for selective testing are too general to be interpreted or applied in specific clinical situations. In addition, the language of current recommendations is imprecise. For example, "advanced age" is often used as an indication for testing without defining a clear minimum age. In addition, recommendations are often based on the ASA physical status classification system, a system for assessing fitness of patients before surgery. The ASA classification system has been criticized as inaccurate because it is based on anesthesiologists' judgment, and different providers often assign different ASA classes to the same patient [20–22].

There also are differences in recommendations between societies (Table 1). For example, the CAS does not recommend preoperative testing for "advanced age." The ASA recommends CBC and ECG only, and the OPTG additionally recommend creatinine level, electrolytes, and chest radiography (CXR). In all 3 cases, no clear definition of advanced age is provided. These differences in recommendation between societies are also seen among other conditions and test types.

CURRENT DATA FOR USE OF SPECIFIC TESTS

Testing in older patients

As the United States population ages and the criteria for ambulatory surgery expand, older patients represent an increasing proportion of patients undergoing ambulatory surgery. The overall mortality rate following ambulatory surgery is 4 to 8 deaths per 100,000 procedures [23], and this risk increases to approximately 41 per 100,000 procedures in patients older than 65 years [2]. Older patients have been shown to be at increased risk for intraoperative complications [24], postoperative admission [2], and pulmonary complications [8]. However, in the absence of significant comorbidities, most surgeons do not consider age a contraindication for ambulatory surgery. Although older patients are at increased risk for abnormal tests, preoperative testing has not been shown to decrease adverse outcomes in this high-risk population [5]. There are advocates of testing in all older patients [18,25] and strong arguments against this practice [5,14,26,27]. However, minimum age cutoffs are often not stated, and when stated, vary from study to study. In addition, studies arguing against testing in all older patients fail to provide unambiguous indications for testing [5,14,26,27].

Electrocardiography

Because cardiac complications after surgery can be devastating, the use of routine preoperative ECG has been extensively debated. The incidence of ECG abnormalities increases with age, male gender, higher ASA class, and a preexisting diagnosis of heart disease, hypertension, diabetes, or peripheral vascular disease [28]. ECG abnormalities have been shown to predict postoperative ischemic events and arrhythmias [25,29]. However, the indications for and role of preoperative ECG testing in low-risk ambulatory surgery remain unclear [29–36]. The ASA Task Force reviewed 12 studies evaluating routine ECG use and 17 studies reviewing ECG use for specific indications [6]. A wide range of ECG abnormalities were noted in both groups: 7% to 43% of routine ECG and 5% to 78% of ECG done for specific indications. In patients with abnormal findings, management was changed in 9% of patients receiving routine ECG (based on only one study) and 2% to 20% of patients having ECG done for specific indications. Based on these data, the ASA

Task Force did not reach a consensus on a specific minimum age for obtaining preoperative ECG in patients without specific risk factors, and recognized that age alone might not be an indication for an electrocardiogram. In addition, the Task Force agrees that an ECG may be indicated for patients with known cardiovascular risk factors or for patients with risk factors identified in the course of a preoperative evaluation, but again, they are not specific regarding these risk factors.

Chest radiography

The ASA Task Force reviewed 20 studies evaluating routine preoperative CXR and 9 studies evaluating preoperative CXR done for indications [6]. There was a wide range of CXR abnormalities detected in the various studies and a wide range in the incidence of subsequent changes in management based on these findings. CXR abnormalities were detected in 3% to 60% of routine CXR and 8% to 65% of CXR done for indications. These studies demonstrated changes in management based on preoperative CXR in 0% to 51% of routine CXR and 0.5% to 74% of indicated CXR. The Task Force concluded that clinical characteristics to consider in obtaining preoperative CXR include smoking, recent upper respiratory infection, chronic obstructive pulmonary disease (COPD), and cardiac disease. The investigators recognized that CXR abnormalities may be higher in such patients, but do not conclude that extremes of age, smoking, stable COPD, stable cardiac disease, or resolved recent upper respiratory infection should be considered unequivocal indications for chest radiography.

Hemoglobin/hematocrit

The incidence of anemia in healthy adults is low [37,38]. The ASA Task Force [6] recommends against routine Hb and hematocrit testing before surgery, and recommend selective testing in patients with liver disease, extremes of age (age limits not specified), history of anemia, bleeding, or other hematologic disorders.

Olson and colleagues [39] performed a retrospective analysis of 9584 patients classified as ASA class 1 or 2 who underwent elective low-risk surgery. Using a hemoglobin cutoff for clinically significant anemia of less than 9 g/dL, only 75 patients (0.8%) were identified as anemic, with 4 presenting with values of less than 7 g/dL, in all cases with clinical indicators. All 4 of the 9584 patients identified as anemic required perioperative transfusion. Given the low incidence of anemia and the presence of symptoms when the anemia was clinically significant, Olson and colleagues recommend against routine Hb/hematocrit testing. Testing should only be performed if signs and symptoms suggestive of anemia are present.

Narr and colleagues [40] reported abnormal Hb or hematocrit values (defined as <10.0 g/dL) in 0.8% of 3782 patients in whom preoperative testing was performed. Only in 0.1% of all patients did Hb testing change preoperative management.

Table 1
Summary of current ASA, CAS, and OPTG recommendations for specific tests in patients undergoing ambulatory surgery

	Test							
Indication	Hb/CBC	Creatinine	Electrolytes	LFTs	Albumin	Coagulation parameters	CXR	ECG
Advanced age	ASA[a] OPTG	OPTG	OPTG				OPTG	ASA[a] OPTG (>45 y)
Anemia	ASA CAS							
Bleeding disorders	ASA					ASA CAS OPTG		
Other hematologic disorders	ASA					OPTG		
Cardiovascular disease	CAS OPTG						ASA CAS	ASA CAS OPTG
Pulmonary disease	CAS OPTG						ASA CAS OPTG	ASA
Renal disease	CAS OPTG	CAS OPTG	ASA CAS OPTG			ASA		OPTG
Liver disease	CAS OPTG			OPTG		ASA CAS OPTG		
Endocrine disease		CAS	ASA					
Malignancy	CAS OPTG						CAS OPTG	

Hypertension	OPTG	CAS OPTG	CAS OPTG			OPTG	CAS OPTG
Diabetes		OPTG	CAS OPTG				CAS
Recent upper respiratory infection			CAS			ASA	
Smoking	OPTG					ASA OPTG	OPTG
Alcohol abuse	OPTG			OPTG	OPTG		
Diuretic use		CAS OPTG	ASA CAS OPTG				OPTG
ACE inhibitor use		OPTG					OPTG
Digoxin use		CAS OPTG	ASA CAS OPTG				OPTG
Steroid use			OPTG				
Anticoagulant therapy	OPTG				ASA CAS OPTG		
Risk factors for cardiac disease							CAS

Abbreviations: ACE, angiotensin-converting enzyme; ASA, American Society of Anesthesiologists; CAS, Canadian Anesthesiologists' Society; CBC, complete blood count; Hb, hemoglobin; LFT, liver function test; OPTG, Ontario Preoperative Testing Grid.

[a]Though recommended for advanced age by ASA, specific age guidelines are not given.

Modified from Benarroch-Gampel J, Sheffield KM, Duncan CB, et al. Preoperative laboratory testing in patients undergoing elective, low-risk ambulatory surgery. Ann Surg 2012;256(3):519; with permission.

Chemistry

The ASA Task Force [6] recommends selective use of chemistry tests, such as electrolytes, glucose, and liver and renal function tests, in patients receiving preoperative diuretics, steroids, or digoxin, diabetic patients, and patients with renal or liver dysfunction.

In a systematic review of the literature performed by Munro and colleagues [15], in studies when routine testing was evaluated the incidence of abnormal results was less than 1.4% of cases for sodium or potassium, less the 2.5% for blood urea nitrogen (BUN) and creatinine, and less than 5.2% for glucose, and abnormal results rarely changed the preoperative management of these patients. Similar results were obtained in a more recent systematic review by Smetana and Macpherson [8].

Coagulation studies (prothrombin time, partial thromboplastin time, and platelets)

The ASA Task Force [6] recommends obtaining coagulation tests for patients with bleeding disorders, on anticoagulation medication, and with renal or liver disease. Routine testing is not recommended because the incidence of abnormal results is low; change in management occurs in fewer than 5.3% of patients; the incidence of adverse events in patients with abnormal results is very rare (lower than 0.6%); and the positive predictive value for postoperative bleeding is low [41]. It is unlikely that a significant bleeding disorder would remain undiagnosed into adulthood.

Hemoglobin A_{1c}

Previous studies have shown that patients with diabetes and elevated preoperative HbA_{1c} have worse postoperative outcomes after cardiac [42,43], colorectal [44], and vascular surgery [45]. The ASA Task Force [6] does not comment on the use of HbA_{1c} as part of the preoperative laboratory evaluation for elective surgery. There are no data evaluating the effect of long-term poor glucose control on outcomes following ambulatory surgery. If HbA_{1c} has not been obtained in the 30 days before surgery and glucose control is reportedly poor, one may consider testing and delay of elective surgery until blood glucose is better controlled. However, studies are needed to provide evidence for policy regarding HbA_{1c} testing in ambulatory surgery.

Pregnancy test

As anesthesia and surgery pose potential risk to the unborn fetus [46], especially during the first trimester when the history and physical findings are unclear and the risk of miscarriage is increased [47], pregnancy tests are recommended in females of reproductive age (who have not had hysterectomy) undergoing elective surgery. Previous studies have shown that positive results (ranging between 0.3% and 2.2% of cases) led to changes in management in 100% of the cases [48–52]. Although not unequivocal, the ASA Task Force [6] recommends considering pregnancy tests for all female patients of child-bearing age.

CURRENT USE OF TESTING IN NORTH AMERICA

Because of the lack of consensus regarding clear indications for testing, preoperative testing is often based on provider preference and historical institutional protocols. Often surgeons, anesthesiologists, and even patients expect that there will be some tests performed before any operative procedure, and testing is often performed out of routine or habit. Moreover, inappropriate use of testing may result from lack of communication between multiple providers (surgeons, anesthesiologists, and primary care physicians) caring for ambulatory surgery patients. For example, most recommendations regarding preoperative testing originate in the anesthesia literature. However, a Canadian study found that 80% of preoperative tests were ordered by surgeons, suggesting that lack of communication between specialties may account for a large portion of noncompliance [12].

Uncertainty regarding the indications for testing leads to high rates of unnecessary testing. Single-institution studies in the United States and Canada demonstrate that up to two-thirds of preoperative laboratory tests obtained are not indicated, based on current recommendations for selective testing [12,14,26,53]. Even after implementation of the OPTG checklist in Canada, noncompliance ranged from 5% to 98% depending on the test or guideline analyzed [12].

A recent study using National Surgical Quality Improvement Program (NSQIP) data evaluated preoperative testing in 73,596 patients undergoing elective inguinal hernia repair [54]. At least 1 preoperative laboratory test (CBC, electrolytes, LFTs, or coagulation parameters) was performed in 63.8% of patients, with at least 1 abnormal test recorded in 61.6% of these patients. In a subgroup analysis of 25,149 patients with no comorbidities and no clear indications for testing, 54% had at least 1 preoperative test. Rates of individual tests for the overall cohort and the subgroup with no comorbidities are shown in Table 2. Also, preoperative testing increased with increasing age, even in the subgroup with no comorbid conditions, rising from 34% in patients younger than 20 years to 75% in patients 81 years and older.

Further analysis performed by the authors of Medicare beneficiaries using 100% Texas Medicare claims data (unpublished data, 2008–2009) undergoing hernia repair (inguinal, femoral, epigastric, and umbilical) or knee/shoulder arthroscopy, demonstrated similar findings, with more than 70% of older patients with no comorbidities undergoing at least 1 test (Table 3) before surgery. Rates of tests varied only slightly across procedure types. In patients with no documented comorbid conditions in the year before surgery, CXR rates exceeded 35% and ECG rates exceeded 50%.

Uncertainty regarding indications for preoperative testing is also reflected in the wide geographic and hospital/facility-level variation in use of tests. Using 100% Medicare claims data for Texas (2008–2009), the authors examined variation at the level of the facility and health service area (HSA) in patients undergoing hernia repair and knee/shoulder arthroscopy. An HSA is a collection of ZIP codes whose residents receive most of their inpatient care from the

Table 2
Use of preoperative laboratory testing and abnormal results in patients undergoing hernia repair from the National Surgical Quality Improvement Program database, 2005–2010

	Total	%	Abnormal	%[a]
Overall Cohort (N = 73,596)				
Any test	46,977	63.8	28,938	61.6
Hematology	43,153	58.6	16,944	39.3
Chemistry	39,402	53.5	15,824	40.2
Coagulation	13,746	18.7	1556	11.3
LFT	17,433	23.7	3974	22.8
All	7291	9.9	5419	74.3
Subgroup Without Comorbidities (N = 25,149)				
Any test	13,591	54.0	7361	54.1
Hematology	13,018	51.8	4708	36.2
Chemistry	10,504	41.8	3460	33.0
Coagulation	3720	14.8	220	5.9
LFT	4931	19.6	905	18.4
All	2038	8.1	1348	66.1
Labs Performed the Day of Surgery (N = 7209)				
Any test	7209	100.0	4443	61.6
Hematology	6198	86.0	2595	41.9
Chemistry	5516	76.5	2257	40.9
Coagulation	2554	35.4	586	22.9
LFT	1859	25.8	618	33.2
All	971	13.5	808	83.2

Abbreviation: LFT, liver function tests.
[a]Among patients with specific test.
Reproduced from Benarroch-Gampel J, Sheffield KM, Duncan CB, et al. Preoperative laboratory testing in patients undergoing elective, low-risk ambulatory surgery. Ann Surg 2012;256(3):522; with permission.

hospitals in that area [55]. The percentage of patients undergoing preoperative CXR ranged from 10% in the lowest HSA to 90% in the highest (Fig. 1A). ECG use ranged from 15% to 95%, with the lowest decile using preoperative ECG in fewer than 40% and the highest decile in greater than 80% of cases (see Fig. 1B). A map showing HSA-level variation in rates of CXR use before hernia repair is shown in Fig. 2. Similar variations in other tests (CBC, electrolytes, creatinine, LFTs, and coagulation tests) were seen across patients undergoing hernia repair or knee/shoulder arthroscopy.

Similar variation in the use of preoperative testing was seen at the facility level. In patients undergoing hernia repair, preoperative CXR use varied from 0% to 95% between facilities doing at least 30 procedures in the time period. The bottom decile of facilities performed CXR in fewer than 10% of cases and the top decile of facilities performed CXR in more than 80% of cases. Likewise, preoperative ECG was performed less than 40% of the time in the bottom decile and greater than 90% of the time in the top decile of facilities.

It can be argued that patients may differ in severity of chronic illness and other factors among different facilities and providers. However, it is reasonable

Table 3
Preoperative testing before hernia repair or arthroscopy in Texas Medicare beneficiaries (>65 years)

	% Overall patients undergoing test[a]		% Patients with no comorbidities[b] undergoing test[a]	
Test	Hernia repair N = 13,029	Arthroscopy[c] N = 21,993	Hernia repair N = 3187	Arthroscopy[c] N = 5515
Hb/Hematocrit	53.1	57.3	49.6	49.1
Platelet count	51.8	54.1	48.3	46.0
Creatinine	27.0	29.9	23.2	24.9
Electrolytes	53.6	60.6	48.2	50.4
LFTs	35.2	35.9	30.9	27.9
Albumin	32.4	33.4	28.1	25.9
Coagulation parameters	16.2	18.8	9.2	12.4
CXR	43.5	41.0	38.1	34.9
ECG	62.0	57.6	59.5	51.0
Any of above tests	84.5	81.2	78.9	73.4

[a]In the 30 days before surgery.
[b]Patients with none of 30 Elixhauser comorbidities.
[c]Knee and shoulder arthroscopy only.
Data from 100% Texas Medicare claim data, 2008–2009.

to postulate that patient characteristics would vary much less across HSAs, especially patients undergoing low-risk, elective ambulatory surgery. As such, the authors hypothesize that the observed HSA-level variation in testing arises because of uncertainty in the appropriateness of current guidelines and subsequent practice variation, rather than selection based on patient characteristics.

EVIDENCE FOR FURTHER REFINEMENT/DEFINITION OF CURRENT GUIDELINES

Better evidenced-based criteria are needed to guide selective preoperative testing in the ambulatory setting. The current guidelines are directed to guide the preoperative evaluation of patients undergoing any surgical procedure, including inpatient procedures. Usually, patients undergoing relatively simple procedures with low complication rates performed in the ambulatory setting are healthy or have stable chronic disease. These procedures are not done emergently, and guidelines applicable to all complex inpatient surgical procedures may not be relevant in this setting. For example, a patient with well-controlled diabetes or stable cardiac disease and good functional status may be a candidate for testing before major abdominal or vascular surgery, but the same patient might not need testing before low-risk ambulatory procedures.

There is evidence to suggest that the current guidelines can be refined for the ambulatory setting. Multiple studies of patients undergoing elective surgery find that abnormal tests lead to changes in management in only 0% to 9% of cases (Table 4) [13,14,26,27,33,35,40,54,56–61]. Kaplan and colleagues [14]

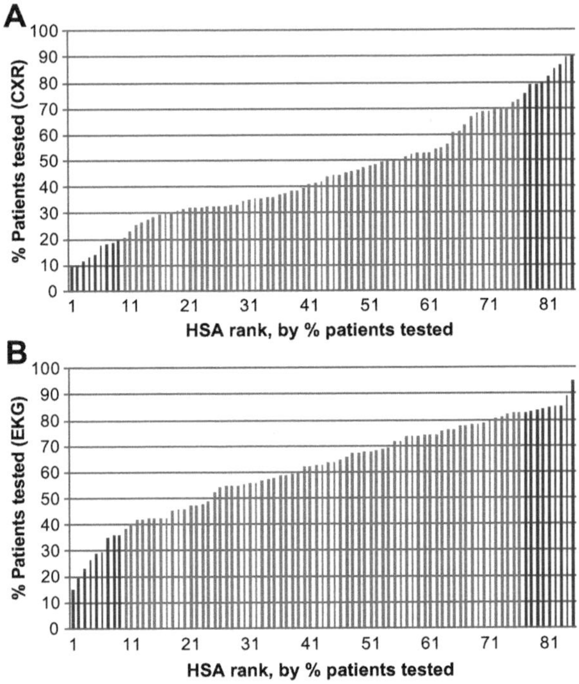

Fig. 1. For each test type, the graphs show the proportion of Texas Medicare beneficiaries in each health service area (HSA) undergoing hernia repair who underwent preoperative testing. (*A*) Chest radiograph (CXR). (*B*) Electrocardiogram (EKG). CXR use varied from 10% to 90% between HSAs. EKG use varied from 15% to 95%. (*Data from* 100% Texas Medicare claim data, 2008–2009.)

evaluated 2000 patients who underwent 6200 routine preoperative tests, and found that 60% of tests were not indicated and only 0.2% had clinically relevant abnormal results. The presence of abnormal results was not associated with change in management or worse postoperative outcomes. Likewise, Narr and colleagues [40] reported abnormal results in 4% of 3782 patients who underwent ambulatory surgery, and found no association between abnormal results and worse postoperative outcomes. In addition, no change in perioperative care management was attributed to the abnormal testing results. Smetana and Macpherson [8] reported similar results after performing a systematic review of the literature. Changes in management were seen in fewer than 0.1% of patients with abnormal CBC results, to up to 2.6% of the cases with abnormal chemistry results.

In 1987, Turnbull and Buck [57] studied 1010 healthy patients undergoing open cholecystectomy for cholelithiasis. In more than 5000 tests ordered, they found that only 4 patients potentially benefited from the battery of tests and concluded that, when compared with the information obtained during the preoperative history and physical examination of patients undergoing

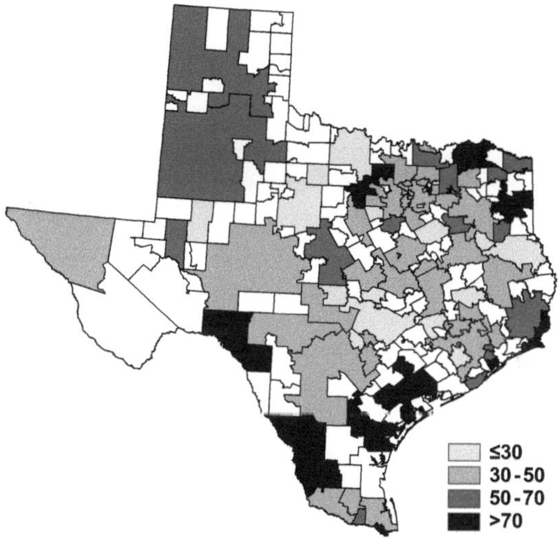

Fig. 2. Percentage of Texas Medicare beneficiaries receiving a preoperative chest radiograph before hernia repair by HSA in Texas. No clear pattern in the use of preoperative chest radiography was seen across HSAs, and variation in the use of chest radiography is evident, even between contiguous HSAs. Colors indicate percentages. (*Data from* 100% Texas Medicare claim data, 2008–2009.)

Table 4
Summary of previous studies evaluating unnecessary testing, incidence of abnormal results, and impact on management

Authors [Ref.], year	N	% Unnecessary	% Abnormal	% Clinical impact
Delahunt and Turnbull [27], 1980	803	NR	21.4	NR
Kaplan et al [14], 1985	2000	61[a]	4.1[b]	0.2[c]
Turnbull and Buck [57], 1987	2570	NR	4.5[b]	0.3
Charpak et al [13], 1988	3866	NR	30[b]	9[c]
Narr et al [40], 1991	3782	NR	4.2	1.2
Macpherson et al [60], 1993	111	NR	0.81	0
Perez et al [61], 1995	3131	NR	27	1.2
Allison and Bromley [26], 1996	61	65.4	NR	NR
Muskett and McGreevy [33], 1986	200	NR	35.5[b]	5.9[c]
Wattsman and Davies [59], 1997	142	58.4[a]	30.6[b]	1.3[c]
Dzankic et al [58], 2001	526	NR	6.8[b]	NR
Benarroch-Gampel et al [54], 2012	73,596	NR	61.6	NR

Abbreviation: NR, not reported.
[a]Percentage of unnecessary tests.
[b]Percentage of abnormal tests.
[c]Percentage of tests that change management.

ambulatory surgery, preoperative testing did not provide additional information that altered the management of otherwise healthy patients.

In a population-based study using the NSQIP participant use data file [54], the authors found that surgery was performed despite abnormal results in 61.6% of patients undergoing same-day testing (see Table 2). Neither preoperative testing nor abnormal results across test types were associated with increased perioperative morbidity and mortality.

In a multicenter landmark study by Schein and colleagues [35], 19,557 patients undergoing cataract surgery were randomized to 2 groups: (1) no preoperative testing or (2) a standard battery of routine tests including ECG, CBC, electrolytes, BUN, creatinine, and glucose. Overall incidence of perioperative complications (including hospital admission and death) did not differ between these 2 groups even after stratifying by patient demographics or ASA class. Although the study design is strong, its generalizability might be limited by the low-risk nature of cataract surgery. Cataract surgery requires a very short period of general anesthesia and sedation, so the findings may not be widely applicable to all ambulatory surgical procedures. Also, the investigators excluded patients who had an indication for testing in the previous 28 days. It is possible that the results were similar in the 2 groups because patients had been optimally evaluated by a complete history and physical examination. In an editorial, Roizen [18] points out that many preoperative assessments for ambulatory surgery are done within 7 days of surgery and may not be adequate for assessing and acquiring needed tests.

In Canada, Chung and colleagues [56] evaluated postoperative outcomes in 1061 patients undergoing ambulatory surgery who were randomly assigned to receive preoperative laboratory testing or not. Although the investigators applied strict exclusion criteria, with only relatively healthy patients undergoing randomization, their study shows no difference in postoperative complications at 7 and 30 days after surgery between tested and untested patients.

Previously, Narr and colleagues [62] performed a retrospective review of 1044 patients undergoing surgical and diagnostic procedures at the Mayo Clinic, randomly selected from a pool of 5120 patients in whom no preoperative laboratory testing was obtained. It was concluded that patients who are assessed by careful history and physical examination, and deemed to have no indication for testing, could safely undergo low-risk elective surgery without preoperative testing.

Other studies have evaluated the utility of "selective" testing. In a 1988 study, Charpak and colleagues [13] evaluated the usefulness of 12 selectively ordered tests based on current indications. The study included 15,920 tests performed in 3866 patients. Thirty percent of performed tests were not indicated according to their preoperative testing protocol. In addition, test results were abnormal 30% of the time. Surgery was delayed or canceled for 19 patients and modified in 1 case, and a treatment was instituted or anesthetic management influenced in 9%. When assessed by the anesthesiologists/anesthetists, 22% of recommended tests and 5% of nonrecommended tests were found useful. The investigators concluded that although the usefulness of selectively ordered preoperative tests may be higher, better criteria for their indications are needed, because some nonrecommended tests in their protocol were found to be useful.

SUMMARY

Current recommendations from the 2002 ASA Task Force on Preanesthesia Evaluation are not specific to ambulatory surgery and are not based on strongly designed and adequately powered studies. Furthermore, although the ASA does not advocate routine testing or testing without indication, the guidelines for "selective" or "indicated" testing are unclear. As a result, preoperative testing in the United States is overused relative to the current ASA Task Force recommendations. Uncertainty regarding indications leads to wide variation in the use of preoperative testing across providers.

There is evidence to suggest that current guidelines may recommend testing more than is necessary. Several studies reviewed in this article have shown that the elimination of routine testing and more selective use based on patient history and physical examination findings would decrease cost and increase patient satisfaction without detriment to patient care. Future studies should evaluate the effectiveness of testing in specific clinical situations, allowing for identification of clear conditions under which preoperative testing should be performed. This approach would allow the promulgation of clear guidelines, the development of which should involve surgeons (as members of a multidisciplinary team), anesthesiologists, and hospital administrators, together with governing bodies such as the ASA and American College of Surgeons that offer support for the dissemination and broad adoption of guidelines.

In the future, studies should focus not only on identifying specific clinical situations whereby preoperative testing will be beneficial but also on determining current barriers to improving adherence to guidelines. Potential barriers include institutional policies for testing, physician reluctance to change practice, problems in communication between members involved in perioperative care, and legal consequences of not ordering preoperative tests. Identification of reasons for overuse of testing is the first step toward changing practice. Once clear guidelines are developed, the creation of preoperative clinics that centralize preoperative care, or promoting the use of clinical pathways and/or checklists for determining appropriate tests, may improve the adequate use of preoperative tests. It will be critical for quality improvement measures to include surgeons, anesthesiologists, hospital administrators, and governing bodies such as the ASA and American College of Surgeons to achieve success.

References

[1] Apfelbaum JL. Current controversies in adult outpatient anesthesia. ASA refreshers courses in Anesthesiology 2003;31(1):1.

[2] Fleisher LA, Pasternak LR, Herbert R, et al. Inpatient hospital admission and death after outpatient surgery in elderly patients: importance of patient and system characteristics and location of care. Arch Surg 2004;139(1):67–72.

[3] Mezei G, Chung F. Return hospital visits and hospital readmissions after ambulatory surgery. Ann Surg 1999;230(5):721–7.
[4] Owings MF, Kozak LJ. Ambulatory and inpatient procedures in the United States, 1996. Vital Health Stat 13 1998;(139):1–119.
[5] Richman DC. Ambulatory surgery: how much testing do we need? Anesthesiol Clin 2010;28(2):185–97.
[6] American Society of Anesthesiologists Task Force on Preanesthesia Evaluation. Practice advisory for preanesthesia evaluation: a report by the American Society of Anesthesiologists Task Force on Preanesthesia Evaluation. Anesthesiology 2002;96(2):485–96.
[7] Hepner DL. The role of testing in the preoperative evaluation. Cleve Clin J Med 2009;76(Suppl 4):S22–7.
[8] Smetana GW, Macpherson DS. The case against routine preoperative laboratory testing. Med Clin North Am 2003;87(1):7–40.
[9] Velanovich V. Preoperative laboratory evaluation. J Am Coll Surg 1996;183(1):79–87.
[10] Fischer SP. Cost-effective preoperative evaluation and testing. Chest 1999;115(Suppl 5): 96S–100S.
[11] Johnstone RE, Martinec CL. Costs of anesthesia. Anesth Analg 1993;76(4):840–8.
[12] Bryson GL, Wyand A, Bragg PR. Preoperative testing is inconsistent with published guidelines and rarely changes management. Can J Anaesth 2006;53(3):236–41.
[13] Charpak Y, Blery C, Chastang C, et al. Usefulness of selectively ordered preoperative tests. Med Care 1988;26(2):95–104.
[14] Kaplan EB, Sheiner LB, Boeckmann AJ, et al. The usefulness of preoperative laboratory screening. JAMA 1985;253(24):3576–81.
[15] Munro J, Booth A, Nicholl J. Routine preoperative testing: a systematic review of the evidence. Health Technol Assess 1997;1(12):i–iv, 1–62.
[16] Ajimura FY, Maia AS, Hachiya A, et al. Preoperative laboratory evaluation of patients aged over 40 years undergoing elective non-cardiac surgery. Sao Paulo Med J 2005;123(2): 50–3.
[17] Apfelbaum J. Preoperation evaluation, laboratory screening, and selection of adult surgical outpatients in 1990s. Anesthesiol Rev 1990;17(Suppl 2):4–12.
[18] Roizen MF. More preoperative assessment by physicians and less by laboratory tests. N Engl J Med 2000;342(3):204–5.
[19] Merchant R, Bosenberg C, Brown K, et al. Guidelines to the practice of anesthesia: revised edition. Can J Anaesth 2011;58(1):74–107.
[20] Haynes SR, Lawler PG. An assessment of the consistency of ASA physical status classification allocation. Anaesthesia 1995;50(3):195–9.
[21] Little JP. Consistency of ASA grading. Anaesthesia 1995;50(7):658–9.
[22] Owens WD, Felts JA, Spitznagel EL Jr. ASA physical status classifications: a study of consistency of ratings. Anesthesiology 1978;49(4):239–43.
[23] Warner MA, Shields SE, Chute CG. Major morbidity and mortality within 1 month of ambulatory surgery and anesthesia. JAMA 1993;270(12):1437–41.
[24] Chung F, Mezei G, Tong D. Adverse events in ambulatory surgery. A comparison between elderly and younger patients. Can J Anaesth 1999;46(4):309–21.
[25] Velanovich V. The value of routine preoperative laboratory testing in predicting postoperative complications: a multivariate analysis. Surgery 1991;109(3 Pt 1):236–43.
[26] Allison JG, Bromley HR. Unnecessary preoperative investigations: evaluation and cost analysis. Am Surg 1996;62(8):686–9.
[27] Delahunt B, Turnbull PR. How cost effective are routine preoperative investigations? N Z Med J 1980;92(673):431–2.
[28] Velanovich V. Preoperative laboratory screening based on age, gender, and concomitant medical diseases. Surgery 1994;115(1):56–61.
[29] Velanovich V. Preoperative screening electrocardiography: predictive value for postoperative cardiac complications. South Med J 1994;87(4):431–4.

[30] Bhuripanyo K, Prasertchuang C, Viwathanatepa M, et al. The impact of routine preoperative electrocardiogram in patients age ≥40 years in Srinagarind Hospital. J Med Assoc Thai 1992;75(7):399–406.
[31] Goldberger AL, O'Konski M. Utility of the routine electrocardiogram before surgery and on general hospital admission. Critical review and new guidelines. Ann Intern Med 1986;105(4):552–7.
[32] Murdoch CJ, Murdoch DR, McIntyre P, et al. The pre-operative ECG in day surgery: a habit? Anaesthesia 1999;54(9):907–8.
[33] Muskett AD, McGreevy JM. Rational preoperative evaluation. Postgrad Med J 1986;62(732):925–8.
[34] Rabkin SW, Horne JM. Preoperative electrocardiography effect of new abnormalities on clinical decisions. Can Med Assoc J 1983;128(2):146–7.
[35] Schein OD, Katz J, Bass EB, et al. The value of routine preoperative medical testing before cataract surgery. Study of Medical Testing for Cataract Surgery. N Engl J Med 2000,342(3):168–75.
[36] Sommerville TE, Murray WB. Information yield from routine pre-operative chest radiography and electrocardiography. S Afr Med J 1992;81(4):190–6.
[37] Recommendations to prevent and control iron deficiency in the United States. Centers for Disease Control and Prevention. MMWR Recomm Rep 1998;47(RR-3):1–29.
[38] Pasternak LR. Preoperative assessment: guidelines and challenges. Acta Anaesthesiol Scand Suppl 1997;111:318–20.
[39] Olson RP, Stone A, Lubarsky D. The prevalence and significance of low preoperative hemoglobin in ASA 1 or 2 outpatient surgery candidates. Anesth Analg 2005;101(5):1337–40.
[40] Narr BJ, Hansen TR, Warner MA. Preoperative laboratory screening in healthy Mayo patients: cost-effective elimination of tests and unchanged outcomes. Mayo Clin Proc 1991;66(2):155–9.
[41] Suchman AL, Mushlin AI. How well does the activated partial thromboplastin time predict postoperative hemorrhage? JAMA 1986;256(6):750–3.
[42] Halkos ME, Puskas JD, Lattouf OM, et al. Elevated preoperative hemoglobin A1c level is predictive of adverse events after coronary artery bypass surgery. J Thorac Cardiovasc Surg 2008;136(3):631–40.
[43] Hudson CC, Welsby IJ, Phillips-Bute B, et al. Glycosylated hemoglobin levels and outcome in non-diabetic cardiac surgery patients. Can J Anaesth 2010;57(6):565–72.
[44] Gustafsson UO, Thorell A, Soop M, et al. Haemoglobin A1c as a predictor of postoperative hyperglycaemia and complications after major colorectal surgery. Br J Surg 2009;96(11): 1358–64.
[45] O'Sullivan CJ, Hynes N, Mahendran B, et al. Haemoglobin A1c (HbA1C) in non-diabetic and diabetic vascular patients. Is HbA1C an independent risk factor and predictor of adverse outcome? Eur J Vasc Endovasc Surg 2006;32(2):188–97.
[46] Duncan PG, Pope WD, Cohen MM, et al. Fetal risk of anesthesia and surgery during pregnancy. Anesthesiology 1986;64(6):790–4.
[47] Mazze RI, Kallen B. Reproductive outcome after anesthesia and operation during pregnancy: a registry study of 5405 cases. Am J Obstet Gynecol 1989;161(5):1178–85.
[48] Azzam FJ, Padda GS, DeBoard JW, et al. Preoperative pregnancy testing in adolescents. Anesth Analg 1996;82(1):4–7.
[49] Manley S, de Kelaita G, Joseph NJ, et al. Preoperative pregnancy testing in ambulatory surgery. Incidence and impact of positive results. Anesthesiology 1995;83(4):690–3.
[50] Pierre N, Moy LK, Redd S, et al. Evaluation of a pregnancy-testing protocol in adolescents undergoing surgery. J Pediatr Adolesc Gynecol 1998;11(3):139–41.
[51] Twersky RS, Singleton G. Preoperative pregnancy testing: "justice and testing for all". Anesth Analg 1996;83(2):438–9.
[52] Wheeler M, Cote CJ. Preoperative pregnancy testing in a tertiary care children's hospital: a medico-legal conundrum. J Clin Anesth 1999;11(1):56–63.

[53] Macario A, Roizen MF, Thisted RA, et al. Reassessment of preoperative laboratory testing has changed the test-ordering patterns of physicians. Surg Gynecol Obstet 1992;175(6): 539–47.
[54] Benarroch-Gampel J, Sheffield KM, Duncan CB, et al. Preoperative laboratory testing in patients undergoing elective, low-risk ambulatory surgery. Ann Surg 2012;256(3): 518–28.
[55] Wennberg J, Fisher E, Goodman D, et al. Tracking the care of patients with severe chronic illness: the Dartmouth atlas of health care. Lebanon (NH): Bonner; 2008.
[56] Chung F, Yuan H, Yin L, et al. Elimination of preoperative testing in ambulatory surgery. Anesth Analg 2009;108(2):467–75.
[57] Turnbull JM, Buck C. The value of preoperative screening investigations in otherwise healthy individuals. Arch Intern Med 1987;147(6):1101–5.
[58] Dzankic S, Pastor D, Gonzalez C, et al. The prevalence and predictive value of abnormal preoperative laboratory tests in elderly surgical patients. Anesth Analg 2001;93(2):301–8 [302nd contents page].
[59] Wattsman TA, Davies RS. The utility of preoperative laboratory testing in general surgery patients for outpatient procedures. Am Surg 1997;63(1):81–90.
[60] Macpherson CR, Jacobs P, Dent DM. Abnormal peri-operative haemorrhage in asymptomatic patients is not predicted by laboratory testing. S Afr Med J 1993;83(2):106–8.
[61] Perez A, Planell J, Bacardaz C, et al. Value of routine preoperative tests: a multicentre study in four general hospitals. Br J Anaesth 1995;74(3):250–6.
[62] Narr BJ, Warner ME, Schroeder DR, et al. Outcomes of patients with no laboratory assessment before anesthesia and a surgical procedure. Mayo Clin Proc 1997;72(6):505–9.

Advances in Surgery 47 (2013) 99–110

ADVANCES IN SURGERY

Factors Affecting Readmission After Pancreaticoduodenectomy

Callisia N. Clarke, MD, Jeffrey J. Sussman, MD, Daniel E. Abbott, MD, Syed A. Ahmad, MD*

Pancreatic Disease Center, Department of Surgery, University of Cincinnati Medical Center, 234 Goodman Street, ML 0772, Cincinnati, OH 45219, USA

Keywords

• Readmission • Pancreaticoduodenectomy • Complications

Key points

- Pancreaticoduodenectomy is associated with a higher complication rate than other major abdominal surgeries.
- Readmission after pancreaticoduodenectomy is common despite advances in perioperative care.
- Readers should be able to identify possible risk factors for readmission after pancreaticoduodenectomy.

INTRODUCTION

The topic of hospital readmission rates has recently come under considerable scrutiny. The Medicare Payment Advisory Commission (MedPAC) has stated that early hospital readmission rates (30-day or less) can be used as a measure of poor patient outcomes and that early readmission contributed an additional $15 billion in Medicare expenditure in 2005 [1,2]. Furthermore, more than 75% of these readmissions were deemed to be preventable. National efforts such as the Hospital Readmissions Reduction Programs have been implicated to reduce the number of potentially preventable readmissions and the health care costs associated with them. Proposals to reduce hospital reimbursement for an excess of potentially preventable readmissions have been incorporated into the Patient Protection and Affordable Care Act and are scheduled to take effect in October 2012 [1]. Surgical readmissions account for

*Corresponding author. Division of Surgical Oncology, Department of Surgery, University of Cincinnati College of Medicine, 234 Goodman Street, ML 0772, Cincinnati, OH 45219. *E-mail address*: ahmadsy@uc.edu

0065-3411/13/$ – see front matter
http://dx.doi.org/10.1016/j.yasu.2013.02.006

approximately 22.4% of all potentially preventable hospital readmissions [2]. Now more than ever, it is critical that surgeons establish appropriate benchmarks regarding acceptable readmission rates after surgery. Efforts have been made to quantify readmissions after major abdominal surgery and to further delineate readmission rates after common surgical procedures such as hernia repairs, bariatric procedures, foregut surgery, and cholecystectomy [2,3]. Readmissions after pancreatic resection and especially after pancreaticoduodenectomy (PD) certainly require special consideration given the difference in operative complexity, patient demographics, and disease.

PD is being performed with increasing frequency for benign and malignant diseases of the pancreas and periampullary region. In the current era, there have been significant improvements in operative outcomes, largely because of advances in perioperative critical care, surgical techniques, and management of common complications [4]. These factors along with regionalization of care to high-volume centers and implementation of clinical pathways to standardize patient care have resulted in improved outcomes after PD. In the current era, the procedure can be performed with acceptable morbidity and mortality, with mortality at high-volume centers less than 5% [5–8]. Despite these advances, complications such as delayed gastric emptying, pancreatic leak, and intra-abdominal infections continue to pose a significant challenge, with reported incidences of 30% to 60% [9,10]. Hospital readmissions after PD are frequent occurrences and represent a significant burden to the health care system.

To understand whether readmission rates after PD can be decreased, baseline rates and factors that predispose to readmission after surgery must be established. Few studies have specifically evaluated readmission rates and correlative factors after PD. Studies that have been completed are single-institution reports and it is difficult to extrapolate their experiences to all patients treated at high-volume pancreas centers because of differences in complexity and variability in postoperative clinical pathways at the various institutions. This article analyzes the current published literature in an effort to determine readmission rates after PD and to identify factors associated with readmission in the early postoperative period. In addition, the recent publication from the Central Pancreatic Consortium is discussed in detail. This is the only multi-institutional study that analyzes prospectively collected data from 6 high-volume pancreatic centers with a mission to establish a benchmark without institutional bias.

METHODS

A literature search was performed of the Medline Current Content and PubMed databases. Search words were "readmission," "unplanned hospitalization," "Whipple," and "pancreaticoduodenectomy." Only articles published in English were included. Studies lacking data on rates of readmission and reasons of readmission were excluded. Case reports/studies were also excluded.

SUMMARY OF THE LITERATURE

Despite the high complication rate and complex patient care required after PD, there is a paucity of reports aimed at assessing or evaluating readmissions and overall outcomes for patients undergoing PD. A review of the current literature showed only a handful of studies, most of them single-institutional retrospective reports. Reported rates of readmission after PD in these studies range from 11% to 60% [6,9,11–14]. The findings of these studies are summarized in Table 1.

Only 7 articles have specifically focused on readmission rates after PD. Five of these studies represented single-institution experiences [11,13–16], 1 represented a multi-institutional analysis, and the seventh a population-based study of a statewide cancer registry [12]. Although these studies attempted to quantify readmission rates specifically related to the procedure, many focused instead on readmission as it related to progression of the patient's disease. These studies do not accurately reflect true readmission rate as it relates to perioperative outcomes and cannot be used to establish a baseline.

Van Geenen and colleagues [11] were the first to quantify rates of readmission after PD. This single-institution study analyzed prospectively collected data of patients undergoing PD over a 7-year period at their center. A total of 283 patients underwent PD during this period. Patients were followed for up to 90 months and readmissions and complications were documented. They reported a readmission rate of 38%, and most of these readmissions were related to complications resulting from disease recurrence or adjuvant therapy. Only 17% of the readmissions could be attributed directly to complications from surgery.

Emick and colleagues [15] published the largest single-institution series reported to date. This study from the Johns Hopkins Medical Institutions was a retrospective review of 1643 patients who underwent PD over a 7-year period. These investigators reported a 26% rate of readmission and identified younger age, blood loss, postoperative complications, and need for vascular reconstruction as independent risk factors for readmission.

Grewal and colleagues [13] then published a single-institutional series from the University of Cincinnati concentrating on early readmission rates, defined as readmission less than 90 days after surgery. This study was one of the first to look specifically at readmissions resulting directly from surgical intervention. The investigators reported a readmission rate of 27% and found that the most common reason for readmission was dehydration or malnutrition and pain.

More recently, Rosemurgy and colleagues [14] reported on their single-center experience with 913 patients undergoing PD over a 10-year period. These investigators assessed the rate of early readmission within 30 days of surgical intervention and reported a rate of 19%. Younger age and increased comorbidities were identified as statistically significant predictors of early readmission.

Yermilov and colleagues [12] were the first to evaluate readmission rates outside a single-institution setting. This group analyzed the California Cancer

Table 1
Factors associated with readmission: a summary of published data

	Rosemurgy et al [14], 2012	Ahmad et al [17], 2012	Grewal et al [13], 2011	Zhu et al [16], 2011	Yermilov et al [12], 2009	Emick et al [15], 2006	van Geenen et al [11], 2001
Cohort (n)	913	1302	124	436	2023	1643	283
Readmission rate (%)	19	19	27	33	59	26	38
≤30 d postoperatively (%)	19	15	14.5	13	19	—	—
≤90 d postoperatively (%)	—	19	27	26	42	—	—
Mortality (%)	—	—	—	—	31	22	—
Race (*P*)	—	NS	NS	—	NS	.01	—
Age (*P*)	<.001	<.02	NS	NS	<.003	<.001	—
CCI (*P*)	<.001	NS	NS	—	<.01	—	—
Cancer stage (*P*)	NS	NS	NS	<.05	<.003	—	—
Chronic pancreatitis (*P*)	—	−.007	−.002	—	—	—	—
Operative time (*P*)	NS	NS	NS	—	—	<.001	—
EBL (*P*)	NS	NS	NS	—	—	.02	—
Transfusion (*P*)	—	.007	.001	—	—	.04	—
Length of stay (*P*)	NS	NS	.01	NS	<.01	.02	—
Postoperative complications (*P*)	—	<.0001	NS	—	—	.03	—

Abbreviation: NS, not significant.

Registry of 2023 patients over a 10-year period who underwent PD and were readmitted to any hospital within 1 year of surgery [12]. The investigators were able to capture all patients who presented to any hospital in the state of California, providing a more comprehensive estimation of readmission rates. This analysis was performed with the realization that many patients travel to high-volume centers for their index procedure but can present to secondary hospitals for complications related to surgery. Single-institution studies likely underestimate readmission rates. These investigators reported a readmission rate of 59%, with almost half (47%) of these patients being admitted at secondary hospitals. T-stage, advanced age, and comorbidities were found on multivariate analysis to be associated with increased rates of readmission. Most secondary hospital readmissions were not directly related to complications of the surgery.

It is difficult to ascertain whether these studies reflect readmission rates after PD. Many of these studies include readmissions more than 1 year after surgery, with many of these admissions being related to recurrent disease rather than the operation itself [11,15,16]. van Geenen and colleagues [11], Zhu and colleagues [16], and Emick and colleagues [15] attributed 60%, 49%, and 23%, respectively, of the readmissions in their series to tumor progression of cancer. In the population-based study by Yermilov and colleagues [12], secondary hospital readmissions were not clearly defined and may not have been related to the surgical procedure.

A recently published study from the Central Pancreas Consortium represents the only multi-institutional study aimed at identifying rates of readmission after PD [17]. Although single-institution studies have given significant insight into the current problem, these experiences are often skewed by institutional bias and may not extrapolate to all patients undergoing PD at other high-volume pancreas centers. By combining experiences at multiple high-volume institutions, the investigators hoped to diminish the effect of institutional variability in management of postoperative complications and criteria for readmission after PD, thereby making the results more applicable to the general population.

SUMMARY OF CENTRAL PANCREAS CONSORTIUM

Ahmad and colleagues [17] sought to determine rates of early readmission (30 days and 90 days postoperatively) after PD and identify factors associated with failed discharge. This multi-institutional research group aimed to minimize the effect of institutional variability in perioperative patient management on outcomes after PD.

These investigators performed a retrospective review of prospectively collected data of patients who underwent PD for any reason over a 5-year period at 6 high-volume pancreatic centers within the Central Pancreas Consortium (University of Cincinnati, University of North Carolina, Emory University, University of Louisville, Northwestern University, University of Wisconsin, Vanderbilt University). Patients undergoing both standard PD and pylorus-preserving PD between January 2005 and January 2010 at these institutions were included in the study. All participating surgeons had completed additional fellowship training in complex pancreatic surgery. Patient demographics, comorbidities, perioperative factors such as preoperative stent placement, and intraoperative factors including operative blood loss and type of PD were analyzed. Readmission was determined at 2 time points and was defined as admission to the primary hospital within 30 days or within 90 days after surgery. The Charlson Comorbidity Index (CCI) was calculated for each patient [18]. This score takes into account several comorbid conditions and can be used as a predictor of postoperative mortality and a measure for patient disease acuity [18]. Operative technique, patient selection, feeding tube placement, and drain placement were left to the surgeons' discretion. Patients were managed postoperatively according to each institution's previously established post-PD clinical pathway. All participating institutions adhered to the International Study Group of Pancreatic Fistulas definition of pancreatic fistula. A pancreatic fistula was defined as any measurable drain output on or after postoperative day 3 with a drain amylase level greater than 3 times the serum amylase level [19]. Delayed gastric emptying was defined as failure to return to a standard diet by postoperative day 7 or prolonged nasogastric intubation according to the International Study Group of Pancreatic Surgery [20].

Over this 5-year period, a total of 1302 patients underwent PD at the 6 participating Central Pancreas Consortium institutions. Men represented 49% of the cohort (n = 644) and women 51% (n = 658). Readmission rates within 30 days and 90 days after surgery were 15% (n = 189) and 19% (n = 247), respectively. Infectious complications were the most common reason for readmission (Table 2). Gender, race, body mass index, and comorbid conditions such as diabetes, hypertension, and chronic obstructive pulmonary disease did not predispose to readmission. There was no difference in preoperative patient acuity in the readmission group as determined by age-adjusted CCI.

The most common indication for PD was pancreatic adenocarcinoma (n = 701, 54%), followed by ampullary cancer (n = 133, 10%) and chronic pancreatitis (n = 102, 8%). Tumor characteristics, preoperative stenting, neoadjuvant therapy, margin status, or type of PD did not predict need for early readmission.

Factors associated with readmission on univariate analysis included advanced age, diagnosis of chronic pancreatitis, need for transfusion at the time of surgery, presence of pancreatic fistula, intra-abdominal abscess, and wound infection (Table 3). On multivariate analysis, these factors remained significant predictors of readmission (Table 4).

Although patients undergoing PD for chronic pancreatitis represented only a few of the entire cohort (n = 102, 8%), many of these patients failed discharge. These patients were in general younger than those undergoing PD for other causes (56.2 vs 64.6 years, $P<.0001$), and had fewer

Table 2
Reason for readmission at 30 days/90 days

	30-d readmission (n = 161) (%)	90-d readmission (n = 281) (%)
Infection		
Wound infection	32 (19.9)	40 (14.2)
Intra-abdominal abscess	21 (13.0)	35 (12.5)
Line infection	2 (1.2)	4 (1.4)
Urinary tract infection	2 (1.2)	3 (1.1)
Pneumonia	1 (0.6)	2 (0.7)
Clostridium difficile infection	1 (0.6)	3 (1.1)
Fever	3 (1.9)	4 (1.4)
Other infection	3 (1.9)	5 (1.8)
Gastrointestinal		
Delayed gastric emptying	23 (14.3)	28 (10.0)
Small bowel obstruction	6 (3.7)	11 (3.9)
Gastrointestinal bleed	6 (3.7)	10 (3.6)
Nausea/vomiting	6 (3.7)	10 (3.6)
Failure to Thrive		
Dehydration/malnutrition/electrolytes	20 (12.4)	38 (13.5)
Pain control	9 (5.6)	16 (5.7)
Deep vein thrombosis/pulmonary embolism	2 (1.2)	3 (1.1)
Other	24 (14.9)	69 (24.6)

Abbreviation: n, total number of complications.

Data from Ahmad SA, Edwards MJ, Sutton JM, et al. Factors influencing readmission after pancreaticoduodenectomy: a multi-institutional study of 1302 patients. Ann Surg 2012;256(3):529–37.

Table 3
Univariate analysis, postoperative complications

	Readmitted (n = 247) (%)	Not readmitted (n = 1055) (%)	*P*
Infection			
Wound infection	45/247 (18.2)	98/1055 (9.3)	<.0001
Intra-abdominal abscess	33/247 (13.4)	55/1055 (5.2)	<.0001
Pneumonia	8/247 (3.2)	24/1055 (2.3)	.38
Line infection	9/247 (3.6)	21/1055 (2.0)	.12
Clostridium difficile infection	9/247 (3.6)	17/1055 (1.6)	.04
Biliary			
Pancreatic fistula	15/247 (6.1)	26/1055 (2.5)	.004
Bile leak	5/247 (2.0)	12/1055 (1.1)	.34
Gastrointestinal			
Delayed gastric emptying	29/247 (11.7)	82/1055 (7.8)	.04
Small bowel obstruction	4 (1.6)	15 (1.4)	.77
Cardiovascular			
Deep vein thrombosis/pulmonary embolism	9 (3.6)	9 (0.9)	.0007
Arrhythmia	7 (2.8)	18 (1.7)	.25
Other	36/154 (23.4)	112/421 (26.6)	.43

Data from Ahmad SA, Edwards MJ, Sutton JM, et al. Factors influencing readmission after pancreaticoduodenectomy: a multi-institutional study of 1302 patients. Ann Surg 2012;256(3):529–37.

Table 4
Multivariate analysis, predictors of readmission

Factor	Odds ratio	95% confidence interval	*P*
Transfusion	1.875	1.2–2.9	.007
Chronic pancreatitis	2.356	1.3–4.4	.007
Wound infection	2.2	1.5–3.2	.005
Pancreas fistula	2.4	1.2–4.8	.02
Intra-abdominal abscess	1.96	1.1–3.5	.02

Data from Ahmad SA, Edwards MJ, Sutton JM, et al. Factors influencing readmission after pancreaticoduodenectomy: a multi-institutional study of 1302 patients. Ann Surg 2012;256(3):529–37.

comorbidities, with an average CCI of 2 (range 1–3) compared with a CCI of 3 (range 2–3, $P = .0078$) in the remainder of the cohort. These patients also had shorter operative times (269 vs 329 minutes, $P < .05$) and less blood loss (300 vs 450 mL, $P < .05$). Despite these positive prognostic indicators, patients with chronic pancreatitis were more likely to be readmitted because of inadequate pain control (16% vs 3.2%, $P < .05$) when compared with the entire cohort.

This was the first study to present a multi-institutional review of readmission rates after PD, thereby eliminating institutional biases. A readmission rate of 19%, which is lower than previously reported rates from single-institution studies, was reported. This finding may be related to one of the limitations of the studies: their inability to accurately capture secondary hospital readmissions. However, because they focused on early readmissions (within 90 days of surgery), they were able to exclude readmissions because of patient disease and need for treatment including need for chemotherapy or radiotherapy and admissions related to tumor progression. This data set likely gives a good estimation of readmissions directly related to surgical intervention and represents most of what would be deemed as potentially preventable by MedPAC. One in 5 patients readmitted within 90 days after surgery likely represents the most accurate benchmark for acceptable readmission rates in patients undergoing PD.

These results are congruent with other published series that report similar readmission rates when admissions are directly related to PD. The predominate reasons for readmissions throughout all studies were infectious complications related to intra-abdominal abscess or wound infection (20%) and delayed gastric emptying (12%).

DOES FAST TRACKING INCREASE READMISSION RATES?

Clinical pathways for management of surgical patients are now commonly being implemented by surgeons in the postoperative period. These enhanced recovery programs, also known as fast-track pathways, are designed to decrease variability between surgeons for postoperative patient management and to safely hasten the time to recovery and discharge. These pathways use evidence-based medicine to optimize postoperative pain control, ambulation, and nutrition, thereby minimizing postoperative stress responses and subsequent organ dysfunction [21–23]. Similar programs have been successfully implemented in other clinical arenas such as colorectal surgery [24–26]. However, given the complexity of pancreatic surgery, there was significant concern whether fast tracking increased readmission rates after PD.

Berberat and colleagues [27] explored the safety and efficacy of fast-track pathways after major pancreatic resection. Perioperative data were collected prospectively from 255 patients undergoing pancreatic resection over 1 year at the University of Heidelberg. One hundred and fifty-five patients (60%) underwent PD. The investigators reported that fast tracking was successfully implemented at their institution with a decrease in the time to safe discharge home. The median time to discharge was 10 days, and this did not negatively affect readmission rates, with a 30-day readmission rate of only 3.5%. Postoperative mortality and morbidity were also unaffected, at 2% and 25% respectively. Age less than 60 years, decreased operative time, and early extubation were found to be statistically significant predictors of early discharge.

Balazano and colleagues [28] expanded on these data and sought to evaluate the effect of fast tracking specifically on patients undergoing PD. This retrospective study evaluated 252 patients over a 3-year period after implementation of a fast-track program at their institution. Patients were compared with a similarly matched historical control group who underwent PD before implementation of fast tracking and were managed via a traditional program. The investigators found that postoperative complications such as pancreatic fistula and intra-abdominal abscess were similar between groups. However, there was a significant decrease in the incidence of delayed gastric emptying from 24.6% to 13.9% ($P = .005$) in the fast-track group. There was also a decrease in length of stay by 2 days (13 vs 15 days; $P < .001$) without a change in the rate of readmission. Recently, Robertson and colleagues [29] concluded that implementation of a similar fast-track program was safe and effective and did not negatively affect mortality, morbidity, or readmission.

IMPROVING OUTCOMES

As health care cost management becomes a more critical issue for surgeons, it is imperative to answer the following question: how can readmission rates be decreased after PD and maintain a reasonably short length of stay? Although the current data give a good estimate of early remission rates after PD, the number of these readmissions that are preventable is still unclear. Ahmad and colleagues [17] reported that although 19% of patients were readmitted within 90 days after PD, 6% of these patients were admitted within 7 days from discharge. This 6% likely represents a realistic target for improvement. It can be assumed that these patients presented secondary to complications that were not anticipated and appropriately planned for. Efforts to safely reduce readmissions after PD must first be focused on identifying patients at high risk for outpatient failure, and second, they must anticipate potential complications to use resources such as skilled nursing facilities and home health services to manage these complications in an outpatient setting.

It is difficult to assess the number of patients being discharged with skilled nursing either at a facility or at home after PD. Ahmad and colleagues [17] reported that approximately 20% to 30% of patients in their series received skilled nursing after discharge. The data presented in this study suggest that patients with a transfusion requirement at the time of surgery, infectious complications such as wound infections or intra-abdominal abscesses, pancreatic fistula, or a preoperative diagnosis of chronic pancreatitis are at higher risk for readmission. Therefore, these patients may not be suitable candidates for fast-tracking programs. Patients once identified must be counseled regarding realistic postoperative expectations while inpatient as well as after discharge. The plan of care should be tailored to the individual patient and their concomitant risk factor. For example, postoperative pain control should be discussed with patients undergoing PD for chronic pancreatitis both in the preoperative and postoperative setting. A detailed discharge pain plan of care should be clearly established with available resources and contact person (ie, surgeon, physician extender, or office staff) for appropriately guided modifications if previously established parameters are not met. It is also essential that the patient's plan of care be communicated effectively with primary caretakers, home health care providers, and skilled nursing facilities so that a cohesive course of therapy can be implemented. Serious consideration should be given to all patients deemed high risk for failed discharge to receive skilled nursing care either at a facility or at home. Also, these patients may benefit from earlier follow-up with their surgeon so that early intervention using outpatient resources may be used in an effective and timely manner. Patients should not only reach a discharge metric but also remain at that metric for a predetermined period before discharge. Thus, patients should not be discharged as soon as they transfer to oral narcotics but should be kept on the prescribed regimen for at least 24 hours to ascertain if the regimen is efficacious. Similar goals should be set in place for ambulation, oral intake, and infection control.

SUMMARY

PD continues to be associated with a high rate of failed discharges, despite significant improvements in techniques and postoperative care at high-volume centers. Even in the best hands, 1 in 5 patients undergoing PD can be expected to require readmission in the early postoperative period. Efforts to minimize readmissions must be aimed at identifying high-risk patients, addressing patient expectations, establishing patient care plans, and using outpatient resources to address anticipated problems and complications.

References

[1] Averill RF, McCullough EC, Hughes JS, et al. Redesigning the Medicare inpatient PPS to reduce payments to hospitals with high readmission rates. Health Care Financ Rev 2009;30(4):1–15.

[2] Jencks SF, Williams MV, Coleman EA. Rehospitalizations among patients in the Medicare fee-for-service program. N Engl J Med 2009;360(14):1418–28.

[3] Lee TJ, Martin RC 2nd. Readmission rates after abdominal surgery: can they be decreased to a minimum? Adv Surg 2012;46:155–70.
[4] Brooks AD, Marcus SG, Gradek C, et al. Decreasing length of stay after pancreatoduodenectomy. Arch Surg 2000;135(7):823–30.
[5] Crist DW, Sitzmann JV, Cameron JL. Improved hospital morbidity, mortality, and survival after the Whipple procedure. Ann Surg 1987;206(3):358–65.
[6] Balcom JHt, Rattner DW, Warshaw AL, et al. Ten-year experience with 733 pancreatic resections: changing indications, older patients, and decreasing length of hospitalization. Arch Surg 2001;136(4):391–8.
[7] Yeo CJ, Cameron JL, Sohn TA, et al. Six hundred fifty consecutive pancreaticoduodenectomies in the 1990s: pathology, complications, and outcomes. Ann Surg 1997;226(3): 248–57 [discussion: 257–60].
[8] Pellegrini CA, Heck CF, Raper S, et al. An analysis of the reduced morbidity and mortality rates after pancreaticoduodenectomy. Arch Surg 1989;124(7):778–81.
[9] Lin JW, Cameron JL, Yeo CJ, et al. Risk factors and outcomes in postpancreaticoduodenectomy pancreaticocutaneous fistula. J Gastrointest Surg 2004;8(8):951–9.
[10] DeOliveira ML, Winter JM, Schafer M, et al. Assessment of complications after pancreatic surgery: a novel grading system applied to 633 patients undergoing pancreaticoduodenectomy. Ann Surg 2006;244(6):931–7 [discussion: 937–9].
[11] van Geenen RC, van Gulik TM, Busch OR, et al. Readmissions after pancreatoduodenectomy. Br J Surg 2001;88(11):1467–71.
[12] Yermilov I, Bentrem D, Sekeris E, et al. Readmissions following pancreaticoduodenectomy for pancreas cancer: a population-based appraisal. Ann Surg Oncol 2009;16(3):554–61.
[13] Grewal SS, McClaine RJ, Schmulewitz N, et al. Factors associated with recidivism following pancreaticoduodenectomy. HPB (Oxford) 2011;13(12):869–75.
[14] Rosemurgy AS, Luberice K, Paul H, et al. Readmissions after pancreaticoduodenectomy: efforts need to focus on patient expectations and nonhospital medical care. Am Surg 2012;78(8):837–43.
[15] Emick DM, Riall TS, Cameron JL, et al. Hospital readmission after pancreaticoduodenectomy. J Gastrointest Surg 2006;10(9):1243–52 [discussion: 1252–3].
[16] Zhu ZY, He JK, Wang YF, et al. Multivariable analysis of factors associated with hospital readmission following pancreaticoduodenectomy for malignant diseases. Chin Med J (Engl) 2011;124(7):1022–5.
[17] Ahmad SA, Edwards MJ, Sutton JM, et al. Factors influencing readmission after pancreaticoduodenectomy: a multi-institutional study of 1302 patients. Ann Surg 2012;256(3): 529–37.
[18] Hall WH, Ramachandran R, Narayan S, et al. An electronic application for rapidly calculating Charlson comorbidity score. BMC Cancer 2004;4:94.
[19] Bassi C, Dervenis C, Butturini G, et al. Postoperative pancreatic fistula: an international study group (ISGPF) definition. Surgery 2005;138(1):8–13.
[20] Wente MN, Bassi C, Dervenis C, et al. Delayed gastric emptying (DGE) after pancreatic surgery: a suggested definition by the International Study Group of Pancreatic Surgery (ISGPS). Surgery 2007;142(5):761–8.
[21] Fearon KC, Ljungqvist O, Von Meyenfeldt M, et al. Enhanced recovery after surgery: a consensus review of clinical care for patients undergoing colonic resection. Clin Nutr 2005;24(3):466–77.
[22] Kehlet H, Wilmore DW. Evidence-based surgical care and the evolution of fast-track surgery. Ann Surg 2008;248(2):189–98.
[23] Lassen K, Soop M, Nygren J, et al. Consensus review of optimal perioperative care in colorectal surgery: Enhanced Recovery After Surgery (ERAS) Group recommendations. Arch Surg 2009;144(10):961–9.
[24] Spanjersberg WR, Reurings J, Keus F, et al. Fast track surgery versus conventional recovery strategies for colorectal surgery. Cochrane Database Syst Rev 2011;(2):CD007635.

[25] Wind J, Polle SW, Fung Kon Jin PH, et al. Systematic review of enhanced recovery programmes in colonic surgery. Br J Surg 2006;93(7):800–9.
[26] Khoo CK, Vickery CJ, Forsyth N, et al. A prospective randomized controlled trial of multimodal perioperative management protocol in patients undergoing elective colorectal resection for cancer. Ann Surg 2007;245(6):867–72.
[27] Berberat PO, Ingold H, Gulbinas A, et al. Fast track–different implications in pancreatic surgery. J Gastrointest Surg 2007;11(7):880–7.
[28] Balzano G, Zerbi A, Braga M, et al. Fast-track recovery programme after pancreatico- duodenectomy reduces delayed gastric emptying. Br J Surg 2008;95(11):1387–93.
[29] Robertson N, Gallacher PJ, Peel N, et al. Implementation of an enhanced recovery programme following pancreaticoduodenectomy. HPB (Oxford) 2012;14(10):700–8.

Advances in Surgery 47 (2013) 111–118

ADVANCES IN SURGERY

Should Peritoneal Lavage Be Used with Suction During Laparoscopic Appendectomy for Perforated Appendicitis?

Shawn D. St. Peter, MD[a,*], George W. Holcomb III, MD, MBA[b]

[a]Department of Surgery, Center for Prospective Trials, Children's Mercy Hospital, 2401 Gillham Road, Kansas City, MO 64108, USA; [b]Department of Surgery, Children's Mercy Hospital, 2401 Gillham Road, Kansas City, MO 64108, USA

Keywords

• Peritoneal lavage • Laparoscopic appendectomy • Perforated appendicitis

Key points

- Historical operative standards included irrigation for peritoneal contamination.
- Abundant laboratory findings suggest irrigation may not be helpful for peritoneal cleansing.
- Few directly comparative studies have been conducted in a controlled model.
- Recent prospective, randomized data suggest no difference between irrigation versus suction alone during laparoscopic appendectomy for perforated appendicitis.

HISTORICAL DEBATE

The debate over the efficacy of peritoneal irrigation or lavage to treat enteric contamination has persisted for at least a century. Lavage was initially advocated in 1906 when Frank Torek described pouring salt water into all peritoneal recesses and "the hand, by some gentle to-and-fro motions, assists it in washing all parts."[1] Furthermore, he advocated that purulent material should be "dipped out, rather than wiped out, as the latter procedure would be more likely to injure the peritoneum." Surgeons in this era seem to have been working under the assumption that cleansing the peritoneum with fluid was important for controlling contamination. As might be expected, reports followed with the suggestion that antibiotics should be added to the irrigant [2]. The pro-irrigation group of surgeons has long held the mantra that "dilution is

*Corresponding author. *E-mail address:* sspeter@cmh.edu

0065-3411/13/$ – see front matter
http://dx.doi.org/10.1016/j.yasu.2013.04.002

the solution to pollution." Although this phrase is entrenched in debates on environmental pollution, trainees are unlikely to complete their surgical residency without hearing it in reference to contamination in the peritoneal cavity, usually when a surgeon is irrigating the abdomen with fervency. This group sees contamination as a simple mechanical problem that can be cleansed like dishes.

On the other side of the debate, many surgeons think the peritoneal cavity is a clever organ that has the capacity to wall off and control contamination [3]. If this is true, normal saline irrigation may also spread contamination to uncontaminated portions of the peritoneal cavity and cause abscesses to form. As early as 1910, Deaver stated, "abdominal irrigation I avoid… it is most important not to spread infection beyond the limit at which we find it."[4] Later, near the middle of the last century, Rodney Maingot stated in a textbook that, "Irrigation of the peritoneal cavity for cleansing purposes is, in my opinion, never justified, even in the presence of gross fecal contamination."[5]

These previously described thoughts were in the setting of contamination from any source. Regarding appendicitis, publications purporting the benefits of peritoneal irrigation during appendectomy for perforated appendicitis began appearing in the literature more than 3 decades ago [6–8]. The early era of this debate was based largely on anecdotal, philosophic, and noncomparative data. Representing the lowest level of evidence, even a large number of publications in favor of one camp or the other should not be used to form an impression without sound comparative evidence. Due to the paucity of such data, the debate continues today with strong arguments coming from both sides of this issue.

BASIC SCIENCE OF IRRIGATION

The premise of irrigation is based on the idea of mobilizing the microbiological pathogens into a solution that can be suctioned out, which results in a more complete cleansing than would be achieved with suction alone or with manual removal. In order for this concept to be plausible, the organisms need to be quite soluble. If that were the case, the peritoneal cavity should be cleansable like any inanimate object that is soiled with particulate matter. However, microorganisms have been shown to adhere to the peritoneal lining by attaching to mesothelial cells [9]. Others have shown that fecal contamination is resistant to intraperitoneal lavage as it results in only brief reductions in microbial density followed by rapid bacterial recovery [10]. Thus, antimicrobial lavage produces only transitory decreases in the number of bacteria bound to the mesothelial cells. In addition to demonstrating inadequate local control of bacteria with irrigation, others have shown irrigation can cause diffuse or remote inoculation after local contamination [11]. These findings in animal models provide data that counter the logic of irrigation. The microbes may not be able to be washed off mesothelial surfaces with irrigation and the impact of decreasing the population density of microbes may be transient and therefore not clinically meaningful.

The previously mentioned studies are focused solely on the microbial invasion component of fecal contamination. The other side of this biologic power struggle is the immune response to the presence of these foreign invaders. Proponents of suction alone (without irrigation) will muse that "macrophages can't swim." There turns out to be some truth to this statement. Phagocytes use opsonic proteins, immunoglobulins, and other inflammatory mediators to attach to a surface and carry out bacterial phagocytosis [12]. Peritoneal irrigation with normal saline may potentially remove or dilute the mediators of phagocytosis [13]. Although the overall phagocytic activity has been shown to be similar after the use of irrigation, the dominant phagocytic cell line becomes neutrophils instead of macrophages [14]. These observations have led to a more accurate phrase, "phagocytes can swim and eat, but not at the same time."

In addition to the cellular response mobilizing leukocytes for phagocytosis, there is the local peritoneal response to consider. Mesothelial cells are thought to be sensitive to exposure from all sources including atmospheric air and touching, accounting for the adhesions that develop postoperatively in most patients. The peritoneal lining is damaged with peritonitis. Mesothelial cells repopulate the lining to repair the damage. Irrigation has been shown to temporarily slough mesothelial cells [15,16], and also attenuate mesothelial cell regrowth and healing [17].

CLINICAL DATA FROM OPEN ERA

Under the assumption that cleansing the abdomen with irrigation will decrease complications, then logically, continuous lavage for a period of time after the operation should cleanse the abdomen more thoroughly. In the chemistry laboratory, it is known that an increasing number of rinses for a glass container will progressively decrease the remaining milimoles of any soluble substrate. The use of continuous irrigation in humans after an abdominal operation is obviously cumbersome and relatively morbid, but the clinical impact of such practice is germane to this conversation. There is a fair amount of comparative clinical data through 3 prospective, randomized trials comparing continuous peritoneal lavage for 24 hours postoperatively to intraoperative lavage for perforated appendicitis [18–20]. In 2 of the trials, there were no differences in outcomes [18,19], while the other found an increase in infectious complications with ongoing lavage [20]. These trials provide some insight that more irrigation is not better, but none of the trials address the question as to whether suction is better than irrigation and suction. However, from these trials, it seems that continuous irrigation does not provide superior outcomes.

A bolus of irrigation, usually with normal saline, at the end of the operation is the typical practice for those who believe that irrigation is beneficial. However, if saline is effective in reducing complications by washing the abdomen, then intuitively saline with antibiotic irrigation should be at least as effective, if not more so. During the prelaparoscopic era, there were a multitude of prospective randomized trials investigating generous irrigation with antibiotics in the fluid in patients with peritoneal contamination from a variety of clinical scenarios [21–28]. These trials encompassed a wide variety of methodologies and patients, with inconsistencies in the lavage technique in the control group, the use of systemic antibiotics, inclusion criteria, and definitions of infectious complications, which makes cumulative evaluation difficult. However, a meta-analysis in 2000 that reviewed 7 of these trials, 6 of which focused on adults, found that patients not receiving antibiotic lavage had a slight increased risk of infectious complications, but no increase in mortality [29]. The main methodological concern in evaluating these trials was the lack of consistency of adequate systemic antibiotic coverage in all patients. In this meta-analysis and literature review, the authors concluded that there is also no appreciable advantage to be gained by using lavage solutions that contain antibiotics if the patient is also receiving systemic antibiotics. In addition, the authors stated that evidence to date suggested that maneuvers in excess of the removal of gross contamination may be a ritual devoid of biologic advantage.

CURRENT CLINICAL DATA

The abundance of data from prior generations has failed to demonstrate a clinical role for irrigation in the face of peritoneal contamination. Despite the lack of compelling data in all the previous studies looking at the role of irrigation, in a survey of North American pediatric surgeons published in 2004, only 7% the respondents reported not using irrigation [30]. Thus, information gained from careful evaluation of the studies on irrigation during the open appendectomy era has not translated into practice habits in the current laparoscopic era. Unfortunately, comparative data in the laparoscopic era are also severely lacking. Although this debate over irrigation continues to occur during discussions at morbidity and mortality conferences, the debate has not translated into many publications. Recently, 2 retrospective studies comparing irrigation and suction to suction alone during appendectomy, mostly laparoscopic, demonstrated an increase in abscess development in patients undergoing irrigation [3,31]. Both author groups recommended against irrigation.

To answer this question more clearly, the authors recently completed a prospective, randomized trial comparing normal saline irrigation followed by suction to suction alone during laparoscopic appendectomy for perforated appendicitis in children [32]. In this study, perforation was defined as a hole in the appendix or fecalith in the abdomen (Fig. 1). Thus, these patients had irrefutable proof of contamination instead of clinical suggestions of perforation. Previously, it was shown that this definition was highly effective. A postoperative abscess rate of about 20% was found in these patients with either a hole in the appendix or a fecalith when compared with an abscess rate of less than 1% in patients without these features [33]. This definition eliminates variation in the cause of contamination while reducing the heterogeneity in the severity of contamination and risk of adverse events.

Based on previously known abscess rates derived from prospective randomized trials [33–35], and using a power of 0.80 and α of 0.05 in a 2-tailed model, a sample size of 220 patients was established in the authors' most recent trial

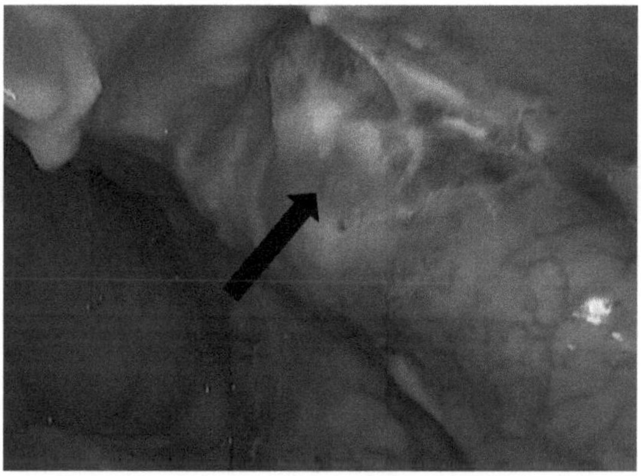

Fig. 1. Appendix with a hole as evidenced by small fecaliths extruding from the appendix (*arrow*).

[32]. Randomization occurred in a computer-generated sequence with allotment concealed from the staff surgeon. All patients underwent standard 3-port laparoscopic appendectomy using a 12-mm umbilical cannula via a vertically oriented transumbilical incision with 2 additional 5-mm ports in the left lower abdomen. The mesoappendix and appendix were ligated and divided using an endoscopic stapler and the appendix was protected during removal with either a bag or the umbilical cannula. The same model battery-powered suction/irrigation device was used in all cases to eliminate variation in suction capacity. In the irrigation arm, a 1-L bag of sterile normal saline was attached to the irrigation device. A minimum of 500 mL saline was required with no maximum volume limit. The surgeons were not given instructions on the style or extent of irrigation to incorporate the range of practice among the surgeons for generalizability. In the suction-only group, no saline was attached and the suction/irrigation device was used only for suction.

All patients were managed with the same antibiotic regimen and protocol as established from a prior trial [34]. Nasogastric tubes were not used; patients were not given raniditine, and diphenhydramine was used only for allergic reactions [36,37].

There were 110 patients treated in each arm of this recent study. On presentation, there were no differences in age, weight, body mass index percentile, gender distribution, duration of symptoms, presenting leukocyte count, or temperature between the 2 groups.

There were no conversions to an open appendectomy and no major intraoperative complications. The mean volume of irrigation used in this trial was 867 $\pm$ 327 mL (500–2000 mL). In only 1 patient was there a protocol violation and irrigation was used when it should not have been.

Outcomes are listed in Table 1. The primary outcome variable was the development of a postoperative abdominal abscess. In patients undergoing

Table 1
Outcome data

	Suction only (N = 110)	Irrigation and suction (N = 110)	*P* value
Abscess rate	19.1%	18.3%	1.0
Operative time (min)	38.7 ± 14.9	42.8 ± 16.7	.056
Time to clear liquids (days)	2.6 ± 1.5	2.5 ± 1.3	.70
Time to regular diet (days)	3.4 ± 1.7	3.5 ± 1.5	.63
Postoperative hospitalization (days)	5.5 ± 3.0	5.4 ± 2.7	.93
Hospital charges ($)	48.1 ± 20.1 K	48.1 ± 18.2 K	.97

suction only, an abscess developed in 19.1%. An abscess developed in 18.3% of patients in which irrigation and suction were both used ($P = 1.0$). There was no difference in time to starting clear liquids, advancement to a regular diet, or discharge. Hospital charges were the same. There was also no difference in mean maximum daily temperatures.

These data clearly demonstrate that the outcome in patients with perforated appendicitis will not be affected by the use of a moderate amount of irrigation during laparoscopic appendectomy. It is natural to speculate whether irrigation has an influence on the size, number, and location of abscesses. More importantly, it is unknown whether irrigation affects the clinical severity of the abscess. Impressively, there was no difference in the location and number of abscesses in this study. Furthermore, there was no difference in any aspect of their management, hospital course, or longer term outcomes (Table 2).

This trial demonstrates that irrigation does not have an impact on the clinical course following laparoscopic appendectomy for perforated appendicitis in children. Taking these data in the context of previous retrospective studies using irrigation and antibiotic irrigation, it would seem that a higher yield will be generated from investigating other operative and postoperative management variables.

Table 2
Outcomes in patients who developed a postoperative abscess

	Suction only (N = 21)	Irrigation (N = 20)	*P* value
Drain placed (%)	52%	40%	.54
Days of drainage	2.3 ± 2.2	1.8 ± 2.8	.58
Postoperative hospitalization (days)	8.7 ± 4.4	9.4 ± 3.8	.56
Days of intravenous antibiotics	19.5 ± 3.9	21.4 ± 8.6	.37
Days of home health care	10.4 ± 4.5	13.0 ± 7.4	.20
Abscess-related charges ($)	28.3 ± 22.7 K	24.6 ± 13.8 K	.54

References

[1] Torek F. The treatment of diffuse suppurative peritonitis following appendicitis. Med Rec 1906;70:849–58.
[2] Burnett WE, Brown GR Jr, Rosemond GP, et al. The treatment of peritonitis using peritoneal lavage. Ann Surg 1957;145:675–82.
[3] Hartwich JE, Carter RF, Wolfe L, et al. The effects of irrigation on outcomes in cases of perforated appendicitis in children. J Surg Res 2013;180(2):222–5.
[4] Deaver J. The diagnosis and treatment of peritonitis of the upper abdomen. Boston Med Surg J 1910;162:485–90.
[5] Maingot R. Abdominal operations. 6th edition, vol. II. New York: Appleton-Century Crofts; 1974. p. 1416.
[6] Stewart DJ, Matheson NA. Peritoneal lavage in appendicular peritonitis. Br J Surg 1978;65:54–6.
[7] Gilbert SR, Emmens RW, Putnam TC. Appendicitis in children. Surg Gynecol Obstet 1985;161:261–5.
[8] Matheson NA. Perforated appendix–a plea for lavage. Br J Surg 1979;66:293–4.
[9] Haagen IA, Heezius HC, Verkooyen RP, et al. Adherence of peritonitis-causing staphylococci to human peritoneal mesothelial cell monolayers. J Infect Dis 1990;161: 266–73.
[10] Edmiston CE Jr, Goheen MP, Kornhall S, et al. Fecal peritonitis: microbial adherence to serosal mesothelium and resistance to peritoneal lavage. World J Surg 1990;14:176–83.
[11] Wood W, Smith M, Watson B. Studies on the mechanism of recovery in pneumococcal pneumonia: IV. The mechanism of phagocytosis in the absence of antibody. J Exp Med 1976;84:387–403.
[12] Lamperi S, Carozzi S. Immunologic patterns in CAPD patients with peritonitis. Clin Nephrol 1988;30(Suppl 1):S41–4.
[13] Abbasoglu O, Sayek I, Hascelik G. The effect of peritoneal lavage on peritoneal cellular defense mechanisms. Acta Chir Belg 1994;94:321–4.
[14] Yaacobi Y, Goldberg EP, Habal MB. Effect of Ringer's lactate irrigation on the formation of postoperative abdominal adhesions. J Invest Surg 1991;4:31–6.
[15] Thoroughman J, Walker L, Collins J. Spreading organisms by peritoneal lavage. Am J Surg 1968;115:339–40.
[16] Breborowicz A, Rodela H, Oreopoulos DG. Toxicity of osmotic solutes on human mesothelial cells in vitro. Kidney Int 1992;41:1280–5.
[17] Tolhurst Cleaver C, Hopkins A, Kee Kwong K, et al. The effect of postoperative peritoneal lavage on survival, wound healing and adhesion formation following fecal peritonitis: an experimental study in the rat. Br J Surg 1974;61:601–4.
[18] Buanes TA, Andersen GP, Jacobsen U, et al. Perforated appendicitis with generalized peritonitis. Prospective, randomized evaluation of closed postoperative peritoneal lavage. Eur J Surg 1991;157:277–9.
[19] Olesen A, Jorgensen F, Bikde T, et al. Peritoneal lavage in diffuse peritonitis originating from perforated appendix. Ugeskr Laeger 1980;14:1415–8.
[20] Hallerback B, Andersson C, Englund N, et al. A prospective randomized study of continuous peritoneal lavage postoperatively in the treatment of purulent peritonitis. Surg Gynecol Obstet 1986;163:433–6.
[21] Schein M, Gecelter G, Freinkel W, et al. Peritoneal lavage in abdominal sepsis. A controlled clinical study. Arch Surg 1990;125:1132–5.
[22] Nomikos IN, Katsouyanni K, Papaioannou AN. Washing with or without chloramphenicol in the treatment of peritonitis: a prospective, clinical trial. Surgery 1986;99:20–5.
[23] Rambo W. Irrigation of the peritoneal cavity with cephalothin. Am J Surg 1972;123: 192–5.
[24] Fowler R. A controlled trial of intraperitoneal cephaloridine administration in peritonitis. J Pediatr Surg 1975;10:43–50.

[25] Sauven P, Playforth M, Smith G, et al. Single-dose antibiotic prophylaxis of abdominal surgical wound infection: a trial of preoperative latamoxef against preoperative tetracycline lavage. J R Soc Med 1986;79:137–41.
[26] Noon G, Beall A, Jordan G, et al. Clinical evaluation of peritoneal irrigation with antibiotic solution. Surgery 1967;62:73–8.
[27] Silverman S, Ambrose N, Young D, et al. The effect of peritoneal lavage with tetracycline solution on postoperative infection. Dis Colon Rectum 1986;29:165–9.
[28] Shurman JO, Luck SR, Borger JA. Irrigation of the peritoneal cavity for appendicitis in children: a double blind study. J Pediatr Surg 1976;11:371–4.
[29] Platell C, Papadimitriou JM, Hall JC. The influence of lavage on peritonitis. J Am Coll Surg 2000;191:672–9.
[30] Muehlstedt SG, Pham TQ, Schmeling DJ. The management of pediatric appendicitis: a survey of North American Pediatric Surgeons. J Pediatr Surg 2004;39:875–9.
[31] Moore CB, Smith RS, Herbertson R, et al. Does use of intraoperative irrigation with open or laparoscopic appendectomy reduce post-operative intra-abdominal abscess? Am Surg 2011;77:78–80.
[32] St. Peter SD, Adibe OO, Iqbal CW, et al. Irrigation versus suction alone during laparoscopic appendectomy for perforated appendicitis: a prospective randomized trial. Ann Surg 2012;256:581–5.
[33] St. Peter SD, Sharp SW, Holcomb GW III, et al. An evidence based definition for perforated appendicitis derived from a prospective, randomized trial. J Pediatr Surg 2008;43:2242–5.
[34] St Peter SD, Tsao K, Spilde TL, et al. Single daily dosing ceftriaxone and metronidazole vs. standard triple antibiotic regimen for perforated appendicitis in children: a prospective randomized trial. J Pediatr Surg 2008;43:981–5.
[35] Fraser JD, Aguayo P, Leys CM, et al. A complete course of intravenous antibiotics versus a combination of intravenous and oral antibiotics for perforated appendicitis in children: a prospective, randomized trial. J Pediatr Surg 2010;45:1198–202.
[36] St. Peter SD, Little DC, Calkins CM, et al. Does routine nasogastric tube placement after an operation for perforated appendicitis make a difference? J Surg Res 2007;143:66–9.
[37] St. Peter SD, Sharp SW, Ostlie DJ. Influence of histamine receptor antagonists on the outcome of perforated appendicitis: analysis from a prospective, randomized trial. Arch Surg 2010;145:143–6.

Advances in Surgery 47 (2013) 119–140

ADVANCES IN SURGERY

ELSEVIER
MOSBY

Appendicitis: Changing Perspectives

Pedro G.R. Teixeira, MD, Demetrios Demetriades, MD, PhD*

Division of Trauma and Acute Care Surgery, LAC and USC Medical Center, University of Southern California, 2051 Marengo Street, IPT, Room C5L 100, Los Angeles, CA 90033-4525, USA

Keywords

• Appendicitis • Laparoscopy • Nonoperative • Imaging

Key points

- Neoplasms are uncommon, occurring in less than 1% of appendectomies.
- A negative ultrasound is not adequate to rule out appendicitis and should be followed by CT scan.
- During pregnancy, MRI is a reasonable alternative to CT scan.
- Nonoperative management with antibiotics is a safe initial treatment of uncomplicated appendicitis, with less complications but high failure rate.
- Open and laparoscopic appendectomies provide similar results overall.
- A negative appendectomy is associated with a significant incidence of fetal loss.
- The increased morbidity associated with appendectomy delay suggests that prompt surgical intervention remains the safest approach.
- Routine incidental appendectomy should not be performed.
- Interval appendectomy is not indicated because of risks of complications and lack of clinical benefit.
- Patients older than 40 years treated nonoperatively should have a colonoscopy to rule out cancer or alternative diagnosis.

INTRODUCTION

Despite remarkable advances in medicine and surgery, appendicitis continues to fascinate and challenge surgeons. Although records of the initial anatomic illustrations and descriptions of the vermiform appendix date back more than 500 years, it was not until the late nineteenth century that the inflammatory process occurring in the right lower quadrant and its association with the appendix were systematically described by Dr Reginald H. Fitz [1]. In his 1886 address to the first meeting of the Association of the American Physicians, Dr Fitz presented

*Corresponding author. *E-mail address:* demetria@usc.edu

0065-3411/13/$ – see front matter
http://dx.doi.org/10.1016/j.yasu.2013.02.002

an elegant article entitled, "Perforating Inflammation of the Vermiform Appendix; With Special Reference to Its Early Diagnosis and Treatment," [1] and used the term, *appendicitis*, for the first time [2]. Soon after, a series of important articles by McBurney contributed significantly to consolidate appendicitis as a surgical condition [3,4]. After several generations, McBurney's remarks remain true: "I know of no localized disease which is capable of presenting such a variety of pathologic processes. The real difficulty lies in estimating at an early period the probable behavior of each individual case" [3].

More than 120 years later, significant scientific and technological progress has revolutionized the field of surgery and resulted in a major improvement in outcomes. In 1955, Cantrell and Stafford described the Johns Hopkins 25-year experience with appendicitis management [5]. The steady decrease in mortality during that period was associated not only with the advent of antibiotics but also with better understanding of the physiopathology of sepsis and of the importance of fluid and electrolyte resuscitation and the role of early ambulation in prevention of pulmonary complications and venous thromboembolic events. By the end of the 1950s, mortality for perforated appendicitis was in the single digits and virtually no deaths occurred as a result of a nonperforated appendicitis [5,6].

Despite these significant advances, however, there are still many unresolved and controversial issues regarding the optimal diagnostic evaluation, need for an operation, timing and operation technique, indication for incidental and interval appendectomies, and optimal management strategy during pregnancy. This article addresses these issues (Box 1).

EPIDEMIOLOGY

Appendectomy is the most commonly performed emergent abdominal operation in the United States [7]. The estimated incidence of acute appendicitis has been reported as 11 per 10,000 population per year, with male and female lifetime risks of appendicitis of 8.6% and 6.7%, respectively [8]. A more recent epidemiologic investigation performed in California estimated a 9.0% lifetime risk of appendicitis [9]. Overall, the peak incidence of appendicitis occurs during the second decade of life [8,9]. There is a gender difference, however, with

Box 1: Controversial issues

- Optimal diagnostic evaluation
- Nonoperative management versus appendectomy
- Appendectomy timing
- Open versus laparoscopic technique
- Interval appendectomy
- Incidental appendectomy
- Optimal management strategy during pregnancy

earlier male peak incidence between 10 and 14 years of age compared with female peak incidence at ages 15 to 19 [8].

The risk of perforation is higher at the extremes of age [9]. Patients younger than 8 years or older than 45 years have an overall perforation incidence of 48% compared with 20% for patients between 8 and 45 years of age ($P<.001$) [10].

INCIDENTAL MALIGNANCIES

After appendectomy for suspected acute appendicitis, the incidence of unexpected findings in histopathologic examination of the surgical specimens is low. The overall incidence of malignancy is approximately 1%, with carcinoid the most frequent [11–25].

In a recent study from the University of Southern California, a neoplasm was identified in 31 of 4108 (0.75%) appendectomy specimens. Carcinoid was the most common tumor, identified in 27 (87%) of the specimens with a malignancy (Table 1).

DIAGNOSTIC ADVANCES AND CONTROVERSIES

History and physical examination remain powerful tools for the diagnosis of acute appendicitis and in many instances may be enough to warrant surgical exploration without additional imaging [26]. Alvarado described a scoring system to predict the diagnosis of acute appendicitis based on symptoms, signs, and laboratory findings [27]. This score, initially proposed to discriminate between patients who should be observed (scores 5 or 6) and those who should be operated on (score 7 or higher), later became a tool to identify patients with intermediate risk for appendicitis who need imaging investigation. A recent systematic review investigated the value of the Alvarado score for predicting acute appendicitis and found that a score less than 5 can accurately rule out appendicitis. It also found, however, that a score of 7 or higher is not specific enough to warrant surgical exploration, suggesting that imaging investigation may be necessary even for patients with a high score [28].

The use of imaging has been found to outperform the Alvarado score [29] and decrease the incidence of negative appendectomies but had no impact in decreasing perforation rate [30]. Currently, the imaging modalities most

Table 1
Neoplasms found in 4108 surgical specimens of patients undergoing appendectomy for acute appendicitis at LAC + USC Medical Center

Neoplasms	Appendectomies for acute appendicitis (N = 4108)
Neoplasms overall	31/4108 (0.75%)
Carcinoid tumor	27/31 (87%)
Mucinous tumor or uncertain malignant potential	2/31 (7%)
Mucinous adenocarcinoma	1/31 (3%)
Granular cell tumor	1/31 (3%)

commonly used for the diagnosis of acute appendicitis include ultrasonography, CT scan, and MRI.

On ultrasound, a normal appendix can be visualized at the right lower quadrant as a blind-ended tubular structure arising from the cecum. Its normal diameter is 6 mm to 7 mm or less and the normal wall thickness is 2 mm or less. When inflamed, the appendix becomes dilated, with thickened wall, immobile, and noncompressible (Fig. 1) [31], which can be demonstrated applying graded compression with the ultrasound probe (Fig. 2). Periappendicular fluid and a fecalith may also be present (Figs. 3 and 4).

Ultrasound was found 78% to 83% sensitive and 83% to 93% specific for the diagnosis of acute appendicitis [32,33]. Not being associated with ionizing radiation remains the most important advantage of ultrasound compared with CT scan. Ultrasound can be used for patients in whom additional imaging investigations is considered necessary and is particularly valuable in women for evaluation of gynecologic problems, which have a clinical presentation similar to appendicitis. Due to its lower sensitivity, however, a negative ultrasound should not be relied on to exclude the diagnosis, and further imaging with CT scan is advisable [34]. Poortman and colleagues [35] prospectively investigated a diagnostic pathway in which ultrasound was the initial investigation and was followed by CT scan if it was negative or inconclusive. This pathway was 100% sensitive and 86% specific for appendicitis, suggesting that ultrasound can be safely used as the initial assessment of patients presenting with right lower quadrant pain.

The most current iteration of the American College of Radiology Appropriateness Criteria for right lower quadrant pain and suspected appendicitis suggests that for adults CT scan provides higher sensitivity and specificity

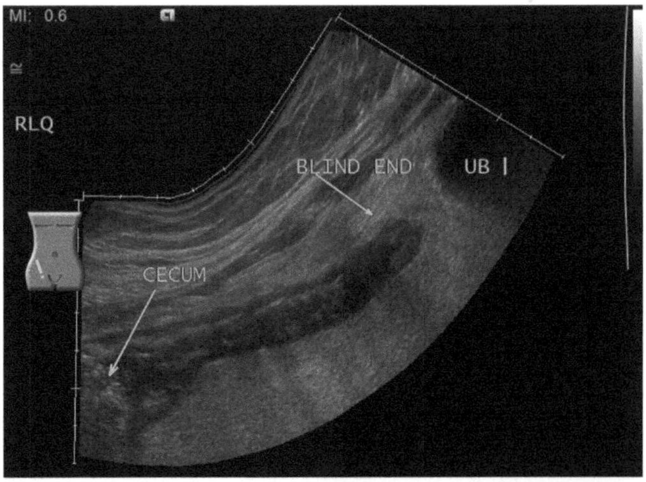

Fig. 1. Ultrasound image demonstrating a sagittal section of a dilated, blind-ended structure arising from the cecum, suggestive of acute appendicitis.

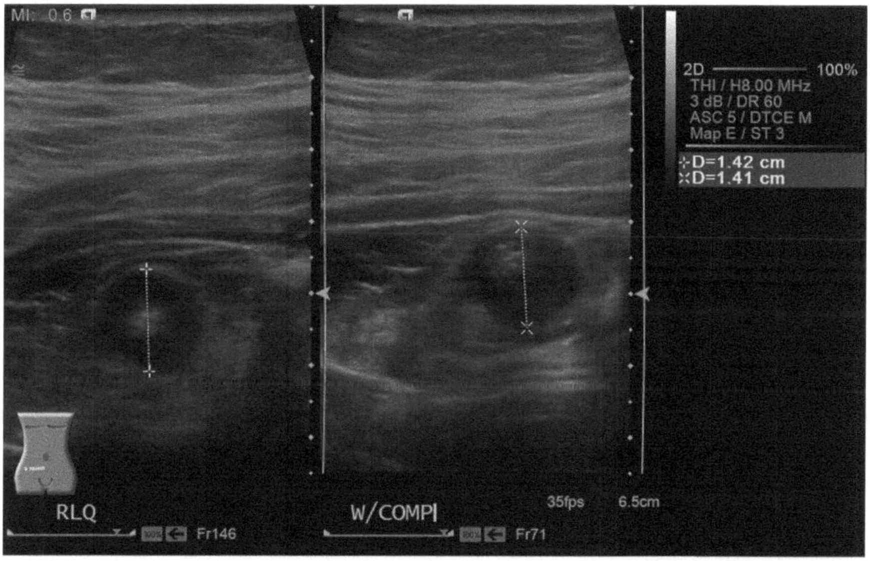

Fig. 2. Ultrasound image demonstrating transverse section of a noncompressible tubular structure in the right lower quadrant. The increased diameter and noncompressibility suggest acute appendicitis.

compared with ultrasound and decreases the incidence of negative appendectomies. In children, graded-compression ultrasonography has sensitivity and specificity comparable to those from CT scan without the potential harm of ionizing radiation [36].

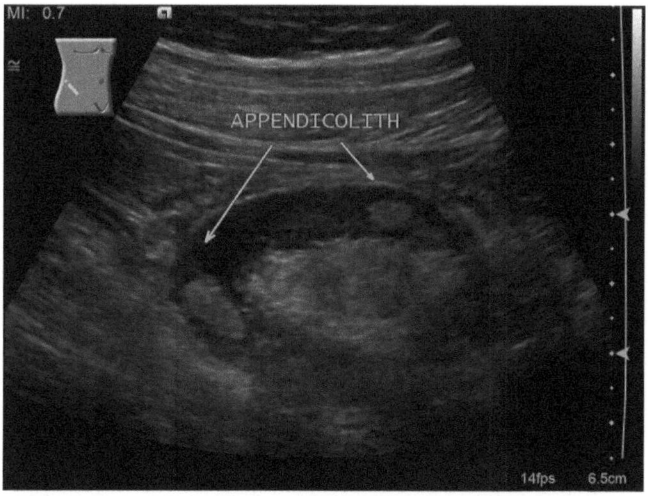

Fig. 3. Ultrasound image of a dilated appendix containing fecaliths.

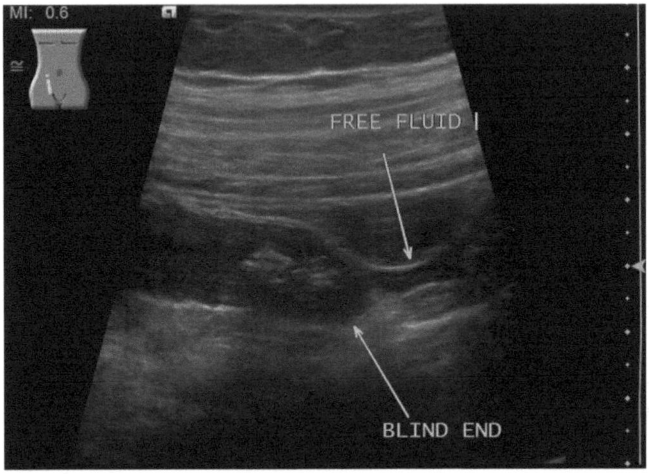

Fig. 4. Ultrasound image of a dilated appendix with adjacent free fluid, suggestive of acute appendicitis.

The CT scan findings of acute appendicitis include a dilated appendix, with no luminal contrast or gas, associated with periappendicular fluid and fat stranding (Fig. 5). CT scan is particularly useful in elucidating an alternative diagnosis or identifying complications associated with appendicitis, such as rupture, phlegmon, and abscess (Figs. 6 and 7).

Although MRI has been reported highly sensitive and specific for appendicitis [37,38] as well as cost effective [39], the value of this imaging modality in the general population presenting with right lower quadrant pain and

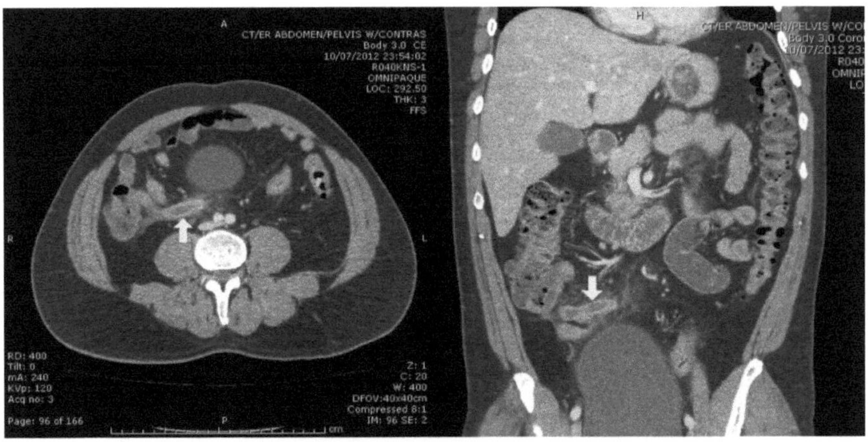

Fig. 5. CT scan images (axial and coronal sections) demonstrating a dilated appendix, with adjacent fat stranding, suggestive of acute appendicitis. Arrows, dilated appendix.

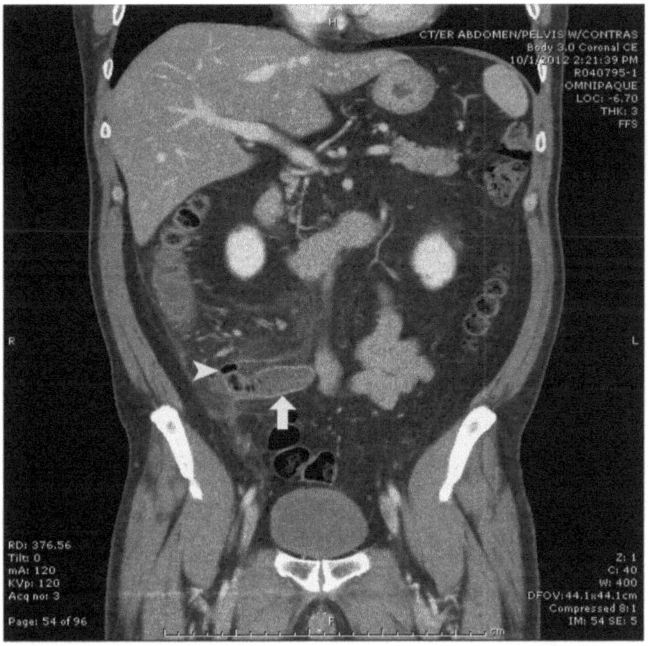

Fig. 6. CT scan coronal section image demonstrating a dilated appendix, with periappendicular fat stranding and extraluminal gas, suggestive of perforated appendicitis. Arrow, dilated appendix. Arrowhead, extraluminal gas.

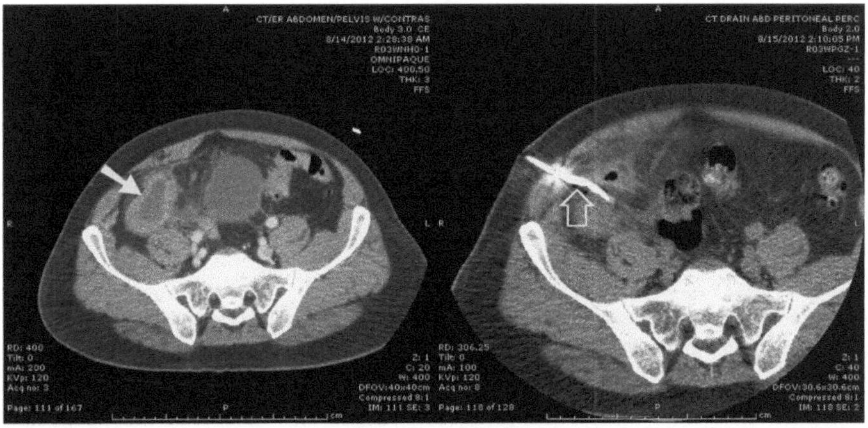

Fig. 7. CT scan axial images demonstrating perforated appendicitis with abscess (*left*) and percutaneous CT-guided drainage of the abscess (*right*). Arrow, abscess. Empty arrow, percutaneous catheter insertion.

suspicion for appendicitis remains to be determined. For pregnant patients, however, MRI seems a reasonable alternative to CT scan when ultrasound is negative or inconclusive [36].

Table 2 highlights a comparison of ultrasound, CT scan, and MRI diagnostic capabilities for the diagnosis of acute appendicitis. The appendicitis management algorithm is described in Fig. 8.

MANAGEMENT ADVANCES AND CONTROVERSIES

Nonoperative management

Nonoperative management is the preferred approach in cases of diagnosis of an appendiceal mass or abscess [40]. In uncomplicated cases, appendectomy has been considered the only acceptable therapeutic option. Recent studies have challenged this concept, however, and support a definitive role of nonoperative management [41–47]. It has been suggested that the adoption of nonoperative management for uncomplicated appendicitis is safe and can avoid an operation in approximately two-thirds of patients [48].

Two recent meta-analyses summarized the findings of prospective randomized trials comparing the efficacy of antibiotics versus appendectomy for the treatment of acute uncomplicated appendicitis [41,47]. According to Mason and colleagues [47], the nonoperative group had significantly lower risk of complications at 12% compared with 18% for the appendectomy group (odds ratio [OR] 0.54; 95% Confidence Interval [CI] 0.37–0.78; $P = .001$), which is in agreement with Varadhan and colleagues [41], who demonstrated a complication risk ratio of 0.69 (95% CI, 0.54–0.89; $P = .004$) for antibiotics compared with appendectomy. Appendectomy, however, outperformed the nonoperative management in terms of overall treatment failure rate. In the antibiotic group, the treatment failure rate was 40% compared with 9% in the appendectomy group (OR 6.72; 95% CI 3.48–12.99; $P < .001$) [47].

After analysis of similar pooled data sets, both studies agree that antibiotics are safe as initial treatment of uncomplicated appendicitis, with a significant decrease in complications but a significant failure rate.

Open versus laparoscopic

Initially described by Semm [49], laparoscopic appendectomy became widely accepted and currently is the most frequent technique for removal of the appendix (Fig. 9) [50–52]. Although laparoscopy offers several theoretic advantages

Table 2
Comparison of ultrasound, CT scan, and MRI diagnostic capabilities for the diagnosis of acute appendicitis

	Sensitivity	Specificity	Accuracy	PPV	NPV
Ultrasound [119]	75%–90%	86%–100%	87%–96%	91%–94%	89%–97%
CT scan [119]	90%–100%	91%–99%	94%–98%	92%–98%	95%–100%
MRI [37,38]	97%–100%	92%–98%	92%–99%	98%	100%

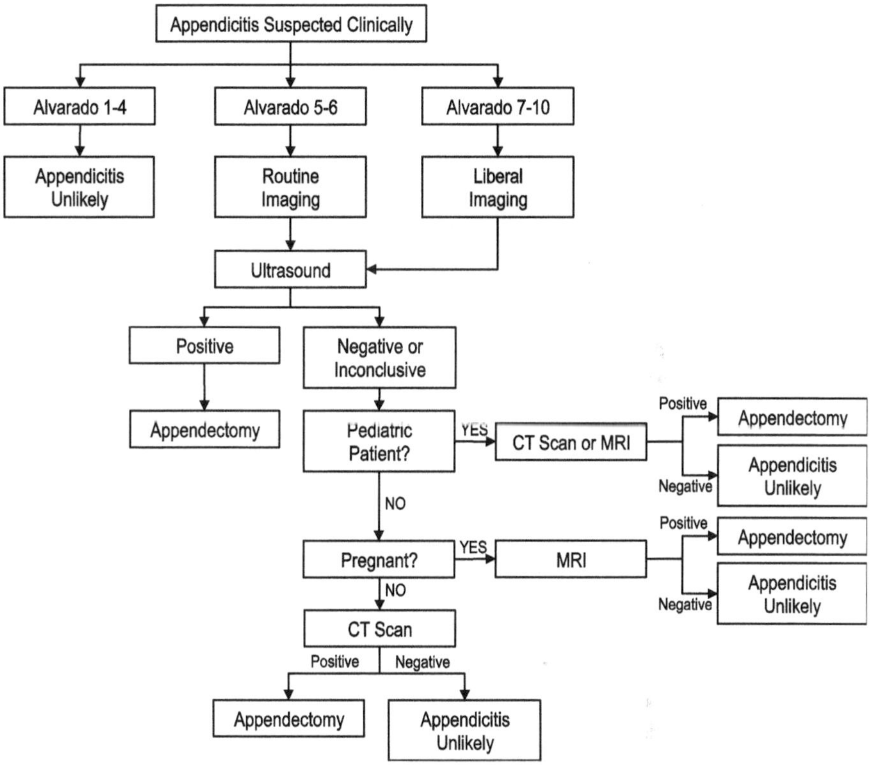

Fig. 8. LAC + USC Medical Center appendicitis management algorithm.

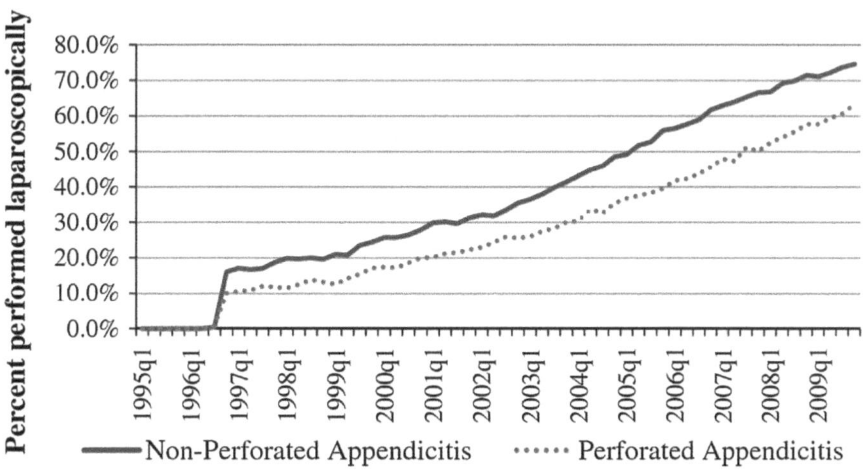

Fig. 9. Trend in the use of laparoscopic technique for appendectomies in California. (*Data from* Anderson JE, Bickler SW, Chang DC, et al. Examining a common disease with unknown etiology: trends in epidemiology and surgical management of appendicitis in California, 1995-2009. World J Surg 2012;36:2787–94.)

compared with open procedures, such as less pain, shorter recovery time, quicker return to work, and decreased inflammatory response, several studies have failed to demonstrate the superiority of laparoscopic appendectomy.

Studies using the *American College of Surgeons National Surgical Quality Improvement Program (NSQIP)* database have consistently demonstrated that laparoscopic appendectomy is associated with significantly lower incidence of wound infections compared with open appendectomy. The risk of intra-abdominal abscess increases, however, if laparoscopy is used [52–54]. Ingraham and colleagues [52] performed a robust analysis of this large database using propensity score to minimize the bias associated with the lack of randomization in the study and found that although laparoscopy was associated with a lower risk of overall complications, both techniques were comparable in terms of risk of serious complications. Using the same database, other groups found that the laparoscopic technique was associated with fewer complications in obese patients [55] and elderly patients [56].

At the Los Angeles County + University of Southern California (LAC + USC) Medical Center, from July 2003 to June 2011, 41% of 4108 appendectomies were performed laparoscopically [57]. Compared with the open procedures, laparoscopic appendectomies were associated with a decreased risk of wound infection (OR 0.57; 95% CI 0.34–0.97; $P = .038$).

A recent Cochrane review compiled and analyzed 67 randomized clinical trials comparing laparoscopic with open appendectomy. Laparoscopy was associated with significantly lower rates of wound infections (OR 0.43; 95% CI 0.34–0.54) but with a significantly higher incidence of intra-abdominal abscess (OR 1.77; 95% CI 1.14–2.76). The laparoscopic technique was found beneficial for postoperative pain level, hospital stay, and return to work; however, significant heterogeneity among the studies included makes the significance of these findings weaker. Although the investigators conclude with a recommendation in favor of laparoscopic appendectomy, they note that the benefits of laparoscopy compared with the conventional open technique are small and of questionable clinical significance [58].

Although laparoscopic technique is associated with a decreased risk of postoperative adhesive bowel obstruction compared with most open abdominal operations, this advantage was not confirmed for appendectomies, as suggested by a recent systematic review demonstrating no difference in the incidence of this complication after laparoscopic or open appendectomies (1.4% vs 1.3%) [59].

In summary, approximately 30 years after Semm's first laparoscopic appendectomy, the surgical community has embraced the technique but the true advantages compared with conventional surgery remain unclear.

Appendicitis during pregnancy

Appendicitis during pregnancy carries unique diagnostic and management challenges and can have a negative impact on outcomes for both mother and fetus. Low birth weight, preterm birth, small for gestational age, low Apgar scores, and preeclampsia/eclampsia have all been associated with acute appendicitis during pregnancy [60–62]. If perforation develops, fetal mortality increases from 7% to 10% to as high as 24% [63,64].

A wide spectrum of conditions can present as acute abdominal pain in pregnant women and significantly broaden the differential diagnosis. Although the reported incidence of appendicitis during pregnancy is low, appendicitis is the most common nonobstetric condition requiring emergent surgery during pregnancy [65], occurring during the second trimester in approximately half of cases [61].

A shift of the anatomic position of the appendix as the uterus size increases, gestational symptoms, frequent lack of febrile response, and the physiologic changes of pregnancy, which include leukocytosis, make a diagnosis of acute appendicitis a dilemma. The diagnostic challenges and the urge to proceed expeditiously to the operating room may lead to rates of negative explorations as high as 25% to 50% [10,62,66]. A recent large population-based study identified that the rate of negative appendectomy in pregnant women is significantly higher than in nonpregnant women (23% vs 18%; $P<.05$) [67]. Preoperative diagnostic accuracy is of utmost importance because a negative surgical exploration is not inconsequential. An overall fetal loss rate of 4% after negative appendectomy has been reported. Among pregnant women undergoing appendectomy who sustained a fetal loss or early delivery, almost 1 in 3 had a negative appendectomy [67].

Ultrasonography is an attractive imaging modality during pregnancy because of its lack of ionizing radiation, but it is highly operator depended. When the performance of the study is technically optimal, ultrasonography has an overall reported sensitivity of 100%, specificity of 96%, and accuracy of 98% [68]. In instances, however, when obesity or a large uterus limits the ability to perform graded compression, the ultrasonography findings may be equivocal. CT scan of the abdomen and pelvis has a reported negative predictive value of 99% for appendicitis [69]. The risk of irradiation to the fetus is of major concern, however, and most surgeons and emergency physicians use alternative methods. When presented with the scenario of imaging appendicitis or abscess in a pregnant patient during the second and third weeks of gestation, radiologists from 183 academic radiology departments in the United States chose CT scan over MRI. In patients in the first trimester of pregnancy, however, the same radiologists were more likely to use MRI [70]. This finding likely reflects the higher level of concern regarding potential teratogenic effects of ionizing radiation during the early phase of pregnancy.

It has been suggested that MRI may be a better second-line investigation compared with CT scan for cases when ultrasonography is equivocal or nondiagnostic [38,71]. Despite several reports of MRI's high sensitivity, specificity, and diagnostic accuracy for acute appendicitis, the exact role of this imaging modality in assessment of pregnant patients with suspected appendicitis remains unclear [72–75]. Although no report exists of human teratogenic or carcinogenic effects of MRI, the safety of MRI for the human fetus has not been completely proved. The Society for Magnetic Resonance Imaging safety committee has suggested that MRI should be avoided in the first trimester [76]. More recent recommendations from the American College of Radiology state that MRI is acceptable for pregnant patients at any stage of pregnancy if warranted by the risk/benefit assessment and waiting until the pregnancy is over to obtain the test is not possible [77].

As nonoperative management emerges as a valid and safe approach to acute noncomplicated appendicitis, this concept must be applied with caution to pregnant patients. This unique population was not included in the studies investigating the safety and efficacy of the nonoperative strategy and extrapolation of those findings may be problematic [78].

The enlarged uterus may present significant technical challenges for the laparoscopic approach as pregnancy approaches term. The choice of surgical approach has traditionally been guided by the individual institutional expertise because both open and laparoscopic techniques have been successfully applied to appendectomy during pregnancy [79–83]. Experimental work, however, demonstrated the development of fetal acidemia during pneumoperitoneum using CO_2, with fetal pH falling below 7.20 from its normal 7.33 $\pm$ 0.02, with P_{CO_2} rising above 55 mm Hg [84]. The implications in human fetal physiology are not fully known. Recent evidence suggests that the laparoscopic technique may be associated with a significantly higher incidence of fetal loss compared with open surgery [85]. In that systematic review, including 3415 pregnant patients undergoing appendectomy, the pooled relative risk of fetal loss for laparoscopic appendectomy compared with open surgery was 1.91 (95% CI, 1.31–2.77). These data must be interpreted with caution because all the studies included in the review were observational and no risk adjustment was possible, which may lead to significant bias. Notwithstanding, an almost 2-fold increase in fetal loss is worrisome and warrants proper investigation with randomized trials (Box 2).

TIMING OF OPERATION

Historically, time has been considered an important factor in the management of acute appendicitis, and emphasis on early diagnosis and immediate surgical intervention has been an important principle for the successful treatment of this condition [1,3,5,6,86,87].

Box 2: Appendicitis challenges during pregnancy

- Enlarged uterus, gestational symptoms, and physiologic changes of pregnancy make diagnosis difficult.
- Negative appendectomy is associated with significant incidence of fetal loss.
- Fetal mortality increases with perforation.
- CT scan is potentially harmful to the fetus.
- It is unclear if nonoperative management is safe.
- Laparoscopic technique may be associated with increased risks for the fetus.

Recent studies have suggested that prompt antibiotic followed by a semielective appendectomy is a safe strategy for the management of appendicitis [51,88–91]. Those findings are in contrast, however, with several studies demonstrating a negative impact of appendectomy delay [92–94].

Ingraham and colleagues [51] used the *NSQIP* database to investigate the effect of appendectomy delay in outcomes and found that appendectomies performed less than or equal to 6 hours, 6 to 12 hours, and greater than 12 hours after admission had no significant difference in complications. A closer look at the findings of another group that supported a semielective approach to appendicitis reveals that the incidence of abscesses requiring drainage increased from 3% to 6% in patients who were operated on more than 6 hours after admission [88].

Ditillo and colleagues [93] reviewed 1081 patients undergoing appendectomy and found that delay to appendectomy had a significant impact both on worsening pathology and on the development of complications, concluding that delay in appendectomy is unsafe. In another review of 1675 patients undergoing appendectomy for appendicitis, Busch and colleagues [92] found that delay of 12 hours or more was associated with a significantly higher perforation rate and longer hospital stay.

More recent data support the negative impact of appendectomy delay. Over an 8-year period, 4108 appendectomies for acute appendicitis were performed at the LAC + USC Medical Center. Perforated appendicitis was found in 23% of the surgical specimens. No deaths occurred; 64% of the patients underwent appendectomy more than 6 hours after admission, with an overall average time to appendectomy of 11 hours and 50 minutes, and 58% of the operations were performed during nighttime. Logistic regression found that appendectomy delay did not increase the risk of perforation. The independent predictors of perforation identified were age greater than or equal to 55 years old, white blood cell count greater than 16,000, and female gender. Fig. 10 demonstrates the incidence of surgical site infections associated with incremental delay in appendectomy. A delay greater than 6 hours was independently associated with increased incidence of surgical site infections (adjusted OR 1.54; 95% CI, 1.01–2.34; $P = .04$) after adjusting for age, leukocytosis, gender, operative technique (open vs laparoscopic), and perforation. Particularly significant was a delay in appendectomy for patients with a nonperforated appendicitis, as demonstrated in Fig. 11. For these patients, an appendectomy delay greater than 6 hours was associated with an increase in the incidence of surgical site infections from 1.9% to 3.3% (OR 2.16; 95% CI, 1.03–4.52; $P = .03$). Early appendectomy ($\leq$6 hours) for the group of patients without a perforation was associated with a 42% relative risk reduction in the development of surgical site infections. Patients who had their postoperative course complicated with a surgical site infection remained an additional 5 days in the hospital compared with those who did not have this complication (7.9 $\pm$ 5.5 vs 3.4 $\pm$ 3.0 days, mean difference 4.5; 95% CI, 3.5–5.5; $P < .001$ [57].

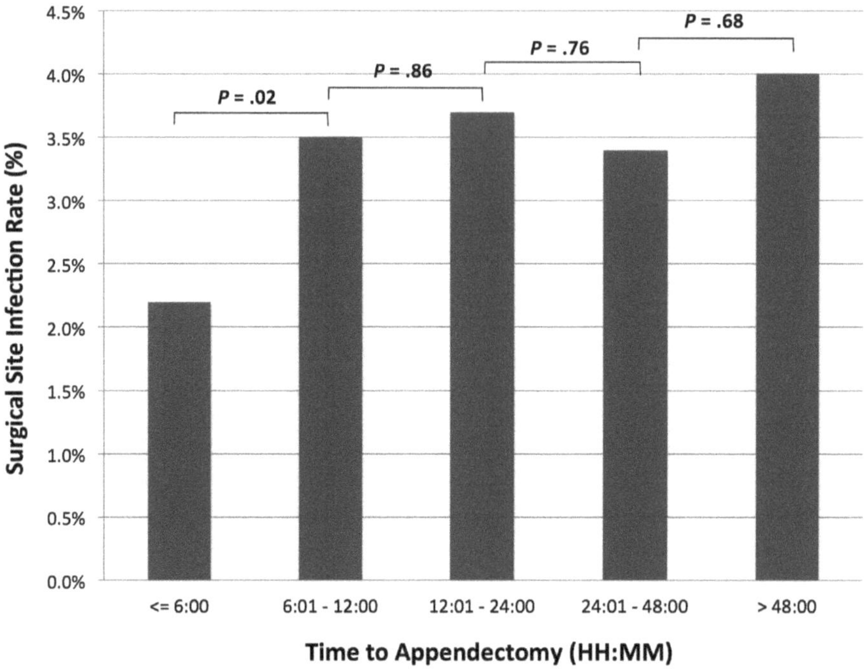

Fig. 10. Incidence of surgical site infections with increasing appendectomy delay. HH:MM, hours:minutes. (*Data from* Teixeira PG, Sivrikoz E, Inaba K, et al. Appendectomy timing: waiting until the next morning increases the risk of surgical site infections. Ann Surg 2012;256(3):538–43.)

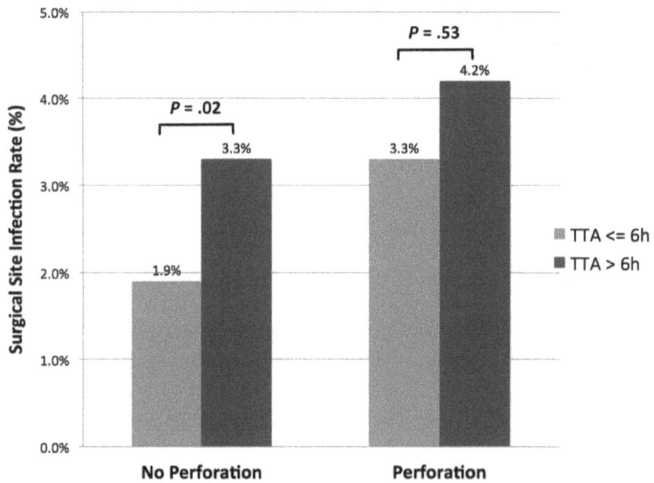

Fig. 11. Effect of appendectomy delay in the incidence of surgical site infections, stratified by perforation presence. TTA, time to appendectomy. (*Data from* Teixeira PG, Sivrikoz E, Inaba K, et al. Appendectomy timing: waiting until the next morning increases the risk of surgical site infections. Ann Surg 2012;256(3):538–43.)

In this era of working-hour limitations and tight health care budgets, emergency surgical services face significant challenges to provide care around the clock. A semielective approach to one of the most frequently performed emergent operation could contribute to optimize hospital resources and personnel use. The increased morbidity associated with appendectomy delay, however, suggests that prompt surgical intervention remains the safest approach.

INCIDENTAL APPENDECTOMY

Supporters of incidental appendectomy during elective or emergency surgery suggest that the risk of adding the appendectomy to the abdominal exploration being performed for another reason would not significantly increase morbidity and potentially avoid the need of a future operation for appendicitis. Young patients, notably those younger than 35 years old, are the age group most likely to benefit from an incidental appendectomy due to their higher lifetime risk of developing acute appendicitis [8,95]. The safety of this practice, however, is questionable. Most studies suggesting that incidental appendectomy is a trivial procedure with no significant additive morbidity reach that conclusion despite a lack of proper risk adjustment in their comparisons, which can underestimate the effect of appendectomy on complications [96–100]. When appropriate scrutiny was used to investigate this issue, Wen and colleagues [101] found that an incidental appendectomy during elective cholecystectomy not only was associated with increased adjusted risk of morbidity but also had a higher mortality (OR 2.65; 95% CI, 1.25–5.64; $P<.001$).

From a cost analysis perspective, incidental appendectomy as a preventive measure has not been found effective [102] and the high cost of laparoscopic equipment contributes negatively to the cost-effectiveness equation in the era of laparoscopic surgery [103].

Controversy exits regarding the function of this otherwise considered vestigial organ. The lymphoid tissue harbored by the appendix is involved in the production of immunoglobulin IgA, suggesting that this organ may participate in the localized intestinal immunity [104,105]. Recent evidence also suggests that appendix may have a role as a reservoir of intestinal commensal bacteria and contribute with recolonization of the colon with its indigenous bacteria [106]. This theoretic role of intestinal recolonization may be important in the recovery after *Clostridium difficile* infection and may also explain the reported association between appendectomy and irritable bowel syndrome [107,108]. The role of appendectomy and the development and progression of ulcerative colitis remains controversial [109].

The combination of potential increase in morbidity, cost inefficacy, and lost of theoretic benefits of preserving the appendix suggest that incidental appendectomy should not be performed except in selected cases.

INTERVAL APPENDECTOMY

The rational for interval appendectomy is the risk of recurrent appendicitis and possible need for emergent appendectomy. A survey of more than 600 pediatric surgeons in North America found that 86% of the responders routinely perform interval appendectomy for children initially treated nonoperatively for perforated appendicitis with phlegmon [110]. Recent data suggest, however, that the majority of these patients do not have a recurrence of appendicitis. Puapong and colleagues [111] found a recurrence rate of 8% after a mean follow-up of 8 years, with all recurrences occurring during the first 3 years. The calculated incidence of recurrence was 21% in a recent meta-analysis [112].

Interval appendectomy is not an innocuous procedure. The reported incidence of complications associated with this procedure varies significantly, ranging from 3% to 18% [112–117]. The indication for this procedure, which may not be necessary in approximately 80% of patients and has a considerable risk of complications, has been challenged. It has been proposed that interval appendectomy is unnecessary [118] and should only be performed if appendicitis recurs. The possibility of a malignancy, however, needs to be carefully excluded in the adult population [114]. Patients older than 40 years with an appendiceal mass or abscess treated nonoperatively should routinely have a colonoscopy as part of their follow-up because approximately 2% have an alternative diagnosis, such as malignancy or Crohn disease, with a majority of cancer cases occurring in patients over age 40 [40].

SUMMARY

1. Neoplasms are an uncommon finding after appendectomy, with malignant tumors occurring in less than 1% of the surgical specimens, and carcinoid being the most frequent malignancy.
2. A negative or inconclusive ultrasound is not adequate to rule out appendicitis and should be followed by CT scan. For pregnant patients, MRI is a reasonable alternative to CT scan.
3. Nonoperative treatment with antibiotics is safe as an initial treatment of uncomplicated appendicitis, with a significant decrease in complications but a high failure rate.
4. Open and laparoscopic appendectomies for appendicitis provide similar results overall, although the laparoscopic technique may be advantageous for obese and elderly patients but may be associated with a higher incidence of intra-abdominal abscess.
5. Preoperative diagnostic accuracy is of utmost importance during pregnancy because a negative appendectomy is associated with a significant incidence of fetal loss.
6. The increased morbidity associated with appendectomy delay suggests that prompt surgical intervention remains the safest approach.
7. Routine incidental appendectomy should not be performed except in selected cases.
8. Interval appendectomy is not indicated because of considerable risks of complications and lack of any clinical benefit.
9. Patients older than 40 years with an appendiceal mass or abscess treated nonoperatively should routinely have a colonoscopy as part of their follow-up to rule out cancer or alternative diagnosis.

References

[1] Fitz RH. Perforating inflammation of the vermiform appendix; with special reference to its early diagnosis and treatment. Am J Med Sci 1886;92:321–46.

[2] Williams GR. Presidential address: a history of appendicitis. With anecdotes illustrating its importance. Ann Surg 1983;197(5):495–506.

[3] McBurney C II. The indications for early laparotomy in appendicitis. Ann Surg 1891;13(4): 233–54.

[4] McBurney C. IV. The incision made in the abdominal wall in cases of appendicitis, with a description of a new method of operating. Ann Surg 1894;20(1):38–43.

[5] Cantrell JR, Stafford ES. The diminishing mortality from appendicitis. Ann Surg 1955;141(6):749.

[6] Egdahl RH. Current mortality in appendicitis. Am J Surg 1964;107(5):757–9.

[7] Owings MF, Kozak LJ. Ambulatory and inpatient procedures in the United States, 1996. Vital Health Stat 13 1998;(139):1–119.

[8] Addiss DG, Shaffer N, Fowler BS, et al. The epidemiology of appendicitis and appendectomy in the United States. Am J Epidemiol 1990;132(5):910–25.

[9] Anderson JE, Bickler SW, Chang DC, et al. Examining a common disease with unknown etiology: trends in epidemiology and surgical management of appendicitis in California, 1995-2009. World J Surg 2012;36:2787–94.

[10] Hale DA, Molloy M, Pearl RH, et al. Appendectomy: a contemporary appraisal. Ann Surg 1997;225(3):252–61.

[11] Khan RA, Ghani I, Chana RS. Routine histopathological examination of appendectomy specimens in children: is there any rationale? Pediatr Surg Int 2011;27(12): 1313–5.

[12] Marudanayagam R, Williams GT, Rees BI. Review of the pathological results of 2660 appendicectomy specimens. J Gastroenterol 2006;41(8):745–9.

[13] Swank HA, Eshuis EJ, Ubbink DT, et al. Is routine histopathological examination of appendectomy specimens useful? A systematic review of the literature. Colorectal Dis 2011;13(11):1214–21.

[14] Jones AE, Phillips AW, Jarvis JR, et al. The value of routine histopathological examination of appendicectomy specimens. BMC Surg 2007;7:17.

[15] Akbulut S, Tas M, Sogutcu N, et al. Unusual histopathological findings in appendectomy specimens: a retrospective analysis and literature review. World J Gastroenterol 2011;17(15):1961–70.

[16] Smeenk RM, van Velthuysen ML, Verwaal VJ, et al. Appendiceal neoplasms and pseudomyxoma peritonei: a population based study. Eur J Surg Oncol 2008;34(2): 196–201.

[17] Blair NP, Bugis SP, Turner LJ, et al. Review of the pathologic diagnoses of 2,216 appendectomy specimens. Am J Surg 1993;165(5):618–20.

[18] Collins DC. 71,000 human appendix specimens. A final report, summarizing forty years'study. Am J Proctol 1963;14:265–81.

[19] Schmutzer KJ, Bayar M, Zaki AE, et al. Tumors of the appendix. Dis Colon Rectum 1975;18(4):324–31.

[20] Ma KW, Chia NH, Yeung HW, et al. If not appendicitis, then what else can it be? A retrospective review of 1492 appendectomies. Hong Kong Med J 2010;16(1):12–7.

[21] Matthyssens LE, Ziol M, Barrat C, et al. Routine surgical pathology in general surgery. Br J Surg 2006;93(3):362–8.

[22] Lohsiriwat V, Vongjirad A, Lohsiriwat D. Value of routine histopathologic examination of three common surgical specimens: appendix, gallbladder, and hemorrhoid. World J Surg 2009;33(10):2189–93.

[23] Connor SJ, Hanna GB, Frizelle FA. Appendiceal tumors: retrospective clinicopathologic analysis of appendiceal tumors from 7,970 appendectomies. Dis Colon Rectum 1998;41(1):75–80.

[24] Deans GT, Spence RA. Neoplastic lesions of the appendix. Br J Surg 1995;82(3): 299–306.
[25] In't Hof KH, van der Wal HC, Kazemier G, et al. Carcinoid tumour of the appendix: an analysis of 1,485 consecutive emergency appendectomies. J Gastrointest Surg 2008;12(8):1436–8.
[26] Wagner JM, McKinney WP, Carpenter JL. Does this patient have appendicitis? JAMA 1996;276(19):1589–94.
[27] Alvarado A. A practical score for the early diagnosis of acute appendicitis. Ann Emerg Med 1986;15(5):557–64.
[28] Ohle R, O'Reilly F, O'Brien KK, et al. The Alvarado score for predicting acute appendicitis: a systematic review. BMC Med 2011;9:139.
[29] Sun JS, Noh HW, Min YG, et al. Receiver operating characteristic analysis of the diagnostic performance of a computed tomographic examination and the Alvarado score for diagnosing acute appendicitis: emphasis on age and sex of the patients. J Comput Assist Tomogr 2008;32(3):386–91.
[30] SCOAP Collaborative, Cuschieri J, Florence M, Flum DR, et al. Negative appendectomy and imaging accuracy in the Washington State Surgical Care and Outcomes Assessment Program. Ann Surg 2008;248(4):557–63.
[31] Parks NA, Schroeppel TJ. Update on imaging for acute appendicitis. Surg Clin North Am 2011;91(1):141–54.
[32] van Randen A, Bipat S, Zwinderman AH, et al. Acute appendicitis: meta-analysis of diagnostic performance of CT and graded compression US related to prevalence of disease. Radiology 2008;249(1):97–106.
[33] Doria AS, Moineddin R, Kellenberger CJ, et al. US or CT for diagnosis of appendicitis in children and adults? A meta-analysis. Radiology 2006;241(1):83–94.
[34] Hernanz-Schulman M. CT and US in the diagnosis of appendicitis: an argument for CT. Radiology 2010;255(1):3–7.
[35] Poortman P, Oostvogel HJ, Bosma E, et al. Improving diagnosis of acute appendicitis: results of a diagnostic pathway with standard use of ultrasonography followed by selective use of CT. J Am Coll Surg 2009;208(3):434–41.
[36] Rosen MP, Ding A, Blake MA, et al. ACR appropriateness criteria® right lower quadrant pain—suspected appendicitis. J Am Coll Radiol 2011;8(11):749–55.
[37] Cobben L, Groot I, Kingma L, et al. A simple MRI protocol in patients with clinically suspected appendicitis: results in 138 patients and effect on outcome of appendectomy. Eur Radiol 2009;19(5):1175–83.
[38] Singh A, Danrad R, Hahn PF, et al. MR imaging of the acute abdomen and pelvis: acute appendicitis and beyond. Radiographics 2007;27(5):1419–31.
[39] Heverhagen JT, Pfestroff K, Heverhagen AE, et al. Diagnostic accuracy of magnetic resonance imaging: a prospective evaluation of patients with suspected appendicitis (diamond). J Magn Reson Imaging 2012;35(3):617–23.
[40] Andersson RE, Petzold MG. Nonsurgical treatment of appendiceal abscess or phlegmon: a systematic review and meta-analysis. Ann Surg 2007;246(5):741–8.
[41] Varadhan KK, Neal KR, Lobo DN. Safety and efficacy of antibiotics compared with appendicectomy for treatment of uncomplicated acute appendicitis: meta-analysis of randomised controlled trials. BMJ 2012;344:e2156.
[42] Vons C, Barry C, Maitre S, et al. Amoxicillin plus clavulanic acid versus appendicectomy for treatment of acute uncomplicated appendicitis: an open-label, non-inferiority, randomised controlled trial. Lancet 2011;377(9777):1573–9.
[43] Styrud J, Eriksson S, Nilsson I, et al. Appendectomy versus antibiotic treatment in acute appendicitis. a prospective multicenter randomized controlled trial. World J Surg 2006;30(6):1033–7.
[44] Hansson J, Körner U, Ludwigs K, et al. Antibiotics as first-line therapy for acute appendicitis: evidence for a change in clinical practice. World J Surg 2012;36(9):2037–8.

[45] Eriksson S, Granström L. Randomized controlled trial of appendicectomy versus antibiotic therapy for acute appendicitis. Br J Surg 1995;82(2):166–9.
[46] Farahnak M, Talaei-Khoei M, Gorouhi F, et al. The Alvarado score and antibiotics therapy as a corporate protocol versus conventional clinical management: randomized controlled pilot study of approach to acute appendicitis. Am J Emerg Med 2007;25(7):850–2.
[47] Mason RJ, Moazzez A, Sohn H, et al. Meta-analysis of randomized trials comparing antibiotic therapy with appendectomy for acute uncomplicated (no abscess or phlegmon) appendicitis. Surg Infect (Larchmt) 2012;13(2):74–84.
[48] Mason RJ. Appendicitis: is surgery the best option? Lancet 2011;377(9777):1545–6.
[49] Semm K. Endoscopic appendectomy. Endoscopy 1983;15(2):59–64.
[50] Bulian DR, Knuth J, Sauerwald A, et al. Appendectomy in Germany-an analysis of a nationwide survey 2011/2012. Int J Colorectal Dis 2013;28:127–38.
[51] Ingraham AM, Cohen ME, Bilimoria KY, et al. Effect of delay to operation on outcomes in adults with acute appendicitis. Arch Surg 2010;145(9):886–92.
[52] Ingraham AM, Cohen ME, Bilimoria KY, et al. Comparison of outcomes after laparoscopic versus open appendectomy for acute appendicitis at 222 ACS NSQIP hospitals. Surgery 2010;148(4):625–35 [discussion: 635–7].
[53] Fleming FJ, Kim MJ, Messing S, et al. Balancing the risk of postoperative surgical infections: a multivariate analysis of factors associated with laparoscopic appendectomy from the NSQIP database. Ann Surg 2010;252(6):895–900.
[54] Tuggle KR, Ortega G, Bolorunduro OB, et al. Laparoscopic versus open appendectomy in complicated appendicitis: a review of the NSQIP database. J Surg Res 2010;163(2): 225–8.
[55] Mason RJ, Moazzez A, Moroney JR, et al. Laparoscopic vs open appendectomy in obese patients: outcomes using the American College of Surgeons National Surgical Quality Improvement Program database. J Am Coll Surg 2012;215(1):88–99 [discussion: 99–100].
[56] Kim MJ, Fleming FJ, Gunzler DD, et al. Laparoscopic appendectomy is safe and efficacious for the elderly: an analysis using the National Surgical Quality Improvement Project database. Surg Endosc 2011;25(6):1802–7.
[57] Teixeira PG, Sivrikoz E, Inaba K, et al. Appendectomy timing: waiting until the next morning increases the risk of surgical site infections. Ann Surg 2012;256(3):538–43.
[58] Sauerland S, Jaschinski T, Neugebauer EA. Laparoscopic versus open surgery for suspected appendicitis. Cochrane Database Syst Rev 2010;(10) CD001546.
[59] Barmparas G, Branco BC, Schnüriger B, et al. The incidence and risk factors of post-laparotomy adhesive small bowel obstruction. J Gastrointest Surg 2010;14(10): 1619–28.
[60] Wei PL, Keller JJ, Liang HH, et al. Acute appendicitis and adverse pregnancy outcomes: a nationwide population-based study. J Gastrointest Surg 2012;16(6):1204–11.
[61] Mazze RI, Källén B. Appendectomy during pregnancy: a Swedish registry study of 778 cases. Obstet Gynecol 1991;77(6):835–40.
[62] Andersen B, Nielsen TF. Appendicitis in pregnancy: diagnosis, management and complications. Acta Obstet Gynecol Scand 1999;78(9):758–62.
[63] Yilmaz HG, Akgun Y, Bac B, et al. Acute appendicitis in pregnancy—risk factors associated with principal outcomes: a case control study. Int J Surg 2007;5(3):192–7.
[64] Ueberrueck T, Koch A, Meyer L, et al. Ninety-four appendectomies for suspected acute appendicitis during pregnancy. World J Surg 2004;28(5):508–11.
[65] Tamir IL, Bongard FS, Klein SR. Acute appendicitis in the pregnant patient. Am J Surg 1990;160(6):571–5 [discussion: 575–6].
[66] Hée P, Viktrup L. The diagnosis of appendicitis during pregnancy and maternal and fetal outcome after appendectomy. Int J Gynaecol Obstet 1999;65(2):129–35.
[67] McGory ML, Zingmond DS, Tillou A, et al. Negative appendectomy in pregnant women is associated with a substantial risk of fetal loss. J Am Coll Surg 2007;205(4):534–40.

[68] Lim HK, Bae SH, Seo GS. Diagnosis of acute appendicitis in pregnant women: value of sonography. AJR Am J Roentgenol 1992;159(3):539–42.
[69] Lazarus E, Mayo-Smith WW, Mainiero MB, et al. CT in the evaluation of nontraumatic abdominal pain in pregnant women. Radiology 2007;244(3):784–90.
[70] Jaffe TA, Miller CM, Merkle EM. Practice patterns in imaging of the pregnant patient with abdominal pain: a survey of academic centers. AJR Am J Roentgenol 2007;189(5): 1128–34.
[71] Long SS, Long C, Lai H, et al. Imaging strategies for right lower quadrant pain in pregnancy. AJR Am J Roentgenol 2011;196(1):4–12.
[72] Pedrosa I, Levine D, Eyvazzadeh AD, et al. MR imaging evaluation of acute appendicitis in pregnancy. Radiology 2006;238(3):891–9.
[73] Cobben LP, Groot I, Haans L, et al. MRI for clinically suspected appendicitis during pregnancy. AJR Am J Roentgenol 2004;183(3):671–5.
[74] Brown JJ, Wilson C, Coleman S, et al. Appendicitis in pregnancy: an ongoing diagnostic dilemma. Colorectal Dis 2009;11(2):116–22.
[75] Basaran A, Basaran M. Diagnosis of acute appendicitis during pregnancy: a systematic review. Obstet Gynecol Surv 2009;64(7):481–8 [quiz: 499].
[76] Shellock FG, Kanal EE. Policies, guidelines, and recommendations for MR imaging safety and patient management. SMRI Safety Committee. J Magn Reson Imaging 1991;1(1): 97–101.
[77] Kanal EE, Borgstede JP, Barkovich AJ, et al. American College of Radiology White Paper on MR Safety. AJR Am J Roentgenol 2002;178(6):1335–47.
[78] Vasireddy A, Atkinson S, Shennan A, et al. Surgical management of appendicitis remains best option during pregnancy. BMJ 2012;344:e3575.
[79] Affleck DG, Handrahan DL, Egger MJ, et al. The laparoscopic management of appendicitis and cholelithiasis during pregnancy. Am J Surg 1999;178(6):523–9.
[80] Sadot E, Telem DA, Arora M, et al. Laparoscopy: a safe approach to appendicitis during pregnancy. Surg Endosc 2010;24(2):383–9.
[81] Kirshtein B, Perry ZH, Avinoach E, et al. Safety of laparoscopic appendectomy during pregnancy. World J Surg 2009;33(3):475–80.
[82] de Bakker JK, Dijksman LM, Donkervoort SC. Safety and outcome of general surgical open and laparoscopic procedures during pregnancy. Surg Endosc 2011;25(5):1574–8.
[83] Fatum M, Rojansky N. Laparoscopic surgery during pregnancy. Obstet Gynecol Surv 2001;56:50–9.
[84] Hunter JG, Swanstrom L, Thornburg K. Carbon dioxide pneumoperitoneum induces fetal acidosis in a pregnant ewe model. Surg Endosc 1995;9(3):272–7 [discussion: 277–9].
[85] Wilasrusmee C, Sukrat B, McEvoy M, et al. Systematic review and meta-analysis of safety of laparoscopic versus open appendicectomy for suspected appendicitis in pregnancy. Br J Surg 2012;99(11):1470–8.
[86] Berry J, Malt RA. Appendicitis near its centenary. Ann Surg 1984;200(5):567–75.
[87] Temple CL, Huchcroft SA, Temple WJ. The natural history of appendicitis in adults. A prospective study. Ann Surg 1995;221(3):278–81.
[88] Yardeni D, Hirschl RB, Drongowski RA, et al. Delayed versus immediate surgery in acute appendicitis: do we need to operate during the night? J Pediatr Surg 2004;39(3): 464–9.
[89] Abou-Nukta FF, Bakhos CC, Arroyo KK, et al. Effects of delaying appendectomy for acute appendicitis for 12 to 24 hours. Arch Surg 2006;141(5):504–7.
[90] Kearney D, Cahill RA, O'Brien E, et al. Influence of delays on perforation risk in adults with acute appendicitis. Dis Colon Rectum 2008;51(12):1823–7.
[91] Stahlfeld K, Hower J, Homitsky S, et al. Is acute appendicitis a surgical emergency? Am Surg 2007;73(6):626–9 [discussion: 629–30].
[92] Busch M, Gutzwiller FS, Aellig S, et al. In-hospital delay increases the risk of perforation in adults with appendicitis. World J Surg 2011;35(7):1626–33.

[93] Ditillo MF, Dziura JD, Rabinovici RR. Is it safe to delay appendectomy in adults with acute appendicitis? Ann Surg 2006;244(5):656–60.
[94] Omundsen M, Dennett E. Delay to appendicectomy and associated morbidity: a retrospective review. ANZ J Surg 2006;76(3):153–5.
[95] Snyder TE, Selanders JR. Incidental appendectomy - Yes or No? A retrospective case study and review of the literature. Infect Dis Obstet Gynecol 1998;6(1):30–7.
[96] Shumake LB. Right inguinal herniorrhaphy and incidental appendectomy. Am Surg 1971;37(5):310–1.
[97] Norton LW, Sweeney M, Eiseman B. Incidental appendicectomy with laparotomy for trauma. Br J Surg 1975;62(6):487–9.
[98] Lowery CH, Lenhardt HF. Incidental appendectomy in gallbladder surgery. Arch Surg 1962;85:476–9.
[99] O'Malley VP, Finch DR, Powley PH. Wound sepsis after cholecystectomy. Influence of incidental appendectomy. J Clin Gastroenterol 1986;8(4):435–7.
[100] Strom PR, Turkleson ML, Stone HH. Safety of incidental appendectomy. Am J Surg 1983;145(6):819–22.
[101] Wen SW, Hernandez R, Naylor CD. Pitfalls in nonrandomized outcomes studies. The case of incidental appendectomy with open cholecystectomy. JAMA 1995;274(21):1687–91.
[102] Sugimoto T, Edwards D. Incidence and costs of incidental appendectomy as a preventive measure. Am J Public Health 1987;77(4):471–5.
[103] Wang HT, Sax HC. Incidental appendectomy in the era of managed care and laparoscopy. J Am Coll Surg 2001;192(2):182–8.
[104] Doe WF. The intestinal immune system. Gut 1989;30(12):1679–85.
[105] Ansaloni L, Catena F, Pinna AD. What is the function of the human vermiform appendix? Eur Surg Res 2009;43(2):67–71.
[106] Randal Bollinger R, Barbas AS, Bush EL, et al. Biofilms in the large bowel suggest an apparent function of the human vermiform appendix. J Theor Biol 2007;249(4):826–31.
[107] Reshetnikov OV, Kurilovich SA, Denisova DV, et al. Prevalence and risk factors of the development of irritable bowel syndrome in adolescents: a population study. Ter Arkh 2001;73(2):24–9 [in Russian].
[108] Sleator RD, Cronin M, Hill C. Why appendectomies may lead to an increased risk of functional gastrointestinal disorders. Med Hypotheses 2008;71(5):814–6.
[109] Gardenbroek TJ, Eshuis EJ, Ponsioen CI, et al. The effect of appendectomy on the course of ulcerative colitis: a systematic review. Colorectal Dis 2012;14(5):545–53.
[110] Chen C, Botelho C, Cooper A, et al. Current practice patterns in the treatment of perforated appendicitis in children. J Am Coll Surg 2003;196(2):212–21.
[111] Puapong D, Lee SL, Haigh PI, et al. Routine interval appendectomy in children is not indicated. J Pediatr Surg 2007;42(9):1500–3.
[112] Hall NJ, Jones CE, Eaton S, et al. Is interval appendicectomy justified after successful nonoperative treatment of an appendix mass in children? A systematic review. J Pediatr Surg 2011;46(4):767–71.
[113] Oliak D, Yamini D, Udani VM, et al. Initial nonoperative management for periappendiceal abscess. Dis Colon Rectum 2001;44(7):936–41.
[114] Willemsen PJ, Hoorntje LE, Eddes EH, et al. The need for interval appendectomy after resolution of an appendiceal mass questioned. Dig Surg 2002;19(3):216–22.
[115] Lugo JZ, Avgerinos DV, Lefkowitz AJ, et al. Can interval appendectomy be justified following conservative treatment of perforated acute appendicitis? J Surg Res 2010;164(1):91–4.
[116] Eriksson S, Styrud J. Interval appendicectomy: a retrospective study. Eur J Surg 2003;164(10):771–4.
[117] Iqbal CW, Knott EM, Mortellaro VE, et al. Interval appendectomy after perforated appendicitis: what are the operative risks and luminal patency rates? J Surg Res 2012;177(1):127–30.

[118] Tekin A, Kurtoğlu HC, Can I, et al. Routine interval appendectomy is unnecessary after conservative treatment of appendiceal mass. Colorectal Dis 2008;10(5):465–8.
[119] Birnbaum BA, Wilson SR. Appendicitis at the millennium. Radiology 2000;215(2): 337–48.

Advances in Surgery 47 (2013) 141–152
ADVANCES IN SURGERY

Readmission After Abdominal Aortic Aneurysm Repair: What Does it Mean?

David Yu Greenblatt, MD, MSPH, Sara Fernandes-Taylor, PhD, K. Craig Kent, MD*

Department of Surgery, University of Wisconsin School of Medicine & Public Health, 600 Highland Avenue, Madison, WI 53792-0001, USA

Keywords

• Readmission • Abdominal aortic aneurysm repair • Vascular surgery • Medicare • Health care reform

Key points

- Thirty-day hospital readmission is common after both open and endovascular abdominal aortic aneurysm (AAA) repair.
- Early readmission is strongly associated with 1-year mortality.
- Preoperative comorbidities have a modest association with readmission after AAA repair; however, postoperative factors, including serious complications leading to prolonged length of stay and discharge to a skilled nursing facility, have a profound influence on the probability of readmission.

INTRODUCTION

Hospital readmissions are common and costly. One in 5 hospitalized Medicare beneficiaries is readmitted within 30 days of discharge, at a cost of more than $17 billion per year [1]. The readmission rate after vascular surgical procedures is nearly 24%, significantly higher than the average of 15.6% for all surgical interventions [1]. The Medicare Payment Advisory Commission (MedPAC) has identified vascular procedures as 1 of 7 categories that account for almost one-third of potentially preventable readmissions, and vascular readmissions are the most costly on a per-patient basis [2].

Early readmission has emerged as a health care reform target as part of the Patient Protection and Affordable Care Act. The Centers for Medicare and

Disclosures: The authors report no conflicts of interest.

*Corresponding author. 600 Highland Avenue, Madison, WI 53792-7375. *E-mail address*: kent@surgery.wisc.edu

0065-3411/13/$ – see front matter
http://dx.doi.org/10.1016/j.yasu.2013.02.007

Medicaid Services (CMS) currently tracks risk-adjusted 30-day hospital readmission rates for several medical conditions, and this information is available to the public on the Hospital Compare Web site (http://www.hospitalcompare.hhs.gov). CMS will reduce total Medicare reimbursements to hospitals with readmission rates that are higher than predicted for these diagnoses, and in the next 3 years vascular procedures will be added to the targeted list. Hospitals that fail to control vascular readmissions will face significant financial penalties.

The majority of extant research on readmission has been performed in patients with medical rather than surgical conditions. To date, there have been few studies on early readmission after vascular surgical procedures such as abdominal aortic aneurysm (AAA) repair. Recent reports, discussed in this review, have shed light on the frequency, causes, risk factors, and consequences of readmission after AAA repair. These findings are relevant to ongoing policy debates and to developing targeted interventions to decrease vascular surgical readmissions.

FREQUENCY OF EARLY READMISSION AFTER AAA REPAIR

There are few studies in the literature that have focused on the policy-relevant outcome of 30-day readmission for AAA repair. To gain a better understanding of early readmission after AAA repair and determine the contemporary rate of 30-day readmission after nonruptured AAA repair, the authors' group analyzed 3 years of data from the CMS Chronic Condition Data Warehouse (http://www.ccwdata.org), a 5% random national sample of Medicare beneficiaries [3]. A total of 2481 patients underwent AAA repair: 1502 endovascular repair (EVAR) and 979 open. Patients who underwent EVAR were older (76.6 ± 6.0 vs 75.5 ± 5.6 years, $P<.001$), more likely to be male (79.1% vs 71.4%, $P<.001$), and had more comorbid illness as measured by the Charlson Comorbidity Index (2.9 ± 1.6 vs 2.6 ± 1.4, $P<.001$) than patients who underwent open procedures. The length of hospital stay associated with EVAR was shorter (3.4 ± 4.2 vs 9.4 ± 7.4 days, $P<.001$).

Of note, the rates of 30-day readmission after EVAR and open AAA repair were similar (13.3% and 12.8%, respectively, $P = .69$) [3]. Consistent with the authors' findings, Vogel and colleagues [4] found 30-day readmission rates of 11.6% for EVAR and 13.1% for open repair in their analysis of a Washington State hospital administrative discharge database. A recent analysis of national Medicare data also showed no difference in the rate of 1-year admissions between EVAR and open repair [5].

By contrast, Jackson and colleagues [6] reported much lower rates of 30-day readmission after AAA repair: 4.9% for EVAR and 10.5% for open repair. However, the single-institution retrospective study design may have resulted in underdetection of readmissions, as patients are not always readmitted to the index hospital where the surgical procedure was performed. In the authors' analysis of Medicare data, 36% of readmissions after AAA repair were to a hospital other than the index surgical hospital, which is much higher than the rate of 22% in the general Medicare population [7]. Nasir and colleagues

[8] also concluded that same-hospital readmission is a poor proxy for true readmission rates. Taken together, these results suggest that single-institution studies using retrospective or administrative data are likely to miss a large proportion of readmissions.

REASONS FOR READMISSION

After determining that the rate of readmission after elective AAA repair in Medicare beneficiaries is approximately 1 in 8, the authors described the diagnoses that lead to readmission. Jencks and colleagues [1] have shown that patients who are hospitalized for a medical condition and then readmitted are most often rehospitalized for the same primary diagnosis; for example, patients with heart failure are readmitted for heart failure, and patients with pneumonia are readmitted for pneumonia. The authors found that most readmissions after AAA repair are due to complications of the procedure. The most common reason for readmission after both EVAR and open repair was wound complication. The relative frequencies of other readmission diagnoses differed between EVAR and open repair. For example, bowel obstruction was common after open repair, whereas graft complications were more frequent after EVAR. The frequencies of readmission diagnoses for each type of procedure are summarized in Table 1.

PREDICTORS OF READMISSION

Designing an intervention to reduce readmission begins by identifying patients who are at highest risk. Therefore, the authors examined patient-related and treatment-related factors that are associated with readmission. Preoperative comorbidities were only weakly associated with early readmission after aneurysm repair. In bivariate analysis (summarized in Table 2) 8 preoperative comorbidities increased the rate of readmission modestly (3%–8%) with the exception of paralysis, which was associated with a 12% increase in readmission rate. Paralysis may predispose patients to complications such as deep venous thrombosis or pneumonia.

Consistent with previous research [9], older patient age was strongly associated with readmission, with an 11% rate of readmission in patients younger than 75, and approximately 17% in those older than 85 years. The authors did confirm an association between diabetes and increased readmission risk that has been reported in previous studies [6,10].

Patients that had any of 9 in-hospital complications had a readmission rate of 17.4% compared with 11.3% in those without complications. In bivariate analysis, 5 complications were associated with readmission: wound complications, renal/urologic, vascular/graft-related, cardiac, and respiratory. Of these, wound complications had the strongest association with readmission; more than 35% of patients with a wound complication were readmitted within 30 days, compared with 12.8% among patients who did not have this complication.

In multivariate analysis (Table 3), wound complications (odds ratio [OR] 2.50) and renal/urologic complications (OR 1.75) were significantly associated

Table 1
Readmission diagnoses after endovascular AAA repair (EVAR) and open nonruptured AAA repair in 2481 Medicare beneficiaries

EVAR (200 Readmissions)			Open (125 Readmissions)		
Rank	Diagnosis	%	Rank	Diagnosis	%
1	Wound complication	15.5	1	Wound complication	17.6
2	Pneumonia and respiratory	11.5	2	GI obstruction	13.6
3	AAA or graft	10.0	3	Pneumonia and respiratory	12.0
4	Congestive heart failure	8.5	4	Sepsis	10.4
5	Sepsis	6.5	5	AAA or graft	5.6
6	MI, cardiac arrest	6.0	6	MI, cardiac arrest	5.6
7	Renal failure	6.0	7	Arrhythmia	4.0
8	GI obstruction	5.5	8	Fluid and electrolyte	4.0
9	Bleeding	3.0	9	Congestive heart failure	3.2
10	Cancer related	3.0	10	Bleeding	2.4
11	Miscellaneous	3.0	11	Cancer related	2.4
12	GI bleeding	3.0	12	Miscellaneous	2.4
13	Stroke	2.5	13	Diabetes	2.4
14	Urinary tract infection	2.5	14	Venous thromboembolism	2.4
15	Arrhythmia	2.0	15	GI inflammation and infection	2.4
16	Diabetes	2.0	16	Renal failure	1.6
17	Hypertension	2.0	17	GI bleeding	1.6
18	Fluid and electrolyte	1.5	18	Stroke	1.6
19	Neurologic	1.5	19	Hypertension	1.6
20	Other	4.5	20	Other	3.2

Abbreviations: GI, gastrointestinal; MI, myocardial infarction.
Data from Greenblatt DY, Greenberg CC, Kind AJ, et al. Causes and implications of 30-day readmission after abdominal aortic aneurysm repair. Ann Surg 2012;256(4):595–605.

with readmission after adjusting for other factors. Prolonged length of stay (LOS) and discharge destination were then removed from the analysis to reduce multicollinearity with complications, and 3 postoperative complications were significantly associated with readmission: wound complication (OR 3.21), renal/urologic (OR 1.97), and vascular/graft (OR 1.55). These results indicate that, as expected, serious postoperative complications are associated with readmission, and LOS and discharge destination mediate this relationship.

Another variable examined that is related to complicated postoperative course was LOS. Surgical patients who experience serious postoperative complications are more likely to have a prolonged LOS and be discharged to skilled nursing care. Accordingly, prolonged LOS during the index hospitalization was associated with 30-day readmission (Fig. 1).

Discharge destination was the strongest predictor of early readmission. After adjusting for potential confounders, the odds of readmission for patients discharged to a skilled nursing facility were 2.50 times those for patients discharged home without nursing care (95% confidence interval [CI] 1.68–3.71). Overall, this analysis suggests that surgical complications leading to prolonged LOS and alternative discharge destinations increase the likelihood of

Table 2
Univariate analysis of factors potentially related to 30-day readmission after nonruptured AAA repair in 2481 Medicare beneficiaries

Factor	% Readmitted if factor present	% Readmitted if factor absent	*P*
Age (y)			<.023
65–74	11.0	n/a	
75–84	14.1	n/a	
≥85	16.7	n/a	
Gender			.048
Male	12.4	n/a	
Female	15.5	n/a	
Race			.99
White	13.1	n/a	
Black	13.3	n/a	
Other	13.8	n/a	
Charlson Comorbidity Score			<.001
1st tertile	10.5	n/a	
2nd tertile	13.9	n/a	
3rd tertile	18.9	n/a	
Comorbid conditions (Elixhauser codes)			
Paralysis	25.0	12.9	.018
Other neurologic disease	19.3	12.7	.020
Anemia	18.9	11.6	<.001
Congestive heart failure	18.4	12.0	<.001
Renal failure	17.8	12.6	.026
Obesity	17.5	13.0	.24
Coagulation disorder	17.4	12.9	.12
History of cancer	16.4	12.4	.028
Hypothyroidism	16.5	12.6	.064
Diabetes mellitus	15.4	12.4	.065
Chronic pulmonary disease	14.9	11.9	.030
Valvular disease	14.3	12.7	.31
Hypertension	13.3	12.2	.52
Weight loss	15.4	13.0	.40
Depression	14.5	13.0	.62
Peripheral vascular disease	12.9	16.8	.26
Fluid or electrolyte disorder	16.8	12.6	.034
Other comorbidity	14.4	12.8	.35
Underwent procedure at high-volume hospital	14.0	12.4	.25
Had in-hospital complication			
Any complication	17.4	11.3	<.001
Wound	35.5	12.8	<.001
Reoperation	25.0	13.0	.11
Renal/urologic	26.0	12.7	.001
Vascular/graft-related	20.1	12.6	.006
Cardiac	20.5	12.7	.015
Respiratory	17.3	12.6	.035
Hemorrhage/shock	16.3	12.8	.12
Neurologic	16.2	13.1	.45
Venous thromboembolism	8.3	13.1	.62

(*continued on next page*)

Table 2
(continued)

Factor	% Readmitted if factor present	% Readmitted if factor absent	P
Prolonged length of stay	19.1	11.2	<.001
Discharge destination			<.001
Home	9.9	n/a	
Home with home care	16.8	n/a	
Skilled nursing facility	27.4	n/a	
Other facility	21.1	n/a	

Abbreviation: n/a, no data available.

Data from Greenblatt DY, Greenberg CC, Kind AJ, et al. Causes and implications of 30-day readmission after abdominal aortic aneurysm repair. Ann Surg 2012;256(4):595–605.

Table 3
Multivariate analysis of predictors of 30-day readmission after elective AAA repair in 2481 Medicare beneficiaries

Factor	Odds ratio (95% CI)
Age (y)	
65–70	Referent
71–75	2.01 (1.35–2.98)[a]
76–80	1.57 (1.05–2.33)[a]
81–85	1.80 (1.18–2.76)[a]
>85	1.76 (0.99–3.10)
Female (vs male)	1.14 (0.86–1.50)
Comorbid conditions	
Paralysis	1.59 (0.73–3.47)
Neurologic disease	1.16 (0.74–1.82)
Anemia	1.39 (1.05–1.85)[a]
Congestive heart failure	1.40 (1.03–1.89)[a]
Renal failure	1.15 (0.78–1.68)
History of cancer	1.40 (1.03–1.90)[a]
Chronic pulmonary disease	1.11 (0.86–1.42)
Fluid/electrolyte disorder	1.05 (0.73–1.50)
Postoperative complications	
Wound	2.50 (1.08–5.79)[a]
Renal/urologic	1.75 (1.01–3.06)[a]
Vascular/graft	1.40 (0.91–2.13)
Cardiac	1.31 (0.78–2.20)
Respiratory	0.84 (0.56–1.25)
Prolonged length of stay (>7 d)	1.26 (0.93–1.72)
Discharge destination	
Home	Referent
Home with home care	1.52 (1.09–2.11)[a]
Skilled nursing facility	2.50 (1.68–3.71)[a]
Other facility	1.72 (1.03–2.88)[a]

Odds ratios are adjusted for the variables shown in the table: age, gender, 8 comorbid conditions, 5 complications, prolonged LOS, and discharge destination.

[a]Denotes a statistically significant association at the $P<.05$ level.

Data from Greenblatt DY, Greenberg CC, Kind AJ, et al. Causes and implications of 30-day readmission after abdominal aortic aneurysm repair. Ann Surg 2012;256(4):595–605.

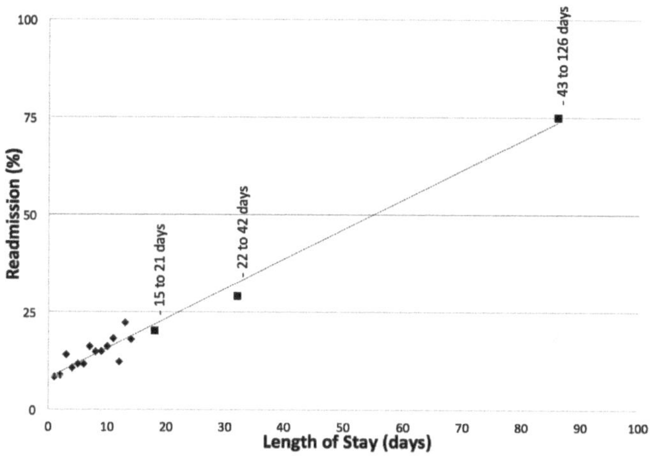

Fig. 1. Index hospital length of stay (LOS) and frequency of readmission after nonruptured AAA repair (N = 2481). The readmission rates for LOS longer than 14 days are aggregates for each of 3 intervals: 15 to 21 days (n = 99), 22 to 42 days (n = 55), and 43 to 126 days (n = 8), using the midpoint and mean rates within each interval. (*From* Greenblatt DY, Greenberg CC, Kind AJ, et al. Causes and implications of 30-day readmission after abdominal aortic aneurysm repair. Ann Surg 2012;256(4):595–605; with permission.)

rehospitalization. The authors' data also suggest that some complications, if recognized and treated, resolve and do not lead to readmission. Other complications, however, lead to increased LOS and the need for nursing care, which, in turn, lead to readmission.

CONSEQUENCES OF READMISSION

After determining the rates, causes, and risk factors of readmission after EVAR and open AAA repair, the authors examined the association between 30-day readmission and mortality. Twenty-one of the 325 readmitted patients died during the readmission inpatient stay, yielding a rehospitalization mortality rate of 6.5%, which was markedly higher than the in-hospital mortality rate of 2.2% for the index stay. The in-hospital mortality for patients who were discharged to a skilled nursing facility and subsequently readmitted was even higher, with 10% dying during the readmission stay.

Remarkably, the unadjusted 1-year mortality in readmitted patients was 23.4%, compared with 4.5% in nonreadmitted patients ($P<.001$). Kaplan-Meier survival analysis confirmed a significant difference in survival based on 30-day readmission status (Fig. 2). After adjusting for age, gender, comorbidity, and procedure type, the odds ratio of readmission for 1-year mortality was 5.76 (95% CI 4.09–8.10); other investigators have also noted a strong association between readmission and mortality for patients undergoing aneurysm repair [10,11].

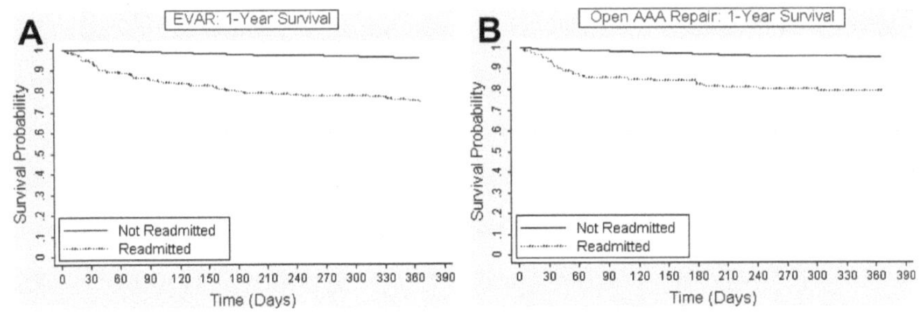

Fig. 2. (*A*) Kaplan-Meier survival curves for patients who were readmitted (n = 200) or were not readmitted (n = 1302) after endovascular AAA repair (EVAR). (*B*) Kaplan-Meier survival curves for patients who were readmitted (n = 125) or were not readmitted (n = 854) after open AAA repair. y-Axis displays probability of survival and x-axis shows days after surgical discharge. (*From* Greenblatt DY, Greenberg CC, Kind AJ, et al. Causes and implications of 30-day readmission after abdominal aortic aneurysm repair. Ann Surg 2012;256(4):595–605; with permission.)

Readmission may be a proxy for patients who have diminished preoperative longevity. Alternatively, events leading to readmission may alter survival, indicating that better postoperative care and interventions to reduce readmissions have the potential to also reduce mortality. The authors hypothesize that postoperative complications, which may occur before or after discharge, are important determinants of both early readmission and long-term mortality after AAA repair. The striking association between readmission and mortality indicates that the problem of readmission is much more than economic.

CONCEPTUAL MODELS OF READMISSION AND EFFORTS TO PREVENT READMISSION

To approach the issue of surgical readmission and to help guide future research, the authors have proposed a conceptual model, shown in Fig. 3. This model builds on a theoretical framework proposed by Kangovi and Grande [12], which includes health policy, quality of and access to inpatient and outpatient care, and patient health status and socioeconomic resources. To these components the authors add the new concept of "complication identification and management failure," which is proposed to be fundamentally important in surgical readmissions. Three major paradigms fall under this rubric. First, a complication develops during the index hospitalization that is not adequately treated, which leads to readmission (eg, a patient is diagnosed with a surgical-site infection and inappropriately treated with antibiotics rather than opening of the wound). Second, a complication develops during the index hospitalization that is not recognized and thus not treated, leading to readmission (eg, a patient with fluid overload is sent home without diuresis and is then readmitted with pulmonary edema). Third, a de novo complication develops following discharge that leads to readmission (eg, a pulmonary embolism). Approximately 38% of readmitted patients in the authors' study had a diagnosis or procedure code corresponding to an in-hospital complication during the

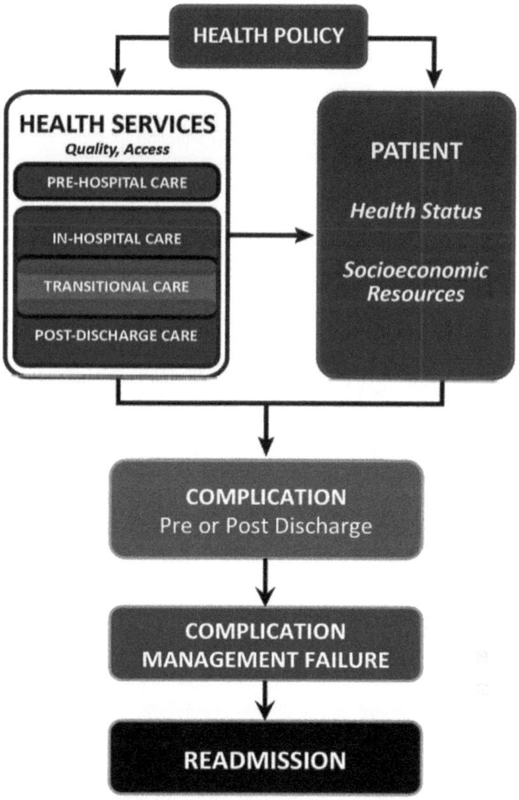

Fig. 3. Model of surgical readmission showing complication management failure as the proximate cause. (*From* Greenblatt DY, Greenberg CC, Kind AJ, et al. Causes and implications of 30-day readmission after abdominal aortic aneurysm repair. Ann Surg 2012;256(4):595–605; with permission.)

surgical hospital stay, suggesting that a significant number of readmissions are due to paradigm 1: inadequate treatment of a recognized complication. The data, however, suggest that about 60% of complications that resulted in readmission were either not diagnosed during the index stay or developed after discharge. Therefore, improved identification and management of postoperative complications, both in hospital and after discharge, are likely to be key elements of any readmission prevention program for patients undergoing AAA repair and other vascular surgical procedures.

Brooke and colleagues [13] have also developed a conceptual model that includes factors related to readmissions in vascular surgery. As shown in Fig. 4, the model divides these factors into 4 phases of care. The investigators argue that variability in clinical pathways and decision making in each of these 4 phases may be associated with the risk of readmission after vascular surgical procedures.

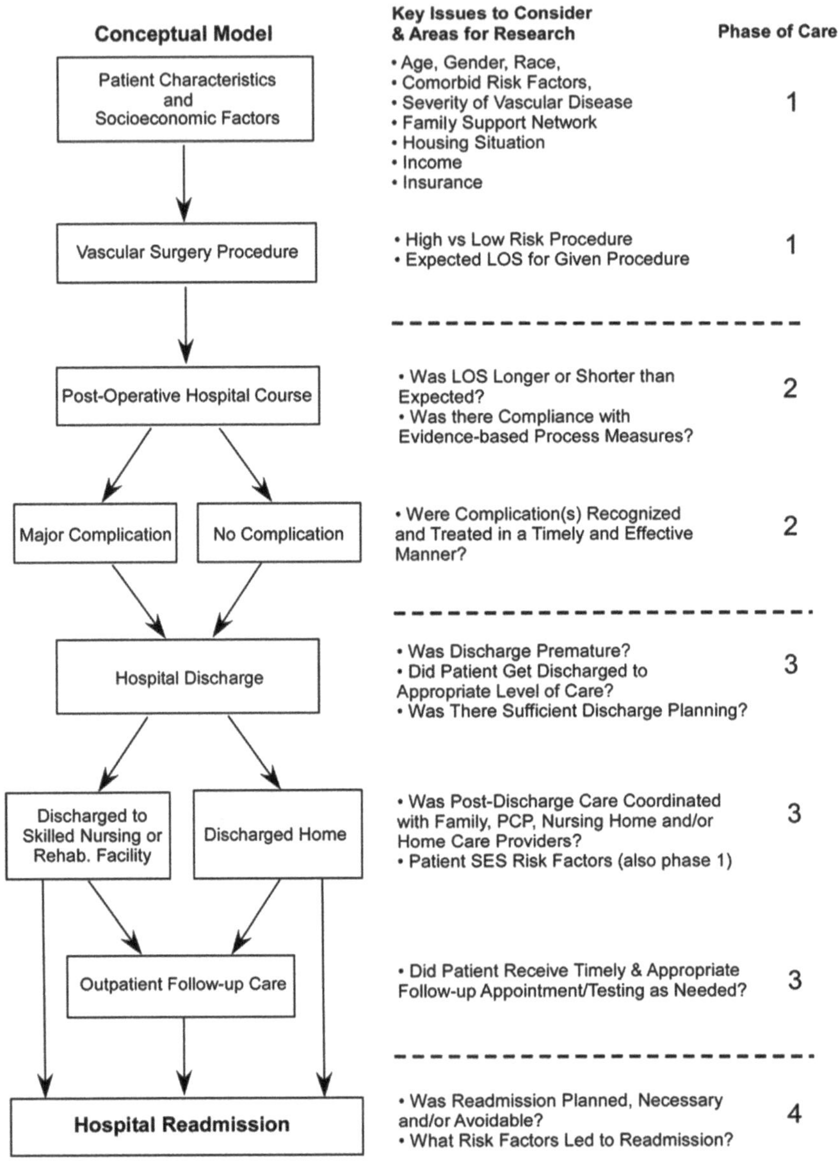

Fig. 4. Conceptual model of preventable readmission in vascular surgery. (*From* Brooke BS, De Martino RR, Girotti M, et al. Developing strategies for predicting and preventing readmissions in vascular surgery. J Vasc Surg 2012;56(2):556–62; with permission.)

At present, no interventions to prevent readmission have been developed specifically for patients undergoing AAA repair. However, several interventions targeting readmissions in medical patients have been evaluated in randomized controlled trials and observational studies [14], some of which are listed here.

Interventions designed to prevent readmissions in patients with medical conditions

- Nurse "transition coach," "discharge advocate," or "transitional care partner" assigned to each high-risk patient to prepare the patient for discharge and help solve problems that arise in the transition-to-home process [15–17]
- In-hospital education to prepare patient for transition home [15–17]
- In-hospital medication reconciliation [17]
- Discharge instruction booklet using simple low-literacy language provided to patient and primary care provider [17]
- Standardized discharge summary document containing expert-recommended components [18–23]
- Postdischarge follow-up phone calls by advanced nurse [15,16]
- Postdischarge follow-up phone calls by clinical pharmacist to review and reconcile medication [17]
- Postdischarge home visits by nurse [15,16]

A toolkit of interventions targeting early readmission after AAA repair will likely incorporate several interventions that have previously been evaluated in medical patients. Other components of an aneurysm repair–specific toolkit may be novel; for example, postdischarge active surveillance for the most common postoperative complications (listed in Table 1) using a variety of methods including phone calls, telemonitoring, early clinic follow-up, and home visits for high-risk patients. As postoperative complications are perhaps the most important determinant of early readmission in surgical patients [24], it is likely that an effective approach to prevent surgical readmissions will differ in important ways in comparison with existing programs for medical patients.

SUMMARY

Thirty-day readmission is common after AAA repair, and postoperative events are strong predictors of readmission after adjusting for comorbidity. In addition, readmission is strongly associated with 1-year mortality. Considering the current evidence for readmission after AAA repair, improved coordination of care across the inpatient, transitional care, and outpatient settings, with active surveillance for procedure-specific (EVAR vs open) postoperative complications, may prevent some early readmissions. Given the pending financial implications and the striking association with 1-year mortality, developing interventions that target readmission after AAA repair is of paramount importance in the landscape of vascular surgery practice.

References

[1] Jencks SF, Williams MV, Coleman EA. Rehospitalizations among patients in the Medicare fee-for-service program. N Engl J Med 2009;360(14):1418–28.

[2] Medicare Payment Advisory Commission. Report to the Congress: Promoting Greater Efficiency in Medicare. Washington, DC: Medicare Payment Advisory Commission; 2007:103.
[3] Greenblatt DY, Greenberg CC, Kind AJ, et al. Causes and implications of readmission after abdominal aortic aneurysm repair. Ann Surg 2012;256(4):595–605.
[4] Vogel TR, Symons RG, Flum DR. Longitudinal outcomes after endovascular repair of abdominal aortic aneurysms. Vasc Endovascular Surg 2008;42(5):412–9.
[5] Jackson RS, Chang DC, Freischlag JA. Comparison of long-term survival after open versus. endovascular repair of intact abdominal aortic aneurysm among Medicare beneficiaries. JAMA 2012;307(15):1621–8.
[6] Jackson BM, Nathan DP, Doctor L, et al. Low rehospitalization rate for vascular surgery patients. J Vasc Surg 2011;54(3):767–72.
[7] Kind AJ, Bartels C, Mell MW, et al. For-profit hospital status and rehospitalizations at different hospitals: an analysis of Medicare data. Ann Intern Med 2010;153(11):718–27.
[8] Nasir K, Lin Z, Bueno H, et al. Is same-hospital readmission rate a good surrogate for all-hospital readmission rate? Med Care 2010;48(5):477–81.
[9] Holt PJ, Poloniecki JD, Hofman D, et al. Re-interventions, readmissions and discharge destination: modern metrics for the assessment of the quality of care. Eur J Vasc Endovasc Surg 2010;39(1):49–54.
[10] Gioia LC, Filion KB, Haider S, et al. Hospital readmissions following abdominal aortic aneurysm repair. Ann Vasc Surg 2005;19(1):35–41.
[11] Giles KA, Landon BE, Cotterill P, et al. Thirty-day mortality and late survival with reinterventions and readmissions after open and endovascular aortic aneurysm repair in Medicare beneficiaries. J Vasc Surg 2011;53(1):6–12, 13.e1.
[12] Kangovi S, Grande D. Hospital readmissions—not just a measure of quality. JAMA 2011;306(16):1796–7.
[13] Brooke BS, De Martino RR, Girotti M, et al. Developing strategies for predicting and preventing readmissions in vascular surgery. J Vasc Surg 2012;56(2):556–62.
[14] Hansen LO, Young RS, Hinami K, et al. Interventions to reduce 30-day rehospitalization: a systematic review. Ann Intern Med 2011;155(8):520–8.
[15] Naylor MD, Brooten DA, Campbell RL, et al. Transitional care of older adults hospitalized with heart failure: a randomized, controlled trial. J Am Geriatr Soc 2004;52(5):675–84.
[16] Coleman EA, Parry C, Chalmers S, et al. The care transitions intervention: results of a randomized controlled trial. Arch Intern Med 2006;166(17):1822–8.
[17] Jack BW, Chetty VK, Anthony D, et al. A reengineered hospital discharge program to decrease rehospitalization: a randomized trial. Ann Intern Med 2009;150(3):178–87.
[18] Kripalani S, LeFevre F, Phillips CO, et al. Deficits in communication and information transfer between hospital-based and primary care physicians: implications for patient safety and continuity of care. JAMA 2007;297(8):831–41.
[19] Sackley CM, Pound K. Stroke patients entering nursing home care: a content analysis of discharge letters. Clin Rehabil 2002;16(7):736–40.
[20] Coleman EA. Falling through the cracks: challenges and opportunities for improving transitional care for persons with continuous complex care needs. J Am Geriatr Soc 2003;51(4): 549–55.
[21] Solomon JK, Maxwell RB, Hopkins AP. Content of a discharge summary from a medical ward: views of general practitioners and hospital doctors. J R Coll Physicians Lond 1995;29(4):307–10.
[22] Tulloch AJ, Fowler GH, McMullan JJ, et al. Hospital discharge reports: content and design. Br Med J 1975;4(5994):443–6.
[23] van Walraven C, Rokosh E. What is necessary for high-quality discharge summaries? Am J Med Qual 1999;14(4):160–9.
[24] Kassin MT, Owen RM, Perez SD, et al. Risk factors for 30-day hospital readmission among general surgery patients. J Am Coll Surg 2012;215(3):322–30.

Advances in Surgery 47 (2013) 153–176

ADVANCES IN SURGERY

ELSEVIER
MOSBY

Duodenal Switch for Morbid Obesity

Is it Safe?

Rodney J. Mason, MD, PhD

Department of Surgery, University of Southern California, 1100 North State Street, Room 6A231, Los Angeles, CA 90033, USA

Keywords

• Duodenal switch • Bariatric procedures • Roux-en-Y gastric bypass
• Postoperative complications • NSQIP • SID • Outcomes

Key points

- The duodenal switch (DS) procedure is associated with the highest short-term and long- term morbidity of any contemporary bariatric procedure.
- More than one-third of DS patients require readmission for a procedure-related complication which is 50% more than associated with the gold standard laparoscopic Roux-en-Y gastric bypass (RYGB).
- Nutritional abnormalities from malabsorption after the DS are 2.5 times more likely to occur compared with after a laparoscopic RYGB.
- Liver abnormalities after DS are 7 times more likely to develop than after a laparoscopic RYGB.

INTRODUCTION

The epidemic of refractory severe obesity and its metabolic consequences has been met with a barrage of efficient surgical procedures aimed at achieving sustained weight loss and improving the accompanying serious comorbidities. Among the procedures, 4 are currently recognized in the United States by the national health agencies, insurances companies, and medical societies. These procedures include the gastric adjustable band, the Roux-en-Y gastric bypass (RYGB), the duodenal switch (DS) with biliopancreatic diversion (BPD) and the newest procedure, the vertical sleeve gastrectomy. All

Disclosures: R.J. Mason has no conflicts of interest or financial conflicts to disclose. The American College of Surgeons National Surgical Quality Improvement Program and the Healthcare Cost and Utilization Project are the source of the data used herein; they have not verified and are not responsible for the statistical validity of the data analysis or the conclusions derived by the author.

E-mail address: Rodney.mason@med.usc.edu

0065-3411/13/$ – see front matter
http://dx.doi.org/10.1016/j.yasu.2013.02.010

procedures are usually performed laparoscopically except for the DS, which in certain centers is still performed using an open approach.

The DS with BPD was first described by Hess and Hess in 1988 [1]. The procedure is the result of a combination of 2 concepts; namely, BPD developed by Scopinaro and colleagues in 1976 [2], which consists of a distal gastrectomy with a 200-mL to 500-mL residual gastric pouch, a long 250-cm alimentary limb with a short common channel of 50 cm to induce fat malabsorption, and the DS developed by DeMeester and colleagues in 1987 for the treatment of primary duodenogastric bile reflux gastritis [3].

Marceau and colleagues [4] published the first report of the DS in 1993. Rabkin and colleagues [5] and later Gagner and colleagues in 2000 described the laparoscopic approach [6]. The first long-term report with a large series of 701 patients operated on at the University of Southern California was published in 2003 [7]. It is universally accepted that the DS is the most effective procedure for achieving weight loss and has the best results among all 4 operations, with sustained long-term outcomes of more than 70% (EBWL) [8,9]. It is also the most effective procedure for achieving resolution of major comorbidities such as type 2 diabetes mellitus, sleep apnea, hypertension, and dyslipidemia [8–10]. However, despite these good functional results, the DS has not gained popularity, and is the least favored procedure, with only 1040 DS (0.95%) having been performed in 2010 compared with 59,191 gastric bypass, 42,989 gastric bandings, and 3353 gastric sleeves (data from the ASMBS-Center of Excellence 2010, which represents roughly half of the total bariatric procedures performed annually in the United States). Reasons include the massive malabsorptive component, which has major metabolic side effects, including protein malnutrition, nutrient and vitamin deficiencies, and the relative technical complexity of the procedure. Furthermore, multiple anastomosis, including the complex duodenoileal anastomosis and the long staple lines of the associated vertical sleeve gastrectomy, have not facilitated its laparoscopic adoption, which increasingly if not exclusively is favored by surgeons and requested by patients.

The fine balance of efficacy and safety is what drives the adoption of a procedure such as the DS. Undesirable consequences can occur after any surgical procedure; however, the overriding question is whether the DS operation for obesity is safe, whether it is associated with an acceptable level of risk and is not associated with excessive procedure-related health issues after the operation. With any surgical procedure there are intraoperative safety-related issues such as bleeding and cardiovascular events. Immediately postoperatively, there are issues such as anastomotic leaks and pulmonary embolism. Following bariatric procedures, there also be long-term safety-related issues such as malnutrition, vitamin deficiencies, and liver abnormalities, which can lead to persistent and long-standing patient safety issues. Level 1 evidence supporting, contrasting, and comparing the DS with other bariatric procedures is almost nonexistent, with only 1 randomized trial [11], and the remaining trials all having small numbers or major selection bias, with short-term follow-up.

Strategy to determine and evaluate safety of the DS

Safety is relative, and in this article, the safety of the DS is compared with the gold standard procedure for weight loss: RYGB. In this article, the strategy for determining whether the DS is safe is to first report both the short-term and long-term outcomes from 1 of the pioneering institutions performing this procedure (University of Southern California [USC]). Second, to compare the intraoperative and early safety and morbidity between the DS and RYGB using the National Safety Quality Improvement Program (NSQIP) database. This database is excellent for 30-day outcomes and is also useful because it provides a means for determining and distinguishing between laparoscopic and open bariatric procedures. The NSQIP dataset for bariatric procedures does have a selection bias in the choice of procedure. To minimize this bias, a matched cohort is analyzed and reported. Third, additional long-term outcomes are determined from analysis of the California State Inpatient Database (SID) and again a comparison made with the gold standard RYGB. The advantages of this overall strategy are that it includes data from 3 different datasets, 2 of which are nationally accredited and audited, and all have sufficient numbers of patients to be representative.

STRATEGY 1: USC DATASET

Materials and methods for USC dataset

A prospective bariatric surgery database and the hospital electronic patient file system were used to extract and review data of all patients who underwent a DS for morbid obesity at the Keck Medical Center of the USC, Los Angeles, over 18 years between January 1993 and January 2011. The procedures were performed by 4 surgeons through an open approach. The preoperative workup and the surgical technique have been described previously [7].

This review consisted of follow-up data of all hospital readmissions (date, reason, duration, laboratory, imaging, and reoperations performed). Systematic telephone interviews using a standardized patient questionnaire were performed when follow-up data were missing and on all patients who were not readmitted for postoperative complications.

The primary outcome measure was hospital readmission and included identification of all major and minor complications associated with the readmission. Major complications included any bleeding, superficial surgical site infection (SSI), deep SSI, organ/space SSI, gastrointestinal (GI) leak, fascial dehiscence, respiratory failure requiring ventilation, pneumonia, fistula, incisional hernia, GI stricture, malabsorption, intestinal obstruction, deep venous thrombosis, pulmonary embolism, acute renal failure, myocardial infarction, rhabdomyolysis, and any organ failure. Subcategories included inpatient, 30-day, and long-term morbidity and mortality. In all patients, a social security number query was performed using the social security death index database via www.ancestry.com, to assess mortality and the duration of time to death. Mortality was classified as perioperative if directly associated with the operation in the early period after the procedure.

Statistical analysis

Patients' demographics, preoperative risk factors, and outcome measures were compared using the Pearson χ^2 test and Mantel-Haenszel odds ratio (OR) for categorical variables and Student *t*-test for continuous variables using STATA 12 (Stata, College Station, TX). A *P* value of .05 was used to determine statistical significance. Summary statistics and time to complication data were performed using the stsum and stdescribe commands in STATA. Overall survival curves and time to complication curves were calculated using the Kaplan-Meier survival and failure functions in STATA. The Institutional Review Board at the Keck School of Medicine at the University of Southern California approved the study.

Results from USC cohort

At USC, which was one of the pioneering institutions for the DS, 1315 patients underwent the procedure for morbid obesity between 1993 and 2010. During follow-up, 153 (12%) patients were lost or missing and 673 (51%) patients presented with a complication. For the primary outcome measure (postoperative readmissions), data were available for 1162 patients at a median follow-up of 115 months (interquartile range [IQR] 99–137 months). This study included 68 (5.9%) patients who had a complication only during the initial hospital admission. The remaining 605 patients with a complication were readmitted a total of 1582 times during the follow-up period for a mean number of readmissions of 2.6 per patient. The overall 30-day morbidity was 7.6% (88 patients). The median time to a complication was 18.7 months (IQR 0.3–32) (Fig. 1).

The incidence of the specific postoperative complications and their associated readmission rates are shown in Table 1. The frequency distribution of the number of reoperations, number of readmissions, and number of

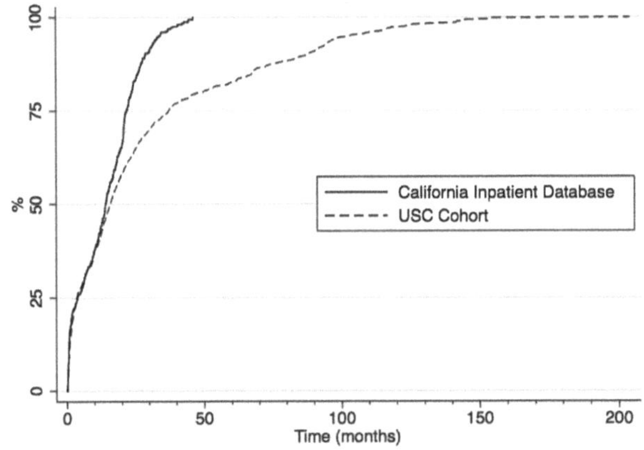

Fig. 1. Cumulative complication rates over time. (*Data from* USC dataset and SID [16].)

Table 1
Incidence of complications and readmissions in USC dataset

	Number of patients with complication (%)	Number of complications (%)	Median time to complication	Reoperative rate (n, %)
Bleeding	15 (1.3)	19 (1)	30 d	6/15 (40)
Infectious complication	104 (9)	177 (9.4)	18 d	none
Leak	27 (2.3)	57 (3)	8 d	16/27 (59)
Dehiscence	33 (2.8)	36 (2)	21 d	18/33 (54.5)
Respiratory failure	49 (4.2)	106 (5.6)	3 d	none
Pneumonia	19 (1.6)	35 (1.9)	8 d	none
Small bowel obstruction	81 (7)	100 (5.3)	26 mo	60/82 (73)
Fistula	14 (1.2)	76 (4)	11 mo	11/14 (78.6)
Hernia	353 (30.4)	398 (21.1)	18 mo	397/398 (99.7)
Stricture	113 (9.7)	206 (10.9)	4 mo	4/113 (3.5)
GERD	64 (5.5)	98 (5.2)	4 y	25/64 (39)
Malabsorption	132 (11.4)	156 (8.3)	16 mo	56/132 (42.4)
Venous thrombotic event	26 (2.2)	27 (1.4)	16 d	none
Other	214 (18.4)	365 (19.3)	4 mo	none
Failure switch	28 (2.4)	31 (1.6)	5 y	25/28 (89)
Wound-related complication	89 (7.7)		17 d	none
None	489 (42.1)			none

complications is shown in Table 2. The overall reoperation rate of patients in this series was 39.7% (461/1162), with 68% (461/673) of patients experiencing a complication requiring a reoperation. Overall, 13.7% (159/1162) of patients required 2 or more reoperations.

Only 489 (42.1%) of DS patients did not experience any postoperative complication. The commonest complication was an incisional hernia, occurring

Table 2
Frequency distribution of the reoperations/readmissions/complications (n = 673 complications)

Frequency	Number of patients with reoperations (%)	Frequency	Number of patients with readmissions (%)	Frequency	Number of patients with complications (%)
1	302 (45)	0	68 (6)	1	347 (30)
2	96 (14)	1	239 (21)	2	166 (14)
3	24 (4)	2	155 (13)	3	75 (6)
4	16 (2)	3	64 (6)	4	45 (4)
5 or more	23 (3)	4	51 (4)	5	16 (1)
		5 or more	96 (8)	6	10 (1)
				7 or more	14 (1)

in 353 (30.4%) patients. This complication was also associated with the most readmissions and the most reoperations (see Table 1). Besides hernia repair, the complication with the highest reoperative rate was fistula formation (see Table 1), and the lowest was in patients developing a postoperative stricture. The commonest sites for stricturing (113 patients had 206 strictures) were in the gastric sleeve (n = 104, 50%), followed by the duodenojejunal anastomosis (n = 61, 30%), at the jejunojejunal anastomosis (n = 5, 2%), and other locations (n = 36, 17%). Most of the bleeding requiring transfusion occurred in the early postoperative period (Fig. 2). Of the 19 episodes with bleeding, 6 were upper GI bleeding (in 2 identified from the anastomosis), 4 lower GI bleeding, and 9 a significantly intra-abdominal or wound bleed. Reoperation for bleeding was necessary in 6 of 15 patients (40%). The commonest site for a GI leak was the gastric staple line in 12 (44%) patients; in 9 (33%) patients, at the duodenojejunal; and in 1 (4%) patient, at the jejunojejunal anastomosis. The leakage site was not identified in 5 (19%) patients. Sixteen (59%) of the 27 patients with a GI leak required a reoperation, with 1 patient requiring 2 reoperations. Wound-related complications, including superficial and deep SSIs, and wound dehiscence occurred in 7.7% (89/1162) of patients. Organ/space SSI occurred in 3.8% (44/1162) of patients. Nineteen (1.6%) patients developed a total of 35 postoperative pneumonias; 18 (51%) pneumonias were classified as aspiration pneumonia. A tracheostomy with a long-term ventilator was necessary in 16.3% (8/49 patients) of patients with postoperative respiratory failure. Thirty-two patients (2.75%), developed new symptoms of heartburn or other reflux symptoms requiring readmission postoperatively, whereas in a further 32 (2.75%) patients symptoms present preoperatively remained persistent or became significantly worse (see Fig. 2). Conversion into a RYGB was necessary for 39% (25/64). Intestinal obstruction occurred in 7% (81/1162) of

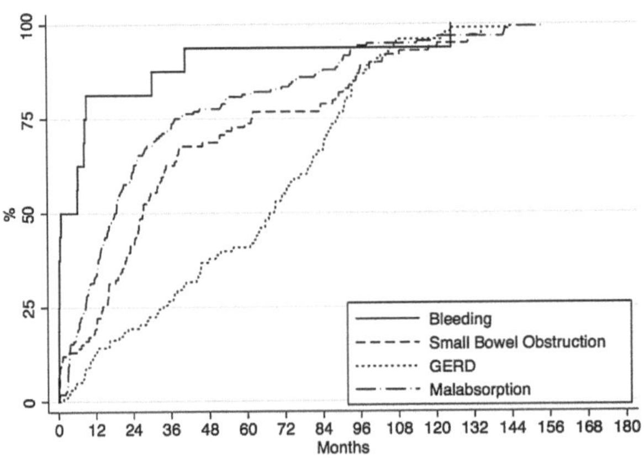

Fig. 2. Cumulative rate of occurrence of bleeding, gastroesophageal reflux disease (GERD), small bowel obstruction, and malabsorption over time.

patients and required an operation with lysis of adhesions in 74% (60/81). The most common forms of malabsorption were hypoalbuminemia (29%), iron deficiency anemia (21%), hypocalcemia (21%), and others (29%). A reoperation to correct the malabsorptive status was required in 42.4% (56/132 patients) for an overall revisional rate for malabsorption of 4.8%. The occurrence over time is shown in Fig. 2. A venous thrombotic event was seen in 2.2% (26/1162 patients): pulmonary embolism in 13 patients and deep venous thrombosis in 13 patients). A total of 2.4% (28/1162) of patients presented with failure of DS defined by either weight gain or no/insufficient weight loss during follow-up, of whom 89% (25/28) required revisional surgery for this complication.

The overall mortality in this series was 7.2% (84/1162 patients). The in-hospital mortality was 0.5% (6 patients). The reasons were fatal cardiac events in 3 patients, pulmonary embolism in 1 patient, and 2 respiratory failures leading to death in 2 patients. Four additional patients died in the perioperative period (<60 days) for causes related to the DS, giving a total perioperative mortality of 0.9%. In the follow-up, 3 deaths were related to severe malnutrition (0.3%).

STRATEGY 2: NSQIP DATASET: 30-DAY MORBIDITY AND MORTALITY

Materials and methods for NSQIP dataset

Data acquisition

Data from the American College of Surgeons (ACS)/NSQIP databases for 2005 to 2009 were analyzed. Patients were included in the analysis if they underwent a DS as their primary procedure (Current Procedural Terminology code (CPT) 43,845) or RYGB (CPT codes 43,846, 43,644, 43,845, 43,846 [open] 43,847 [open >150 cm]) and had a postoperative diagnosis of morbid obesity (*International Classification of Diseases, Ninth Edition* [ICD-9] codes 280.01). Because there is no specific CPT code for laparoscopic DS, these cases were identified if they had secondary procedure codes that were identifiable as a laparoscopic procedure code. The standard NSQIP preoperative risk factors were compared between the 2 groups [12]. Thirty-day outcomes between DS and RYGB patients were compared and the main outcome measures in this section included overall morbidity, serious morbidity, and mortality, as defined in Table 3.

Statistical analysis

Aggregate cohort. Patients' demographics, preoperative risk factors, and outcome measures were compared using the Pearson χ^2 test and Mantel-Haenszel OR for categorical variables and Student *t*-test for continuous variables using STATA MP 12.1. The significance value was set at $P<.05$.

Matched cohort. Because the data from the ACS/NSQIP database are not representative of a prospective study and patients were not randomly assigned to a DS or RYGB, there is a possibility that patients in each group represent a different patient population. To overcome this difference and to reduce the bias caused by this nonrandom assignment, each DS patient was matched with a patient undergoing an RYGB with similar probability of preoperative

Table 3
Association between the main outcome measures and the NSQIP variables. X depicts the variable included in the outcome measure

	Morbidity	Serious morbidity
Superficial SSI	x	
Deep incisional SSI	x	
Organ/space SSI	x	x
Wound disruption	x	x
Pneumonia	x	
Unplanned intubation	x	
Pulmonary embolism	x	x
On ventilator >48 h	x	x
Progressive renal insufficiency	x	x
Acute renal failure	x	x
Urinary tract infection	x	
Cerebrovascular accident/stroke	x	x
Coma >24 h	x	x
Peripheral nerve damage	x	
Cardiac arrest	x	x
Myocardial infarction	x	x
Bleeding transfusions	x	x
Graft prosthesis flap failure	x	
Deep venous thrombosis/thrombophlebitis	x	
Sepsis	x	x
Septic shock	x	x

risk factors and body mass index (BMI, calculated as weight in kilograms divided by the square of height in meters).

The matching was performed using "nearest method" in the MatchIt package [13,14] and the R project for statistical computing (version 2.14.1, The R Foundation for Statistical Computing) [15]. Using MatchIt, the closest match was selected without replacement in the DS for RYGB group. The matching process was performed using all NSQIP preoperative risk factors. One indicator to assess the quality of matching is the standardized bias, which is calculated as the difference in sample means in the duodenal and RYGB group divided by the root average of sample variances. For binomial variables, the mean is replaced by probability. The standardized mean difference before matching and after matching is depicted in Figs. 3 and 4. In addition, as a second measure of quality of matching, none of the preoperative risk factors was different between the 2 groups in the matched cohort. Statistical analysis after matching was performed in similar fashion to the aggregate cohort using STATA MP 12.1.

Results of NSQIP database

A total of 31,758 patients with morbid obesity as the primary diagnostic code who underwent either a DS or RYGB procedure were included in the

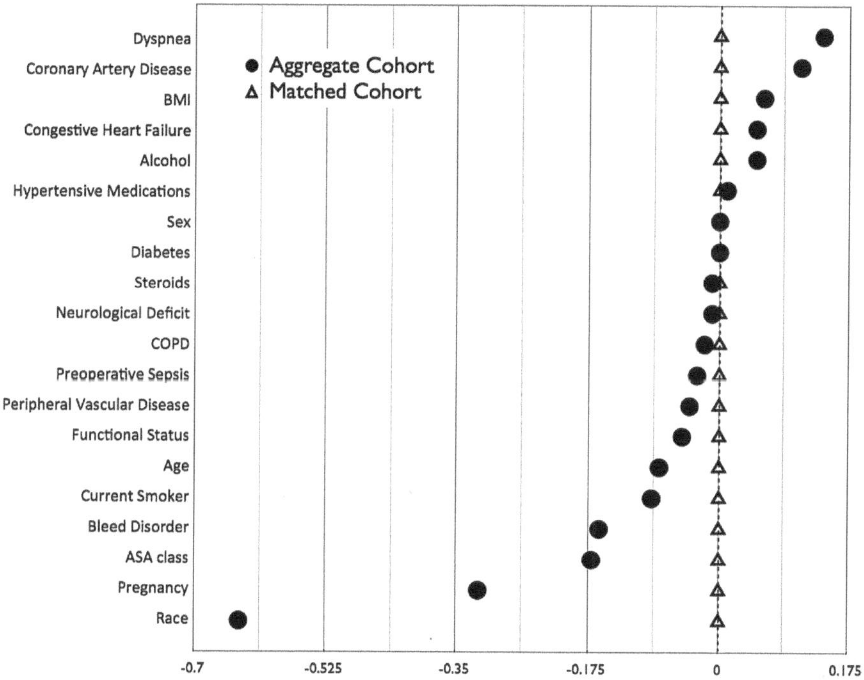

Fig. 3. Standardized mean differences of the preoperative risk factors for the open DS and open RYGB patients, showing results from the aggregate and the matched cohort of patients.

aggregate cohort. A laparoscopic procedure was performed on 27,754 (87%) (72%) patients, and 4184 (13%) patients underwent an open procedure (Fig. 5).

PATIENT CHARACTERISTICS FOR OPEN DS AND OPEN RYGB PROCEDURES

As can be expected, the preoperative risk factor between the open DS patients and the open RYGB patients showed some differences. The mean BMI of the DS patients of 51.3 ± 12.3 kg/m^2 was similar ($P = .27$) to that of the open RYGB patients (50.7 ± 10.6 kg/m^2). In the aggregate cohort, the patients who underwent an open DS tended to be white ($P < .001$), had a lower American Society of Anesthesiologists (ASA) class ($P < .001$), had less dyspnea on exertion ($P = .006$), and had fewer bleeding disorders ($P = .001$) but significantly more coronary artery disease ($P = .031$) than the open RYGB patients. The remaining preoperative risk factors were similar between both groups. However, after matching was performed, there were 326 patients in the DS group and 326 patients in the open RYGB group, with no difference in the 5 risk factors that were originally statistically different between the 2 groups, indicating more comparable groups. A comparison of

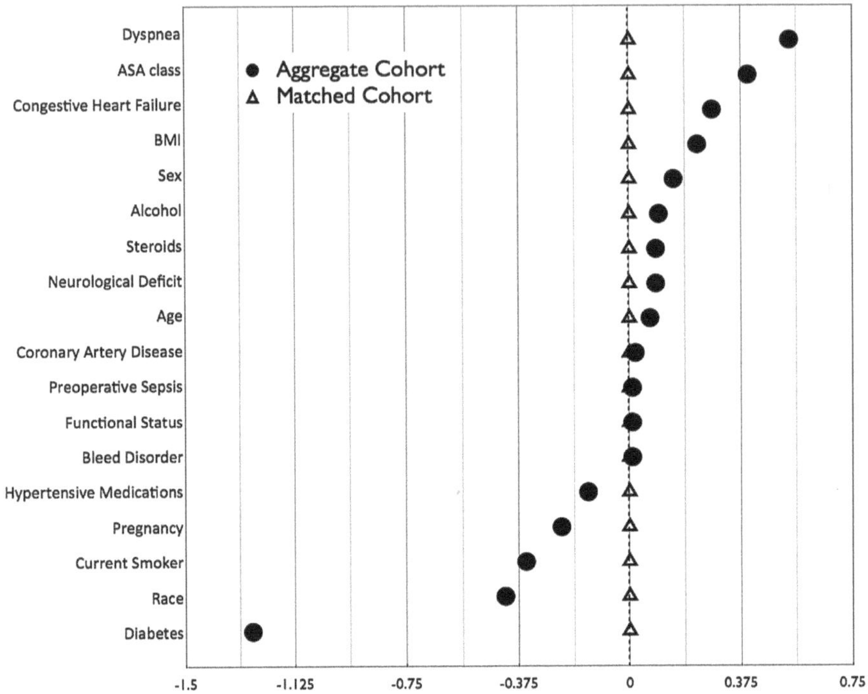

Fig. 4. Standardized mean differences of the preoperative risk factors for the laparoscopic DS and the laparoscopic RYGB patients, showing results from the aggregate and the matched cohort of patients.

the standardized bias between the preoperative and intraoperative risk factors in the aggregate and the matched cohort of open procedures is depicted in Fig. 3.

THIRTY-DAY OUTCOMES: OPEN DS VERSUS OPEN RYGB

In the aggregate cohort of 4178 patients undergoing an open procedure, 495 (11.9%) patients experienced an overall morbidity, 236 (5.7%) a serious morbidity, and 25 (0.6%) patients died. The overall serious morbidity and mortality were similar between the 2 groups (Table 4). However, in the matched cohort with less variation in the risk factors between groups, patients in the open DS had a significantly higher rate of serious morbidity (7.4% vs 3.1%; $P = .014$), higher but not statistically significant rates of overall morbidity (11.0% vs 7.1%; $P = .076$), and similar mortality (2% vs 2%; $P = 1.0$, Fisher exact) (Fig. 6).

In the aggregate cohort, the patients who underwent open DS experienced a higher rate of deep incisional SSI (2.4% vs 1.1%; $P = .014$) and a higher rate of organ/space SSI (3.4% vs 1.8%; $P = .013$, see Table 4). In the matched cohort,

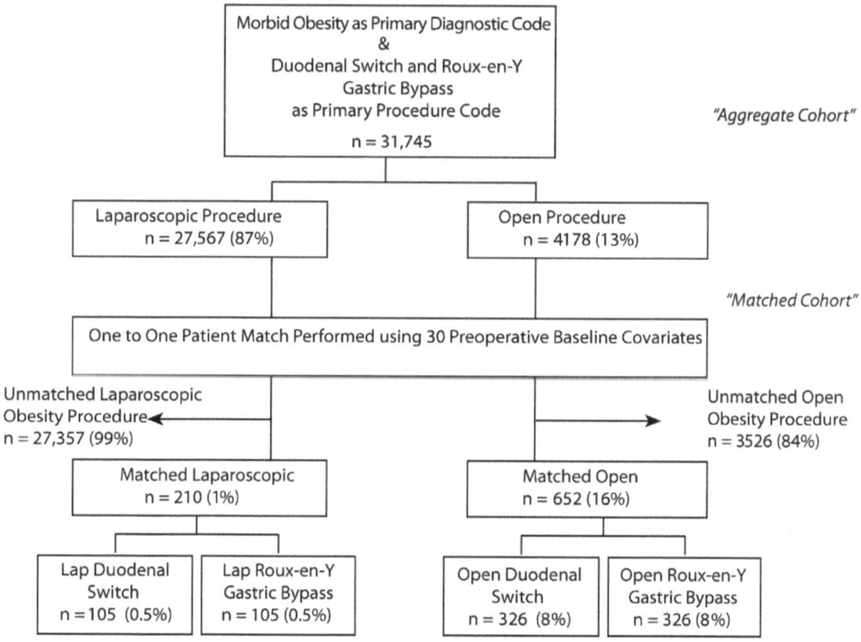

Fig. 5. The study population from the NSQIP dataset [12], showing the derivation of the aggregate and matched cohort of patients.

organ/space SSI remained significantly worse in the DS patients (3.7 vs 0.6; $P = .12$), and return to operating room became statistically significantly worse (4.9% vs 1.5%; $P = .009$) in the DS group. This finding translated to a 5 times greater odds of developing an organ/space SSI (OR: 6.19; 95% confidence interval [CI] 1.37–27.88) and 2 times greater odds (OR 3.31; 95% CI 1.12–5.12) of returning to the operating room for the DS patients.

PATIENT CHARACTERISTICS FOR LAPAROSCOPIC DS AND LAPAROSCOPIC RYGB PROCEDURES

The mean BMI of the laparoscopic DS patients of 49.1 ± 8 kg/m^2 was significantly higher ($P = .013$) than that of the laparoscopic RYGB patients (47.1 ± 8.4 kg/m^2). In the aggregate cohort, the patients who underwent a laparoscopic DS tended to be white ($P < .001$), had a higher ASA class ($P < .001$), had more dyspnea on exertion ($P < .001$), and had a history of congestive cardiac failure ($P = .03$). The remaining preoperative risk factors were similar between both groups. However, after 105 DS patients were matched to 105 patients in the laparoscopic RYGB group, none of the above 4 risk factors, which were originally statistically different between the 2 groups, were different, indicating more comparable groups. A comparison of the standardized bias between the preoperative and intraoperative risk factors in the aggregate and the matched cohort of open procedures is depicted in Fig. 4.

Table 4
Outcomes for open DS versus open RYGB patients (univariate analysis)

	Aggregate cohort			Matched cohort		
	n = 4178			n = 652		
Outcomes	Open DS N = 466	Open RYGB N = 3712	*P* value	Open DS N = 326	Open RYGB N = 326	*P* value
Morbidity	56 (12.02)	439 (11.83)	.904	36 (11.04)	23 (7.06)	.076
Mortality	3 (0.64)	22 (0.59)	.893	2 (0.61)	2 (0.61)	1[a]
Serious morbidity	35 (7.51)	201 (5.41)	.065	24 (7.36)	10 (3.07)	.014
Superficial SSI	13 (2.79)	177 (4.77)	.053	8 (2.45)	11 (3.37)	.643[a]
Deep incisional SSI	11 (2.36)	39 (1.05)	.014	8 (2.45)	4 (1.23)	.383[a]
Organ/space SSI	16 (3.43)	65 (1.75)	.013	12 (3.68)	2 (0.61)	.012[a]
Wound disruption	5 (1.07)	46 (1.24)	1[a]	4 (1.23)	2 (0.61)	.686[a]
Pneumonia	12 (2.58)	65 (1.75)	.202	8 (2.45)	2 (0.61)	.107[a]
Unplanned intubation	7 (1.5)	59 (1.59)	1[a]	4 (1.23)	2 (0.61)	.686[a]
Pulmonary embolism	5 (1.07)	16 (0.43)	.076[a]	4 (1.23)	2 (0.61)	.686[a]
On ventilator >48 h	12 (2.58)	54 (1.45)	.068	7 (2.15)	1 (0.31)	.069[a]
Progressive renal insufficiency	4 (0.86)	30 (0.81)	.78[a]	2 (0.61)	2 (0.61)	1.0[a]
Acute renal failure	2 (0.43)	19 (0.51)	11[a]	2 (0.61)	1 (0.31)	1.0[a]
Urinary tract infection	7 (1.5)	54 (1.45)	.839[a]	2 (0.61)	2 (0.61)	1.0[a]
Cerebrovascular accident/stroke	1 (0.21)	0 (0.0)	14[a]	-	-	
Coma >48 h	(0.0)	4 (0.11)	10[a]	-	-	-
Peripheral nerve damage	0 (0.0)	2 (0.05)	1.0[a]	-	-	
Cardiac arrest	1 (0.21)	20 (0.54)	.503[a]	1 (0.31)	2 (0.61)	1.0[a]
Myocardial infarction	0 (0.0)	1 (0.03)	1.0[a]	-	-	
Bleeding transfusions	0 (0.0)	22 (0.59)	.1642[a]	0 (0.0)	1 (0.31)	1.0[a]
Graft prosthesis flap failure	0 (0.0)	6 (0.16)	1.0[a]	0 (0.0)	1 (0.31)	1.0[a]
Deep venous thrombosis/thrombophlebitis	0 (0.0)	20 (0.54)	.157[a]	-	-	
Sepsis	14 (3.0)	75 (2.02)	.172[a]	9 (2.76)	5 (1.53)	.419[a]
Septic shock	10 (2.15)	48 (1.29)	.141[a]	7 (2.15)	2 (0.61)	.177[a]
Return to OR	25 (5.36)	143 (3.85)	.132[a]	16 (4.91)	5 (1.53)	.024[a]

[a]Fisher exact test.
Data from NSQIP database 2005 to 2009 [12].

THIRTY-DAY OUTCOMES: LAPAROSCOPIC DS VERSUS LAPAROSCOPIC RYGB

In the aggregate cohort of 27,567 patients undergoing a laparoscopic procedure, 1269 (4.6%) patients experienced an overall morbidity, 457 (1.67%) a serious morbidity, and 44 (0.16%) patients died. Overall morbidity was significantly higher in the laparoscopic DS patients (8.8% vs 4.6%, $P = .033$), but serious morbidity and mortality were equivalent between the 2 groups (Table 5). Similarly, in the matched cohort, patients undergoing a laparoscopic

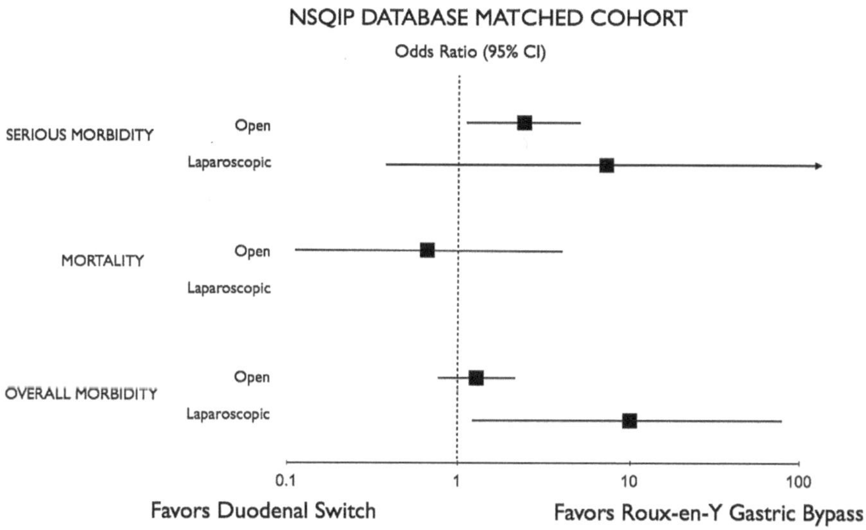

Fig. 6. Comparisons of main outcome measures from the NSQIP for the matched dataset for both open and laparoscopic DS versus open and laparoscopic RYGB cohort of patients. Depicted as ORs with error bars representing the 95% CIs.

DS had significantly higher overall morbidity (8.6% vs 1%; $P = .019$) but equivalent serious morbidity and no mortalities (see Fig. 6). With regard to specific individual NSQIP outcomes, no major differences were seen between the 2 groups in either the aggregate or matched cohort of patients. The adverse event rates were consistently higher in the DS patients, and most probably did not reach significance because of the small numbers of patients.

STRATEGY 3: CALIFORNIA SID: LONG-TERM OUTCOMES AND READMISSIONS

Data acquisition

Data from the California SID from the Healthcare Cost and Utilization Project (HCUP) for 2005 to 2010 were analyzed [16]. Patients were included in the analysis if they underwent a DS identified from the primary ICD-9 procedure code (ICD-9 codes 43.89 plus 45.51 and 45.91) or open RYGB (ICD-9 procedure code 44.39) or laparoscopic RYGB (ICD-9 procedure code 44.38) and had a preoperative primary Clinical Classifications Software (CCS) diagnosis code of 58 (other nutritional disease).

SID outcomes

Readmission rates between the DS and RYGB patients were compared and included: (1) overall hospital readmission rates after the index bariatric operation and (2) procedure-related complications causing the readmission. This categorization was determined from the primary CCS diagnostic codes.

Table 5
Outcomes for laparoscopic DS versus laparoscopic RYGB patients (univariate analysis)

	Aggregate cohort			Matched cohort		
	n = 27,567			n = 210		
Outcomes	Laparoscopic DS N = 114	Laparoscopic RYGB N = 27,453	*P* value	Laparoscopic DS N = 105	Laparoscopic RYGB N = 105	*P* value
Morbidity	10 (8.77)	1259 (4.59)	.033	9 (8.57)	1 (0.95)	.019[a]
Mortality	0 (0.0)	44 (0.16)	1.0[a]	-	-	-
Serious morbidity	3 (2.63)	454 (1.65)	.415	3 (2.86)	0 (0.00)	.246[a]
Superficial SSI	2 (1.75)	476 (1.73)	.987[a]	2 (1.9)	0 (0.00)	.498[a]
Deep incisional SSI	1 (0.88)	64 (0.23)	.236[a]	-	-	-
Organ/space SSI	2 (1.75)	168 (0.61)	.156[a]	2 (1.9)	0 (0.00)	.498[a] 3
Wound disruption	0 (0.00)	40 (0.15)	1[a]	-	-	-
Pneumonia	1 (0.88)	146 (0.53)	.457[a]	1 (0.95)	1 (0.95)	1.0[a]
Unplanned intubation	1 (0.88)	59 (1.59)	1[a]	1 (0.95)	0 (0.00)	1.0[a]
Pulmonary embolism	1 (0.88)	16 (0.43)	.076[a]	1 (0.95)	0 (0.00)	1.0[a]
On ventilator >48 h	0 (0.00)	54 (1.45)	.068	1 (0.95)	0 (0.00)	1.0[a]
Progressive renal insufficiency	0 (0.00)	30 (0.81)	.787[a]	-	-	-
Acute renal failure	0 (0.00)	19 (0.51)	1.0[a]	-	-	
Urinary tract infection	5 (4.39)	246 (0.90)	.04[a]	4 (3.81)	0 (0.00)	.121[a]
Cerebrovascular accident/stroke	0 (0.00)	7 (0.03)	1.0[a]	-	-	
Coma >48 h	0 (0.00)	3 (0.01)	1.0[a]	-	-	-
Peripheral nerve damage	1 (0.88)	13 (0.05)	1.0[a]	-	-	
Cardiac arrest	0 (0.00)	25 (0.09)	10[a]	-	-	-
Myocardial infarction	0 (0.0)	11 (0.04)	1.0[a]	-	-	
Bleeding transfusions	0 (0.0)	83 (0.30)	1.0[a]	-	-	-
Graft prosthesis flap failure	0 (0.0)	2 (0.01)	1.0[a]	-	-	-
Deep venous thrombosis/thrombophlebitis	0 (0.0)	83 (0.30)	1.0[a]	-	-	-
Sepsis	2 (1.75)	198 (0.72)	.201[a]	2 (1.9)	0 (0.00)	.498[a]
Septic shock	0 (0.00)	77 (0.28)	1.0[a]	-	-	-
Return to OR	3 (2.63)	756 (2.75)	1.0[a]	2 (1.9)	0 (0.00)	.498[a]

[a]Fisher exact test.

Data from NSQIP database 2005 to 2009.

Reoperation or reintervention procedures were determined from the primary CCS procedure codes. However, only the CCS codes depicted in Table 6 were considered relevant to this analysis. Total procedure-related readmissions included the sum of only the CCS codes depicted in Table 6.

Results of SID

A total of 65,925 patients were identified in the California SID from 2005 to 2010 with a primary CCS code of 58 who underwent either a DS or RYGB procedure (Fig. 7). A laparoscopic RYGB was performed in 59,869 (91%) patients, 4831 (7%) patients underwent an open RYGB, and 1255 (2%) underwent a DS procedure. The readmission rates for the procedure-associated complications were 342 (27.9%) for the DS patients, 1359 (28.1%) for the open RYGB patients, and 7435 (12.4%) for the laparoscopic RYGB patients. Readmission rates after the index obesity procedure categorized according to relevant CCS codes are depicted in Table 7. Although the incidence of readmission for CCS code 238 ("complication of the procedure") between the DS and open RYGB patients was similar, the DS patients were 38% more likely to undergo a reoperation (OR 0.62; 95% CI 0.40–0.96, Fig. 8) and 39% more likely to be readmitted for a nutritional/endocrine or metabolic disorder (OR 0.61; 95% CI 0.48–0.77, see Fig. 8). The comparison with the laparoscopic RYGB was even more striking, with the DS patients 6 times more likely to be readmitted with a liver disorder (OR 7.5; 95% CI 3.71–15.16) and 2.5 times more likely to be readmitted with a nutritional/endocrine or metabolic disorder (OR 3.42; 95% CI 2.78–4.22, see Fig. 8). The follow-up time from the index bariatric procedure to readmission was 11.4 months (see Fig. 1).

Table 6
HCUP: CCS codes used to identify the primary diagnosis category associated with the procedure-related readmission

CCS code	Description of the CCS code
238	Complication of procedure
143	Abdominal hernia
145	Intestinal obstruction
138	Esophageal disease
55	Fluid electrolyte disease
139	Gastroduodenal disorder
140	Gastritis
153	Upper GI hemorrhage
250	Nausea/vomiting
141	Other disease of stomach
140	Other disease of liver
59	Anemia
135	Intestinal infection
45–58	Nutrition/endocrine/metabolic/immunity

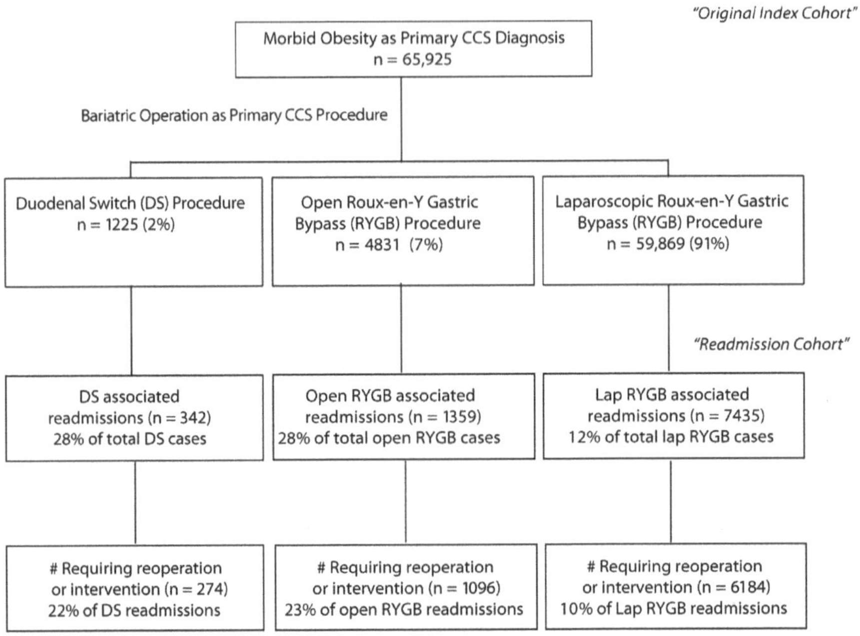

Fig. 7. Flow diagram depicting the study population from the California SID [16] and showing the derivation of the readmission cohort of patients.

DISCUSSION

Short-term morbidity

The overall 30-day morbidity for the open DS is similar to that of the open RYGB. However, the serious morbidity is almost twice that of the RYGB. The main difference in short-term morbidity between the 2 procedures seems related to organ/space SSI, which is most probably an indication of increased anastomotic leakage associated with the open DS. Both the DS and RYGB procedures have 2 intestinal anastomosis, but the DS has a longer gastric staple line as well as a duodenal stump, which is associated with greater incidence of leakage than found in the RYGB patients. Furthermore, the odds of a DS patient having to go back to the operating room in the first 30 days is more than twice that of an RYGB patient (OR 3.31; 95% CI 1.2–9.15). For patients undergoing a laparoscopic procedure, the comparison is even more striking, with the odds of a laparoscopic DS patient having a complication almost 9 times that of a laparoscopic RGYB patient (OR 9.75; 95% CI 1.12–78.4).

Long-term morbidity

After the inferior outcomes associated with the DS in the early postoperative period, there seem to be continuing problems with the significant development of new procedure-related complications. The main outcome from the USC cohort of DS patients was the overall complication rate of 58%. Readmission

Table 7
Primary diagnostic code associated with readmission to hospital after the index bariatric procedure

CCS code	CCS description	DS (n, %) n = 1225	Open RYGB (n, %) n = 4831	Laparoscopic RYGB (n, %) n = 59,869	Mean time to complication (mo)
238	Complication of procedure	103 (8)	424 (9)	2436 (4)	14
	Complication requiring reoperation	46 (3.8)	141 (2.9)	1078 (1.8)	7
143	Abdominal hernia	60 (4.9)	286 (5.9)	799 (1.3)	16
145	Intestinal obstruction	34 (2.8)	120 (2.5)	619 (1)	14
138	Esophageal disease	3 (0.2)	16 (0.3)	127 (0.2)	11
55	Fluid electrolyte disease	27 (2.2)	99 (2)	609 (1)	5
139;141;250;138	Gastroesophageal disorders	12 (1.2)	113 (1.5)	925 (2.3)	9
140	Other liver disease	9 (0.7)	7 (0.1)	59 (0.1)	11
153	Upper GI hemorrhage	1 (0.1)	87 (1.8)	604 (1)	14
59	Anemia	10 (0.8)	23 (0.5)	153 (0.3)	23
45–58	Nutrition/endocrine/metabolic/immunity	102 (8.3)	252 (5.2)	1548 (2.6)	14

Data from the California SID 2010 to 2010.

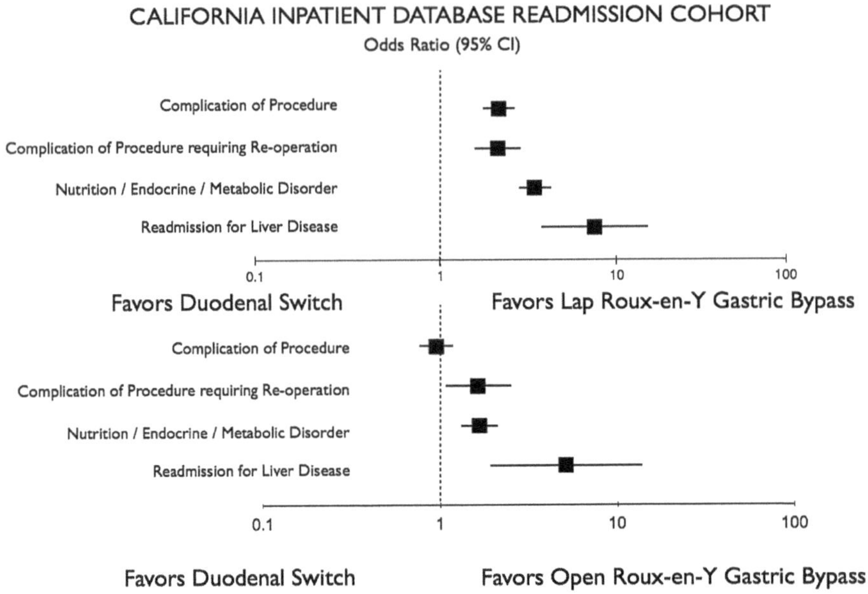

Fig. 8. Comparisons of complications resulting in readmission from the California SID for the DS versus open RYGB and the DS versus laparoscopic RYGB cohort of patients. Depicted as ORs with error bars representing the 95% CIs.

was required for 52% of patients who were readmitted a mean of 2.6 times. Furthermore, there was an overall reoperation rate of 39.7% after the index switch procedure. Analysis of the California SID showed the incidence of readmission after the index bariatric surgery with a procedure-related complication of 28%. The lower readmission rate compared with the USC dataset is most probably related to the shorter follow-up period in the SID dataset, because the analysis of the occurrence of complications from the USC cohort shows an increase over time. The USC dataset was also associated with more incisional hernias after the DS compared with data from the California SID. The USC complication rate excluding patients with the complication of a hernia was 27.5%, which is similar to that of the California SID. Others also concur with this high ongoing morbidity. Sovik and colleagues [17] showed, in a prospective randomized trial comparing laparoscopic gastric bypass with the laparoscopic DS in patients with a BMI between 50 and 60 kg/m^2, a significantly higher adverse events rate (62%) after DS than gastric bypass (32%) after a 2 year follow-up. Dolan and Fielding reported a complication rate of 23% in the laparoscopic group and 35.6% in the open DS group [18]. An outlier study seems to be that from Biertho and colleagues [19,20], who reported the best published results in the literature [21]. In this study, the overall readmission rate related to bariatric surgery was 12.7%, and there was no difference in the reoperation rate between the laparoscopic and open group (6.3% vs

5.2%). Their mean follow-up was only 23 ± 11 months; however, this was longer than the follow-up time of 11.4 months in the California SID analysis, which had higher readmission and reoperation rates. Biertho and colleagues' [20] early complication rate within 30 days was 13% (0.9% intraoperatively), which was similar to that found in the NSQIP dataset.

When the long-term complication rates of the DS are compared with those of the RYGB, a similar inferior outcome is found for the DS patients, which was similar to the inferior outcome found for the short-term comparisons. Finks and colleagues [22], in a study that included 25,469 patients who underwent bariatric surgery in 29 centers, analyzed the predictors for serious complications after bariatric surgery and found that the most significant risk factor for complications was the procedure type, with the DS having the highest OR (9.68). Findings from the California SID showed that 8% of patients were readmitted with the diagnosis code of 238 ("complication of the procedure"), and this incidence was almost double the rate of the laparoscopic RYGB patients. Although the incidence appeared similar to the open RYGB patients, the incidence number of patients requiring a reoperation was significantly higher for the DS patients compared with either the open or laparoscopic RYGB patients. This significantly higher reoperation rate in the DS patients further adds to the high morbidity of the procedure.

Specific complications associated with the DS

Malabsorption occurred in 11.4% of the USC cohort of patients. The median time was 16 months. One-third of these severe malabsorptions were caused by hypoalbuminemia. The rest was divided equally between severe vitamin A and D deficiencies. Reoperation to correct the malabsorptive abnormalities occurred in 42.4% of these patients. The revision performed was a side-to-side enteroenterostomy 100 cm proximal to the junction of the alimentary and biliary limb (kissing X anastomosis) as previously published [23]. Analysis from the California SID showed that readmissions for a nutrition/endocrine/metabolic and immunity disorder occurred in 8.3% of DS patients. This rate was significantly higher than for both open and laparoscopic RYGB patients. Severe persistent malabsorption requiring revisional surgery is a serious complication rarely seen in laparoscopic or open gastric bypass or laparoscopic band procedures. It is more specific to the malabsorptive procedures such as the DS and the BPD and can potentially lead to cirrhosis and death in extreme cases. Baltasar and colleagues in a series of 470 patients with DS reported 10 cases of patients with hepatic impairment that reversed under medical treatment, except 1 patient died while waiting for a liver transplant [24]. Nelson and colleagues [9] showed that in the long-term, 1 of every 24 DS patients developed a major nutritional deficiency, compared with 1 in every 48 people who had had a gastric bypass. Similarly, in the California SID, the odds of readmission for liver disease after a DS were 4 times greater than after an open RYGB and 6.5 times greater than after a laparoscopic RYGB. Baltasar and colleagues' explanation for the hepatic impairment after DS included the negative energy balance, bacterial overgrowth in the biliopancreatic limb, and accumulation of free fatty acids on a predisposed nonalcoholic steatohepatitis fatty liver. Hess and colleagues, who pioneered the DS, published a 4% revision rate for protein malnutrition [25], and Scopinaro warned that the BPD was "a powerful weapon, potentially dangerous if used improperly" [26].

The malabsorptive effects of the DS on pregnancy were studied by Maggard and colleagues [27]. These investigators found that the rates of many adverse maternal and neonatal outcomes may be lower in women who become pregnant after having bariatric surgery compared with the rates of obese pregnant women. These investigators did note an increase in the incidence of macrosomia and lower birth weight, and a higher miscarriage and preterm delivery in the biliopancreatic group, caused by the nutritional deficiencies associated with the malabsorptive nature of the procedure. Parenteral nutrition was used in 20% of pregnancies after BPD. Similar results were reported by Cools [28].

The incidence of gastroesophageal reflux disease (GERD) in the USC cohort was 5.5%. Half of these patients (2.75%) presented with de novo GERD after the procedure. We believe the vertical sleeve gastrectomy to be responsible for this complication. Himpens and colleagues, in a recent review of long-term results after a laparoscopic gastric sleeve procedure, found a preoperative incidence of GERD Of 3.3%, which increased postoperatively to 23% on a 6-year follow-up in the pure sleeve group and to 26% in the sleeve + DS group [29]. Thus, there seem to be 2 peaks of incidence of postoperative GERD after sleeve gastrectomy: one at 1 year, perhaps caused by a narrowing at the gastric incisura that improves over time, allowing for a better gastric emptying; and a second peak at 6 years caused by a neofundus formation near to the angle of His, allowing for an increased gastric acid production and resulting reflux disease. In the SID data, the incidence of gastric and esophageal disorders resulting in a readmission was similar for each of the 3 bariatric procedures. As Himpens and colleagues [29] pointed out, it may be that longer follow-up is needed before noticeable foregut problems develop in the California SID dataset.

Other long-term postoperative complications such as intestinal hernia and intestinal obstruction occurring in the DS patients appeared at a similar rate to those found in the open RYGB patients. Because both these complication rates are significantly lower in the laparoscopic RYGB patients, it seems that these compilations are technique-related and not procedure-related. The only outcome that appeared to be less problematic in the RGYB patients was upper GI hemorrhage. It seems that the gastrojejunal anastomosis is more prone to bleeding than the duodenojeunal anastomosis.

Mortality

The perioperative mortality for the DS patients was 0.9%, 0.6%, and 2% for the USC, NSQIP, and SID cohort of patients. This rate was similar to that of the RYGB patients in the NSQIP and SID cohort. In the USC cohort, rhabdomyolysis was responsible for 3 deaths in 6 patients who presented with this complex condition in the early period, and the lessons learned, such as limiting the duration of the operation, special positioning with additional padding in large male diabetic patients, and better management of postoperative increase of creatine phosphokinase levels, contributed to improved results because this complication has not been encountered in the last 9 years [30]. The early mortality is not different from any published in large series and meta-analysis, which varies between 1.4% and 1.6%. Buchwald and colleagues in a meta-analysis published in 2007 showed an early mortality of 0.9% and 0.7% for the open and laparoscopic DS group, respectively, and a mortality between 30 days and 2 years of 1.7% for the open DS [7,8,31]. Gupta and colleagues in a recent review of the NSQIP data published a risk of death within 30 days of 1.7% for the DS, 0.2% for the laparoscopic RYGB, and 0.7% for open RYGB [32]. Podnos reported similar rates [33].

The effects of the steep learning curve of this relatively complex procedure is evident: the group from Quebec published a recent study with a low 0.1% perioperative mortality in the laparoscopic group for patients operated after 2006, when compared with 1% before 2006 [20]. These investigators attributed the improvements to the high-volume centers that care for high-risk patients, the better preparation and selection of these patients, and the introduction of laparoscopy. The investigators insisted on a potential study bias because the younger, lighter patients were offered a laparoscopic approach, and the heavier and sicker patients were oriented to the laparoscopic sleeve operation (patients who were not included in their study). The complication rate in their laparoscopic group was similar to the open group (7% vs 7.4%), indicating no advantage of the laparoscopic approach for the DS. Similarly, in this review of the NSQIP data, the overall complication rate for the laparoscopic DS was similar to that of the open DS (12% vs 9%, $P = .328$). By contrast, in the NSQIP dataset, the overall complication rates for the laparoscopic RYGB are significantly lower that for the open RYGB (12% vs 5%, $P < .001$). In the series of Topart and colleagues, the learning curve was evaluated at 89 cases [34]. A recent study included data from a group that began offering both open and laparoscopic DS in 2009. These investigators compared their experience with the previous laparoscopic RYGB experience [35]. The conversion from the laparoscopic to the open DS in this series was 25%, and the early major complication rate of the laparoscopic group was 20% when compared with 17% in the open group. These investigators also reported a 45% overall complication rate in the laparoscopic group versus 26% in the open group [35]. This anomaly of the switch procedure, which, unlike other procedures, shows no reduction in morbidity when performed laparoscopically, has and most probably always will hinder more widespread adoption of this operation.

Fazylov and colleagues in 385 patients reported a significantly higher mortality of 7.8% in the supersuperobese (BMI >60 kg/m^2) category compared with 0 in the group between BMI 35 kg/m^2 and BMI 60 kg/m^2 [36]. Kim and colleagues reported a mortality of 7.6% in the laparoscopic DS group versus 3.5% in the open DS group in the same heavy category [37]. A recent study published a 53.8% complication rate and a death rate of 7.2% in the same category of patients with a BMI greater than 60 kg/m^2, and the investigators recommended a 2-stage approach, including a laparoscopic sleeve gastrectomy as the first step [34].

The overall long-term mortality for the USC cohort was 7.2%. This number may not be a true reflection of the deaths directly related to the DS, because there were several patients for whom the reasons for death were unknown. Nevertheless, this mortality is higher than the overall mortality published by several long-term studies that included patients who underwent a gastric bypass. In the Swedish Obese Subjects (SOS) study, the cumulative overall mortality during a follow-up of up to 16 years was 5% in the surgical group when compared with 6.3% in the control nonsurgical group [38]. Adams and colleagues evaluated the long-term mortality from 1984 to 2002 among 9942 patients who underwent a gastric bypass matched to a control nonsurgical group and found a mortality of 2.7% in the surgical RYGB group versus 4.1% in the control [39].

The DS procedure is the most potent operation for weight loss, yielding the highest excess body weight loss among all weight loss procedures. A minimum of 70% EBWL on long-term follow-up is usually obtained and sustained [8,10]; It is also the most powerful in terms of reduction of comorbidities, especially for type 2 diabetes [8,9]. These excellent functional results come with a safety cost, as discussed earlier. It can be argued that the laparoscopic DS can yield better results in terms of morbidity and mortality, but the comparative nonrandomized and randomized studies have failed to show a significant difference and improvement between the 2 approaches [11,18]. Moreover, one would intuitively think that the heavier patients with a BMI more than 50 kg/m^2 might benefit more from a more efficient malabsorptive procedure, but Biron and colleagues found that DS patients with an initial BMI more than 50 kg/m^2 lost less, gained more weight rapidly postoperatively, and at 10 years, 41% still had a BMI greater than 40 kg/m^2 and 70% a BMI of 35 kg/m^2 or greater. More than 50% of the patients in this group were unsatisfied [40]. In addition, the surgical mortality in these super morbidly obese DS patients was higher.

Based on this review, the DS should not be routinely recommended as a primary procedure for morbid obesity. It seems difficult to justify offering this procedure as a surgical option to obese patients given the complications, complexity of the operation, and the high complication rate, which affect more than one-third of patients. One should also be cautious in offering DS to young women of childbearing age because of the potential side effects of nutritional deficiencies on the pregnancies [27,28]. In patients with a high BMI more than 60 kg/m^2, 1 option proposed by some investigators involves a 2-step laparoscopic sleeve gastrectomy followed by a laparoscopic DS in the case of failure of the sleeve [34,41–43]. Relative to the gold standard laparoscopic RYGB procedure, the DS is not safe. It has significantly higher short-term and long-term complications and a higher incidence of readmission and reoperations. Perhaps, the time has come to reevaluate this procedure and relegate it to the status of other abandoned bariatric procedures like the vertical banded gastroplasty.

Acknowledgments

I acknowledge Dr Naila Khalaf and Dr Evgeniya Degnera for their help in data collection of the USC dataset, and Dr Namir Katkhouda and Dr Joerg Zehetner for their input and feedback regarding the USC dataset.

References

[1] Hess DS, Hess DW. Biliopancreatic diversion with a duodenal switch. Obes Surg 1998;8(3):267–82.
[2] Scopinaro N, Gianetta E, Pandolfo N, et al. Bilio-pancreatic bypass. Proposal and preliminary experimental study of a new type of operation for the functional surgical treatment of obesity. Minerva Chir 1976;31(10):560–6 [in Italian].
[3] DeMeester TR, Fuchs KH, Ball CS, et al. Experimental and clinical results with proximal end-to-end duodenojejunostomy for pathologic duodenogastric reflux. Ann Surg 1987;206(4): 414–26.
[4] Marceau P, Biron S, Bourque RA, et al. Biliopancreatic diversion with a new type of gastrectomy. Obes Surg 1993;3(1):29–35.
[5] Rabkin RA, Rabkin JM, Metcalf B, et al. Laparoscopic technique for performing duodenal switch with gastric reduction. Obes Surg 2003;13(2):263–8.
[6] Ren CJ, Patterson E, Gagner M. Early results of laparoscopic biliopancreatic diversion with duodenal switch: a case series of 40 consecutive patients. Obes Surg 2000;10(6):514–23 [discussion: 524].
[7] Anthone GJ, Lord RV, DeMeester TR, et al. The duodenal switch operation for the treatment of morbid obesity. Ann Surg 2003;238(4):618–27 [discussion: 627–8].
[8] Buchwald H, Estok R, Fahrbach K, et al. Weight and type 2 diabetes after bariatric surgery: systematic review and meta-analysis. Am J Med 2009;122(3):248–256.e5.
[9] Nelson DW, Blair KS, Martin MJ. Analysis of obesity-related outcomes and bariatric failure rates with the duodenal switch vs gastric bypass for morbid obesity. Arch Surg 2012;147(9):847–54.
[10] Marceau P, Biron S, Hould FS, et al. Duodenal switch: long-term results. Obes Surg 2007;17(11):1421–30.
[11] Sovik TT, Taha O, Aasheim ET, et al. Randomized clinical trial of laparoscopic gastric bypass versus laparoscopic duodenal switch for superobesity. Br J Surg 2010;97(2):160–6.
[12] ACS-NSQIP. User Guide for the Participant Use Data File 2007. 2012. Available at: http://site.acsnsqip.org/wp-content/uploads/2012/03/ACS-NSQIP-Participant-User-Data-File-User-Guide_06.pdf. Accessed October 12, 2012.
[13] Ho D, Imai K, King G, et al. Matching as nonparametric preprocessing for reducing model dependence in parametric causal inference. Polit Anal 2007;15(3):199–236.
[14] Ho D, Imai K, King G, et al. Matchit: nonparametric preprocessing for parametric causal inference. J Stat Software 2011;42(8):1–28.
[15] Team RDC. R: a language and environment for statistical computing 2011. 2012. Available at: http://www.r-project.org. Accessed October 12, 2012.
[16] Databases H. Healthcare Cost and Utilization Project (HCUP). 2012. Available at: http://www.hcup-us.ahrq.gov. Accessed February 1, 2012.
[17] Sovik TT, Aasheim ET, Taha O, et al. Weight loss, cardiovascular risk factors, and quality of life after gastric bypass and duodenal switch: a randomized trial. Ann Intern Med 2011;155(5):281–91.
[18] Dolan K, HatzifoGs M, Newbury L, et al. A clinical and nutritional comparison of biliopancreatic diversion with and without duodenal switch. Ann Surg 2004;240(1):51–6.
[19] Biertho L, Biron S, Hould FS, et al. Is biliopancreatic diversion with duodenal switch indicated for patients with body mass index <50 kg/m^2? Surg Obes Relat Dis 2010;6(5): 508–14.
[20] Biertho L, Lebel S, Marceau S, et al. Perioperative complications in a consecutive series of 1000 duodenal switches. Surg Obes Relat Dis 2013;9(1):63–8.

[21] Marceau P, Marceau S, Biron S, et al. Long-term experience with duodenal switch in adolescents. Obes Surg 2010;20(12):1609–16.
[22] Finks JF, Kole KL, Yenumula PR, et al. Predicting risk for serious complications with bariatric surgery: results from the Michigan Bariatric Surgery Collaborative. Ann Surg 2011;254(4): 633–40.
[23] Hamoui N, Chock B, Anthone GJ, et al. Revision of the duodenal switch: indications, technique, and outcomes. J Am Coll Surg 2007;204(4):603–8.
[24] Baltasar A, Serra C, Perez N, et al. Clinical hepatic impairment after the duodenal switch. Obes Surg 2004;14(1):77–83.
[25] Hess DS, Hess DW, Oakley RS. The biliopancreatic diversion with the duodenal switch: results beyond 10 years. Obes Surg 2005;15(3):408–16.
[26] Scopinaro N. Biliopancreatic diversion: mechanisms of action and long-term results. Obes Surg 2006;16(6):683–9.
[27] Maggard MA, Yermilov I, Li Z, et al. Pregnancy and fertility following bariatric surgery: a systematic review. JAMA 2008;300(19):2286–96.
[28] Cools M, Duval EL, Jespers A. Adverse neonatal outcome after maternal biliopancreatic diversion operation: report of nine cases. Eur J Pediatr 2006;165(3):199–202.
[29] Himpens J, Dobbeleir J, Peeters G. Long-term results of laparoscopic sleeve gastrectomy for obesity. Ann Surg 2010;252(2):319–24.
[30] Bostanjian D, Anthone GJ, Hamoui N, et al. Rhabdomyolysis of gluteal muscles leading to renal failure: a potentially fatal complication of surgery in the morbidly obese. Obes Surg 2003;13(2):302–5.
[31] Buchwald H, Estok R, Fahrbach K, et al. Trends in mortality in bariatric surgery: a systematic review and meta-analysis. Surgery 2007;142(4):621–32 [discussion: 632–5].
[32] Gupta PK, Franck C, Miller WJ, et al. Development and validation of a bariatric surgery morbidity risk calculator using the prospective, multicenter NSQIP dataset. J Am Coll Surg 2011;212(3):301–9.
[33] Podnos YD, Jimenez JC, Wilson SE, et al. Complications after laparoscopic gastric bypass: a review of 3464 cases. Arch Surg 2003;138(9):957–61.
[34] Topart P, Becouarn G, Ritz P. Should biliopancreatic diversion with duodenal switch be done as single-stage procedure in patients with BMI > or = 50 kg/m^2? Surg Obes Relat Dis 2010;6(1):59–63.
[35] Nelson D, Beekley A, Carter P, et al. Early results after introduction of biliopancreatic diversion/duodenal switch at a military bariatric center. Am J Surg 2011;201(5):678–84.
[36] Fazylov RM, Savel RH, Horovitz JH, et al. Association of super-super-obesity and male gender with elevated mortality in patients undergoing the duodenal switch procedure. Obes Surg 2005;15(5):618–23.
[37] Kim WW, Gagner M, Kini S, et al. Laparoscopic vs. open biliopancreatic diversion with duodenal switch: a comparative study. J Gastrointest Surg 2003;7(4):552–7.
[38] Sjostrom L, Narbro K, Sjostrom CD, et al. Effects of bariatric surgery on mortality in Swedish obese subjects. N Engl J Med 2007;357(8):741–52.
[39] Adams TD, Gress RE, Smith SC, et al. Long-term mortality after gastric bypass surgery. N Engl J Med 2007;357(8):753–61.
[40] Biron S, Hould FS, Lebel S, et al. Twenty years of biliopancreatic diversion: what is the goal of the surgery? Obes Surg 2004;14(2):160–4.
[41] Dapri G, Cadiere GB, Himpens J. Superobese and super-superobese patients: 2-step laparoscopic duodenal switch. Surg Obes Relat Dis 2011;7(6):703–8.
[42] Iannelli A, Schneck AS, Dahman M, et al. Two-step laparoscopic duodenal switch for superobesity: a feasibility study. Surg Endosc 2009;23(10):2385–9.
[43] Silecchia G, Rizzello M, Casella G, et al. Two-stage laparoscopic biliopancreatic diversion with duodenal switch as treatment of high-risk super-obese patients: analysis of complications. Surg Endosc 2009;23(5):1032–7.

Advances in Surgery 47 (2013) 177–197
ADVANCES IN SURGERY

Is Propranolol of Benefit in Pediatric Burn Patients?

Celeste C. Finnerty, PhD[a,b,c], David N. Herndon, MD[a,b,*]

[a]Shriners Hospitals for Children, 815 Market Street, Galveston, TX 77550, USA; [b]Department of Surgery, University of Texas Medical Branch, 301 University Boulevard, Galveston, TX 77550, USA; [c]Institute for Translational Sciences, Sealy Center for Molecular Medicine, University of Texas Medical Branch, 301 University Boulevard, Galveston, TX 77550, USA

Keywords

• Propranolol • Burns • Beta blockade • Hypermetabolic response • Pediatric • Catabolism • Cardiac stress • Safety

Key points

- In severely burned children, propagation of the catecholamine-induced hypermetabolic response can be reduced by propranolol administration.
- The degree of mitigation of the deleterious effects of burn injury depends on the dose of propranolol and duration of administration.
- By achieving a decrease in resting heart rate of 15% to 20%, cardiac work is significantly reduced over time.
- Proteolysis and lipolysis are similarly reduced, as a result of the decrease in resting energy expenditure and potentiation of catecholamine signaling. Instead of the typical net proteolysis that occurs after a severe burn injury, skeletal muscle protein synthesis is increased.

INTRODUCTION

Severe burn injuries result in metabolic and physiologic derangements that persist throughout the acute and rehabilitative stages [1–3]. This hypermetabolic response is driven by supraphysiologic increases in stress hormones,

Funding: This study was supported by grants from Shriners Hospitals for Children (84080, 71001, 71008, 8660, 8760, 8740, 8507 and 9145), National Institutes of Health (R01 GM56687, T32 GM008256, P50 GM60338), and the National Institute for Disabilities and Rehabilitation Research (H133A070026, H133A70019, and H133A120091), CCF is an Institute for Translational Sciences Career Development Scholar supported, in part, by NIH (KL2RR029875 and UL1RR029876). This study is registered at clinicaltrials.gov, NCT00675714.
Disclosure: The authors declare no conflicts of interest.

*Corresponding author. Shriners Hospitals for Children, 815 Market Street, Galveston, TX 77550. *E-mail address*: dherndon@utmb.edu

0065-3411/13/$ – see front matter
http://dx.doi.org/10.1016/j.yasu.2013.02.001

catecholamines, and inflammatory mediators [2,3]. Increased peripheral lipolysis [4], increased muscle wasting [5], increased resting energy expenditure [6], and suppressed immune function [7] characterize the postburn hypermetabolic response. Although the initial catecholamine-induced response is protective and supportive of survival [8], the prolonged stress response can be detrimental and either impedes recovery or leads to organ failure and death [5]. In addition to increasing skeletal muscle catabolism, increased catecholamine levels also cause increases in peripheral lipolysis, resting energy expenditure, and cardiac stress in severely burned patients [9]. The actions of catecholamines on the cardiovascular system are largely mediated by the α and β adrenergic receptors. The effects of chronically increased catecholamine levels on the hypermetabolic response after burn injury have been mitigated through blockade of the β1 and β2 adrenoreceptors with the nonselective β1,2 adrenoreceptor antagonist propranolol [9–17]. Despite the notion that blocking the stress response would negatively affect hemodynamic and metabolic responsiveness [9,10], studies have demonstrated that blockade of catecholamine signaling improves outcomes in pediatric burn patients [9–19]. Reductions in cardiac work and cardiac stress are accompanied by decreased lipolysis, catabolism, and hepatic steatosis, with concurrent increases in skeletal muscle protein anabolism. Few adverse events have been associated with propranolol use [13–15]. Propranolol administration to massively burned patients may be a standard of care for the pharmacologic amelioration of the hypermetabolic response in the not-so-distant future.

THE HYPERMETABOLIC RESPONSE TO BURN INJURY

The extensive hypermetabolic response after a severe burn injury affects many organ systems and persists for up to 2 years after the injury [2,20]. The chances of survival are improved by this adaptive response, enabling increased metabolic demands to be met through stepped up mobilization of energy substrates by tissue catabolism [8]. With current nutritional support regimens meeting the metabolic requirements of the severely burned patient, however, this stress response results in excess tissue catabolism that negatively affects patient outcome [8]. After injury, metabolic activity and tissue perfusion immediately decrease during the early ebb phase, which lasts for 2 to 3 days [21]. This is soon followed by a long-lasting flow phase, which is defined by hypercatabolism and hyperdynamic circulation. Medical support of the flow phase is necessary to avoid physiologic exhaustion and death [1,5,22]. In severely burned children, the hallmarks of this hypermetabolic response include increased metabolic rates, hyperdynamic circulation, lipolysis, catabolism of muscle and bone, hepatic steatosis, infections, insulin resistance, and growth retardation [2,4,20,22–28].

Substrates supporting increased metabolic demands are released by catabolism of tissue fuel stores [5,29]. Lipolysis, glycolysis, and proteolysis lead to excess free substrate that then must be used, eliminated, or stored. In response to increased catecholamine levels, fatty acids and triglycerides are released into the plasma by lipolysis [4,9]. Free fatty acids not used for fuel are typically deposited in the liver or in peripheral muscle, leading to dysfunction in these tissues. Proteolysis releases amino acids, which are either used to build new proteins or, more frequently, catabolized and eliminated, creating a negative nitrogen balance [5,20]. Protein loss and subsequent negative nitrogen balance are proportional to injury severity and the metabolic response. Extensive reduction of lean body mass through the hypercatabolic response has detrimental effects on survival and recovery. After reductions of up to 10% of lean body mass, immune dysfunction occurs. Wound healing is impaired with losses of up to 20% of lean body mass. The risk of pressure sores and pneumonia increases with lean body mass losses of up to 30%. With losses of lean body mass equal to or in excess of 40%, death is almost certain [30]. Nitrogen loss in excess of 20 to 25 g/m^2 of total body surface area (TBSA) per day induces catabolism-associated mortality [5,31]. In pediatric burn patients who survive, protein catabolism significantly retards growth as well [32]. Circumvention or mitigation of the hypermetabolic response is necessary to reduce tissue catabolism [5].

The 10-fold increase in plasma catecholamines after a burn injury induces hyperdynamic, metabolic, catabolic, and inflammatory responses that persist for several years [2]. Chronic increases in epinephrine and norepinephrine continue for ~2 months and a year after injury, respectively [2,33]. Although systemically increased in the plasma, heightened elimination of urinary catecholamines accompanies increased plasma catecholamine levels, demonstrating depletion of catecholamine reserves [9,34]. Severe catecholamine depletion is associated with development of sepsis and death. Attenuation of the postburn catecholamine surge may improve patient outcomes.

EFFECT OF BURN INJURY ON CARDIAC FUNCTION

Increased plasma catecholamines contribute to postburn cardiac stress [3,9]. During the ebb phase, reduced cardiac output is caused by hypovolemia and decreased venous return. Circulating endogenous vasoconstrictors and inflammatory signals worsen cardiac output by decreasing preload along with depressed myocardial contractility. Surges in catecholamines, cortisol, and glucagon during the subsequent flow phase lead to a hyperdynamic cardiovascular state characterized by tachycardia, local myocardial hypoxia, and increased myocardial oxygen consumption. Burn-induced increases in resting heart rate, cardiac output, cardiac work, and resting energy expenditure can lead to physiologic exhaustion unless steps are taken to attenuate this response [28,35]. Significant cardiac morbidity and mortality can occur as a result of chronically increased catecholamine levels that stimulate prolonged cardiac stress [36,37].

In a comparison of severely burned children with normal, age-matched, nonburned children, pathologic increases in average heart rate, rate pressure product, cardiac index, and cardiac output were found to persist for at least 2 years ($P<.05$) [28]. Burn injury did not affect stroke volume or mean arterial pressure, and the ejection fraction was only increased for the first 2 weeks after burn injury before returning to normal levels. Reduced cardiac efficiency was suggested by the increase in rate pressure product, a correlate of myocardial oxygen consumption. Prolonged increases in cardiac work typically decrease the efficiency of oxygen delivery by the heart [38]. Compensatory increases in arterial oxygen content and cardiac output are therefore required to ensure adequate oxygen delivery. Although cardiac function seemed to be preserved, as indicated by normal ejection fraction despite chronic catecholamine stimulation, it is unknown whether this prolonged increase in work eventually results in cardiac failure in these patients. Persistently increased catecholamine levels, resulting in sympathetic overstimulation and cardiac failure, indicate that the cardiovascular response may also exceed the metabolic demands of the patients. Although increases in epinephrine and norepinephrine are typically associated with increased heart rate and stroke volume, this was not the case in children with massive burn injuries. The lack of increase in stroke volume may represent derangements in the β adrenergic receptor signaling pathways, resulting in decreased tissue sensitivity to chronically increased levels of catecholamines [38,39].

BETA BLOCKADE IN SEVERELY BURNED ADULTS

The ability of catecholamines to initiate and propagate the hypermetabolic response was demonstrated by Wilmore and colleagues [9] in 1974. By administering α and β adrenoreceptor blocking agents, the role of the β adrenergic receptor in potentiating postburn increases in metabolic rate, blood pressure, pulse, and free fatty acid levels was demonstrated. The participation of the α adrenergic receptor in these burn-induced responses was ruled out as well. The administration of catecholamines to nonburned volunteers demonstrated that epinephrine infusion was sufficient to induce a partial hypermetabolic response as characterized by nitrogen loss, increased respiration and metabolism, and altered levels of blood glucose, free fatty acids, glucagon, and growth hormone. The role of catecholamines in initiating the hypermetabolic response was clearly established. These early studies suggested the possibility of pharmacologically reducing the hypermetabolic response to burn injury with β blockade.

ADMINISTRATION OF PROPRANOLOL TO REDUCE THE HYPERMETABOLIC RESPONSE IN SEVERELY BURNED CHILDREN

Over the past 25 years, mitigation of the effects of chronically increased catecholamines through β adrenergic receptor blockade has been established as an effective strategy for reducing postburn hypercatabolism and cardiac stress [10–12,14–19]. Propranolol, a nonselective β1, β2 adrenergic receptor antagonist, is commonly used to reduce tachycardia and hypertension by preventing catecholamine binding to β adrenoreceptors. Furthermore, propranolol has been used to treat myriad pediatric conditions with few serious adverse events [14]. From the initial study to determine whether propranolol administration jeopardized metabolic and hemodynamic stability [10], to the recent demonstration of the long-term safety and efficacy of propranolol administration [14], the authors have demonstrated that propranolol administration to decrease the heart rate by 15% to 20% improves outcomes in children with large burn injuries.

To elucidate whether deleterious effects resulted from blunting the catecholamine-induced response to burn injury, our group initiated β blockade for short periods during early experiments. After the safety and efficacy of each evaluation was demonstrated, the duration of propranolol administration was slowly extended from several days to the entire first postburn year. The rest of this article is divided into 2 sections: (1) acute administration during the initial admission to the intensive care unit (ICU) and (2) long-term administration, which was initiated within several days of admission and continued throughout the first year after burn injury. In all of the evaluations presented here, the control and propranolol-treated cohorts were similar, with no differences in age, burn size, time to admission, and other demographic and clinical evaluations performed before propranolol administration.

PROPRANOLOL ADMINISTRATION DURING ACUTE HOSPITALIZATION

Hemodynamic and metabolic stability

The effects of propranolol on hemodynamic and metabolic responsiveness were studied in 40 severely burned children [10]. Twenty-two control and 18 propranolol-treated patients were studied. Propranolol was administered for 5 days at a dose of 2 mg/kg/d. We hypothesized that propranolol would reduce myocardial work, lipolysis, and tremulousness without negatively affecting cardiac output, metabolic rate, or protein breakdown. When administered during the hyperdynamic flow phase, propranolol significantly decreased heart rate, left ventricular work, and the rate pressure product ($P<.05$). Differences in basal resting energy expenditure, PaO_2/FiO_2 ratios, arterial-venous blood oxygen content differences, or oxygen consumption were not found. Adequate oxygen delivery and cardiac output were maintained, and oxygen consumption was not increased after propranolol treatment. Metabolic rate was not affected during this short 5-day infusion protocol either. Tremulousness, agitation, and anxiety were also reduced in those patients treated with propranolol. This study was the first to show that heart rate could be safely reduced by the chronic infusion of propranolol for 5 days in severely burned children without jeopardizing hemodynamic stability.

Cardiac work

Administration of propranolol was then extended to determine whether the positive effects on cardiac work continued with extended administration [19]. Twenty-two patients were studied. Propranolol was administered every 8 hours for 10 days to reduce the heart rate by 10% to 20%. With longer duration of therapy, a sustained decrease in heart rate was observed along with a decrease in the rate pressure product. Cardiac stress was also reduced after propranolol treatment, as indicated by decreased myocardial oxygen consumption. Tachyphylaxis did not result after longer administration of propranolol. Because most children who die as a result of massive burn injuries exhibit myocardial damage (eg, subendocardial ischemia or focal myocardial necrosis), reduction in cardiac stress decreased burn-induced morbidity. This study confirmed that longer administration of propranolol could be used to safely reduce cardiac complications.

Propranolol administration was then extended for the duration of the acute hospitalization period and cardiac function was again assessed [13]. Of the 406 severely burned children enrolled, 235 were randomized to control therapy and 171 were randomized to propranolol therapy. Propranolol was initiated within 24 to 72 hours of admission and given to decrease the heart rate by ~20%. Within 2 days of the initiation of propranolol treatment, significant reductions in resting heart rates occurred ($P<.001$) (Fig. 1). This decrease was noted throughout the study period until the time of discharge. Compared with predicted heart rates for age, the percent of predicted heart rate in the propranolol cohort decreased by 15% compared with the 18% decrease in control patients ($P<.001$). Significant reductions in the rate pressure product and myocardial oxygen consumption throughout the study period were attributed to propranolol administration ($P<.001$). Differences were not found in an age-dependent or sex-dependent manner. By the twentieth postburn day, an increase in propranolol dose to 4 mg/kg/d was necessary to maintain the reduction in heart rate. Cardiac index was not altered with propranolol administration. Significantly greater stroke volumes were found in the propranolol cohort: 112% ± 8% compared with 94% ± 5% in controls ($P<.02$).

These findings demonstrate that administration of propranolol improves cardiac physiology for the duration of acute hospitalization. In the immediate postburn period, cardiac output decreases, whereas myocardial oxygen consumption increases. When hyperdynamic circulation develops, heart rates increase greatly, leading to less time for ventricular filling and reduced stroke volumes. Cardiac output and myocardial oxygen typically increase during this phase. Propranolol administration during the hyperdynamic phase decreased myocardial oxygen consumption. Cardiac stress was further reduced by decreasing heart rate and stroke volumes. Decreasing these parameters greatly decreases cardiac morbidity and the likelihood of physiologic exhaustion. These beneficial effects of propranolol on cardiac parameters demonstrate its clinical usefulness for reducing cardiac stress in severely burned patients.

Fat metabolism

The reduction of free fatty acids in propranolol-treated adults suggested an effect of propranolol on reducing the availability of the primary energy substrate that fuels hypermetabolism. The authors determined whether lipolysis was mediated via the β1 or the β2 adrenergic receptor [40]. Patients were administered either the β1 selective antagonist metoprolol or the nonspecific β1,2 antagonist propranolol during 8-hour intervals for 5 days. Initial dosing with 2 mg/kg/

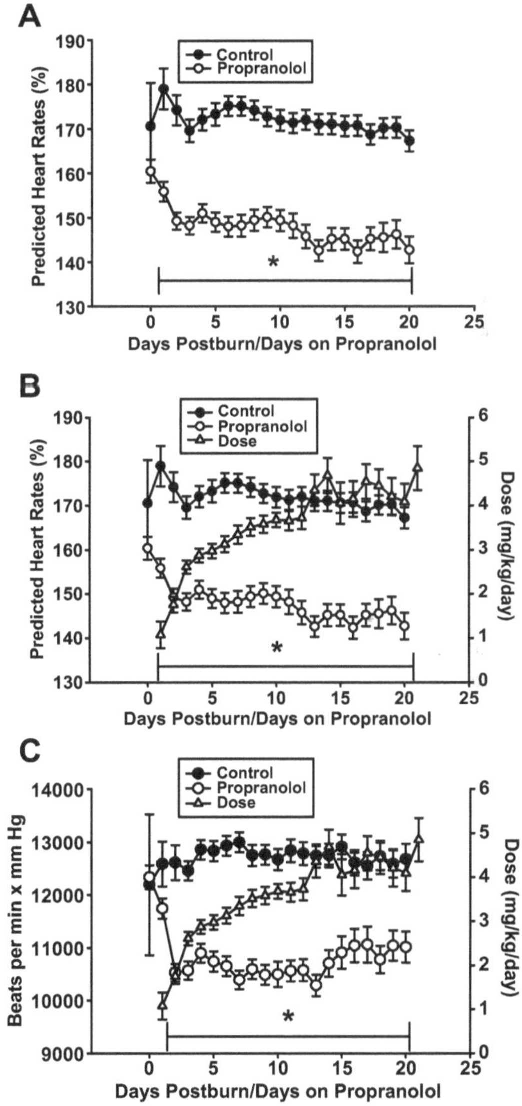

Fig. 1. Heart rate in the acute phase is decreased with propranolol treatment. (*A*) Percent predicted heart rate in control patients and patients receiving propranolol, which was titrated to decrease heart rate by 15–20% from the time of admission. (*B*) Percent predicted heart rate shown with the corresponding upward titration of propranolol dose. A dose of 4 mg/kg/day was required to decrease heart rate by 15–20%. (*C*) Rate pressure product. (*From* Williams FN, Herndon DN, Kulp GA, et al. Propranolol decreases cardiac work in a dose-dependent manner in severely burned children. Surgery 2011;149(2):234.)

d of each drug was titrated to reduce the baseline heart rate by 20%. Both metoprolol and propranolol significantly reduced cardiac work in severely burned children. Lipolysis, however, was only decreased by propranolol administration, demonstrating β2 selective mediation of peripheral lipolysis.

Previous work showed that increased peripheral lipolysis induces greater fatty acid reesterification to triacyglycerols in the liver [4]. In light of the reduction of lipolysis that accompanied propranolol administration, whether propranolol subsequently reduced the incidence of fatty infiltration of the liver was determined next.

Using stable isotope methods, the effects of propranolol on hepatic fat accumulation were determined by measuring the metabolism of splanchnic fatty acid and very low density lipoprotein-triacylglycerol (VLDL-TG) [16]. Fatty acid uptake, oxidation, and secretion in VLDL-TGs across the splanchnic bed were quantitated with and without propranolol treatment. Fatty acid availability and hepatic triacylglycerol storage were greatly reduced with propranolol treatment ($P<.05$). These results demonstrated that hepatic steatosis was reduced after propranolol treatment.

Subsequent studies demonstrated that the percent increase in liver size over expected normal values was also significantly reduced with propranolol treatment [17]. Most control patients (80%) had increases in liver size of 100% or more. Of the propranolol-treated patients, 86% experienced either a decrease or no change in liver size. Lipolysis was assessed by measuring plasma triglyceride levels and determining body composition. Plasma triglyceride levels were significantly reduced in patients receiving propranolol. Lipolysis was significantly greater in the control cohort as apparent by reduced peripheral and truncal fat mass. These studies showed that propranolol decreased lipolysis, availability of free fatty acids for accumulation in the liver, and subsequent development of hepatic steatosis.

Gene expression in adipose tissue from control and propranolol-treated patients was assessed to determine the potential mechanisms behind lipolysis reduction. Biopsies of adipose tissue were taken from control and propranolol-treated patients at 2 time points corresponding to (1) the second surgery and (2) 5 days later. The expression of 147 genes was affected by propranolol treatment; of these, 10 genes involved in lipid metabolism were reduced with propranolol treatment (Table 1). These results indicate that propranolol reduced peripheral lipolysis by decreasing lipid metabolism downstream of the β2 adrenoreceptor. Reduction in lipolysis led to decreased concentrations of circulating triglygerides and subsequent reduction of liver size and steatosis.

Muscle protein catabolism

Decreases in cardiac work, resting energy expenditure, and lipolysis in severely burned children treated with propranolol indicated an overall reduction of the hypermetabolic response, which led to the hypothesis that skeletal muscle catabolism would also be reduced with propranolol administration to reduce the heart rate by 15% to 20%. Patients were randomized to either the control

Table 1
Fat metabolism-related genes differentially expressed between control and propranolol-treated patients

Molecule name	Entrez gene ID for human	Molecule name	Fold change
ACAA2	10449	Acetyl-coenzyme A (CoA) acyltransferase 2	−6.7
ACACA	31	Acetyl-CoA carboxylase 1	−5.5
APOC1	341	Apolipoprotein C1	−5.5
FADS1	3992	Linoleoyl-CoA desaturase	−5.9
GPR137B	7107	G protein-coupled receptor 137B	−4.5
GPX4	2879	Glutathione peroxidase	−3.2
HADH	3033	Hydroxylacyl-CoA dehydrogenase	−5.4
ME1	4199	Malic enzyme 1	−4.8
SCD	6319	Stearoyl-CoA desaturase	−10.5
SCP2	6342	Propanoyl-CoA C-acyltransferase	−3

or propranolol cohort [12]. After 2 weeks of propranolol administration, a significant reduction in oxygen consumption and resting energy expenditure was found, confirming previous results. Stable isotope studies revealed an astounding improvement in the net skeletal muscle protein balance that was the result of a reduction in burn-induced proteolysis with an unexpected increase in muscle anabolism after propranolol administration (Fig. 2). Body

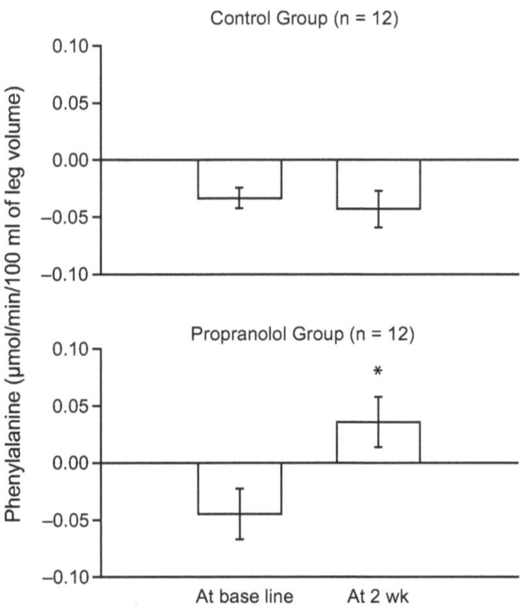

Fig. 2. Reduction in skeletal muscle catabolism accompanies an increase in skeletal muscle anabolism. (*From* Herndon DN, Hart DW, Wolf SE, et al. Reversal of catabolism by beta-blockade after severe burns. N Engl J Med 2001;345:1227; with permission.)

composition studies showed retention of both fat and fat-free mass in patients treated with propranolol, thereby validating the findings from stable isotope studies.

Elucidation of the mechanisms associated with reduction of skeletal muscle catabolism and the concurrent increase in muscle accretion was achieved by studying gene expression in muscle tissue biopsies from patients in each cohort [41]. A significant upregulation of 13 genes related to muscle metabolism was reported in patients treated with propranolol (Table 2). In these same patients, expression of 5 genes related to insulin resistance and gluconeogenesis was decreased. The restoration of metabolic functions in the skeletal muscle by improving cellular transport, prompting mRNA translation, protein export, and downregulation of inflammatory processes may be behind the reduction in catabolism and improved anabolism in skeletal muscle from patients treated with propranolol.

Infections and inflammation

Following reports of increased inflammation and infectious episodes associated with propranolol administration in the critically ill [42,43], the authors examined immune function in children with massive burns randomized to control or propranolol treatment [15]. End points included assessments of systemic cytokine expression, infectious episodes, and incidence of sepsis. Differences in the incidence of sepsis or other infections did not exist between the control and propranolol cohorts. At a single time point, minor alterations in tumor necrosis factor and interleukin-1β concentrations were found with propranolol treatment. Whether

Table 2
Muscle metabolism-related genes differentially expressed between control and propranolol-treated patients

Molecule name	Entrez gene ID for human	Molecule name	Fold change
BCL6	604	B-cell chronic lymphocytic leukemia (CLL) lymphoma 6	−1.7
BLCAP	10904	Bladder cancer associated protein	1.6
CD164	8763	CD164	1.6
DYNC1LI2	1783	Dynein	2.5
FAM127A	8933	Family with sequence similarity 127, member A	1.8
FBP2	8789	Fructose-1,6-bisphosphatase 2	−2.9
GADD45G	10912	Growth arrest and DNA damage inducible, gamma	2.6
HSPA5	3309	Heat shock 70 kDa protein 5	2.2
MAP3K5	4217	Mitogen-activated protein kinase kinase kinase 5	2.1
MDH1	4190	Malate dehydrogenase	1.5
MYL4	4635	Myosin light chain 4	−1.8
TNIP1	10318	TNFAIP3 interacting protein	2.1
VEGFA	7422	Vascular endothelial growth factor	−1.5

these changes have biological importance is unlikely given the small alterations at single time points. These results indicated that propranolol did not suppress immune function or induce inflammation in severely burned children.

Amelioration of the hypermetabolic response in the acute setting

The results of studies performed during the acute hospitalization period demonstrated that propranolol can be administered safely to severely burned children to reduce the postburn hypermetabolic response. Propranolol administration led to reductions in heart rate, cardiac work, lipolysis, hepatic steatosis, and skeletal muscle breakdown as well as increased creation of skeletal muscle. The lack of impact on immune function further supports the use of propranolol during acute hospitalization.

ADMINISTRATION OF PROPRANOLOL FOR 1 YEAR AFTER BURN INJURY

Characterization of the pathophysiologic response to burn injury has shown that the burn-induced hypermetabolic response lasts for at least 1 to 2 years after the injury [2,5]. We therefore extended β blockade with propranolol for a full year after burn injury [3,9,14]. The recent publication of the interim analysis of this ongoing clinical trial demonstrated continued safety and efficacy of long-term propranolol administration to reduce the hypermetabolic response in severely burned children. End points included cardiac function, resting energy expenditure, and body composition.

Patient population

In this randomized controlled trial, 179 patients were enrolled; 89 were randomized to the standard of care treatment group (control) and 90 patients randomized to receive propranolol administration (~4 mg/kg/d) to reduce heart rate by 15%. Propranolol treatment was initiated within 3 $\pm$ 2 days of admission. The patient groups were similar with respect to age, burn severity, incidence of inhalation injury, length of stay, and mortality.

Cardiac function

The percent of predicted heart rate was calculated to determine the effect of β blockade with propranolol on cardiac function [44,45]. During hospitalization, continuous measurements were recorded. After discharge, patients recorded their heart rate 4 times per day. Measurements were also conducted at each follow-up visit (3, 6, 9, and 12 months after burn injury). At the time of acute admission, heart rates were increased ~1.7-fold more than normal for age values in the control and propranolol cohorts (169% $\pm$ 34% predicted and 163% $\pm$ 33% predicted, respectively; $P = .19$) (Fig. 3A). Myocardial oxygen consumption was measured by calculating the rate pressure product (heart rate $\times$ mean arterial pressure) [45]. At the time of admission, both groups had rate pressure products that were increased by ~1.6-fold (control, 11,009 $\pm$ 280 beats per minute [bpm]; propranolol, 11,435 $\pm$ 304 bpm $\times$ mm Hg; $P = .66$). After initiation of propranolol administration, the percent of the

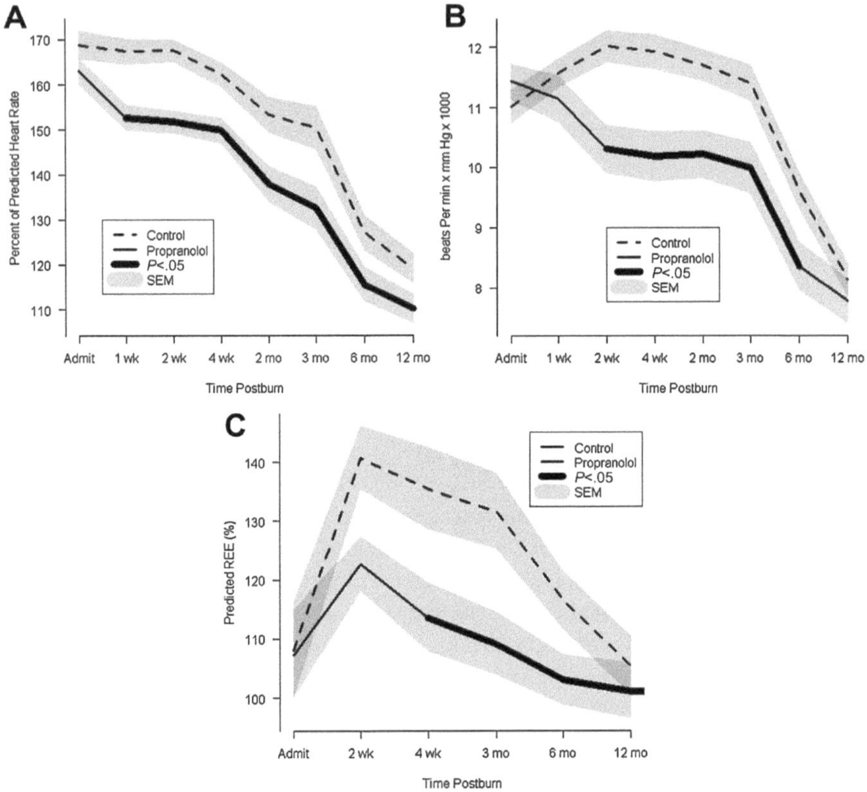

Fig. 3. Reduction in cardiac work and metabolic indices: (*A*) percent predicted heart rate; (*B*) rate pressure product; (*C*) resting energy expenditure (REE), expressed as the percentage of energy expenditure predicted by the Harris-Benedict equation. Data are shown as the Loess-smoothed trend with shading indicating the standard error of the mean (SEM). (*From* Herndon DN, Rodriguez NA, Diaz EC, et al. Long-term propranolol use in severely burned pediatric patients: a randomized controlled study. Ann Surg 2012;256:407; with permission.)

predicted heart rate was significantly decreased during the first postburn week and remained so for the duration of the study. At 1 year after burn injury, the percent of the predicted heart rates in the control cohort compared with the propranolol cohort remained significantly increased (119% ± 2% and 110% ± 2%, respectively; $P = .01$). Decreases in the rate pressure product of approximately 15% were apparent in the propranolol group from 2 weeks until 6 months after burn injury (see Fig. 3B). Mean arterial pressure recordings during the acute hospitalization period were used to determine the incidence of hypotension (<65 mm Hg). Hypotension was not found in either cohort. Although subtle decreases in mean arterial pressure were noted in propranolol-treated patients 2 weeks, 4 weeks, and 2 months after burn injury, the decreases were not significant after adjustments for multiple testing.

Hypermetabolism

As reported in our earlier studies, at the time of admission, all patients were hypermetabolic with increased basal metabolic rates predicted with the Harris-Benedict equation [46,47]. The percent of predicted resting energy expenditure was significantly decreased with propranolol treatment from the second postburn week until 6 months after burn injury ($P<.001$) (see Fig. 3C).

Body composition

Dual-image x-ray absorptiometry was used to measure body composition, including central mass, central fat mass, peripheral lean body mass (PLBM), total bone mineral content (TBMC), and total lumbar bone mineral (TLBMC) content. Total body mass (TBM) increased in both groups from the time of discharge until the 12-month time point. Although nutritional intake was similar between the groups, the control group exhibited significantly higher accretion of central mass. In the propranolol-treated group, as early as 3 months after burn injury, there was a 17% decrease in central mass. These differences remained significantly different throughout the study period ($P<.001$). The propranolol-treated group had significantly lower central fat mass, with a 23% maximal decrease 12 months after burn injury. PLBM increased 11% in the propranolol-treated group compared with the control cohort 6 months after burn injury. Lean body mass was also preserved with propranolol treatment at 3, 6, 9, and 12 months ($P = .02$). Furthermore, at 6 months after burn injury, treatment with propranolol decreased the likelihood of losing more than 5% of TBMC/TBM ($P = .01$). This effect persisted throughout the study (Fig. 4A–C).

Adverse events

Incidences of the following adverse events were collected prospectively: bradycardia, hypotension, hypoglycemia, respiratory arrest, cardiac arrhythmia, and death. There were 5 deaths in the placebo group. In the propranolol-treated group, few incidences of bradycardia (n = 2), hypotension (n = 0), hypoglycemia (n = 1), respiratory compromise (n = 2), cardiac arrhythmia (n = 1), or death (n = 4) were reported. Propranolol administration was halted after the adverse event and then reinitiated at a reduced dose. Sepsis, confirmed by autopsy, was the cause of death for the 5 control patients and 4 propranolol-treated patients.

Prolonged attenuation of the hypermetabolic response with the long-term administration of propranolol in severely burned children

This ongoing randomized controlled study was designed to test the efficacy of propranolol in reducing the hypermetabolic response in children with burns over 30% or more of the TBSA. Propranolol was administered at an approximate dose of 4 mg/kg/d beginning 96 hours after burn injury and ending 1 year later. This interim analysis showed that in severely burned children, the 4 mg/kg/d dose of propranolol was well tolerated with few related adverse events. Significant reductions in heart rate, cardiac work, resting energy expenditure, lipolysis, and catabolism of lean body mass and bone were found during most of the treatment period. The authors also found that although these

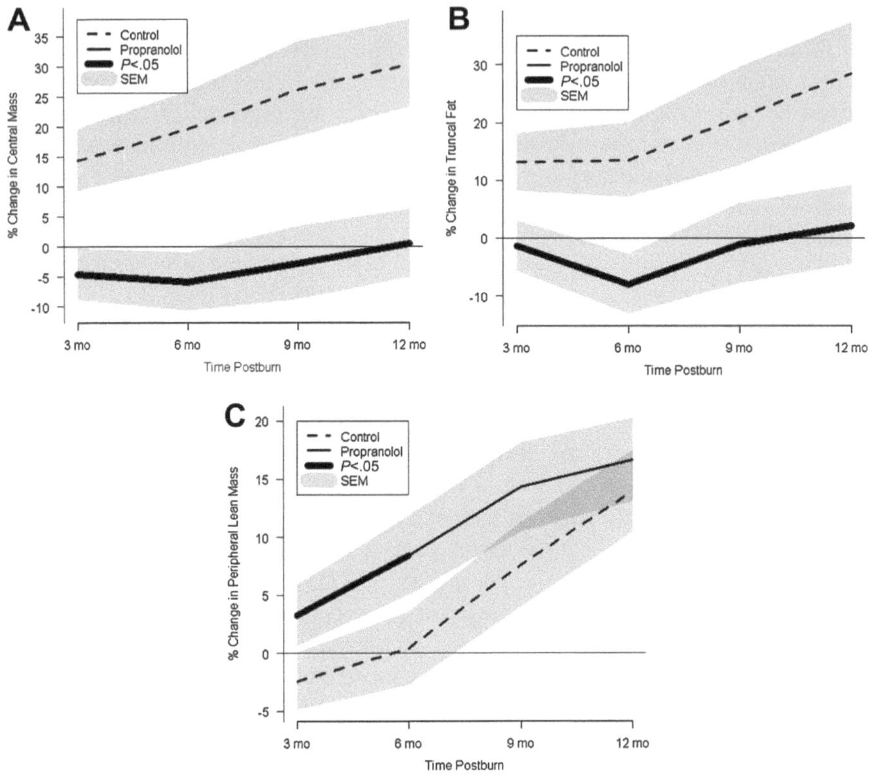

Fig. 4. Effect of propranolol on body composition. (*A*) Percent change in central mass; (*B*) percent change in truncal fat; and (*C*) percent change in peripheral lean mass. Data are expressed as percent change from patient baseline and are shown as the Loess-smoothed trend with shading indicating the standard error of the mean (SEM). *Significant difference at $P<.05$. (*From* Herndon DN, Rodriguez NA, Diaz EC, et al. Long-term propranolol use in severely burned pediatric patients: a randomized controlled study. Ann Surg 2012;256:408; with permission.)

aspects of the hypermetabolic response were attenuated with propranolol treatment, the measured parameters had not returned to normal levels by the time that administration was discontinued. This suggests that larger doses of propranolol, possibly administered for longer periods of time, may achieve even greater improvements in this patient population.

The long-term implications of the persistent postburn hypermetabolic response on cardiovascular morbidity and metabolism are unknown. Continued evaluations of these patients well into the next decades will be necessary to determine the effects of prolonged episodes of tachycardia and increased cardiac work and to evaluate whether the reductions in heart rate with propranolol administration reduce this morbidity. The long-term effects of reducing resting energy expenditure and body composition will be evaluated as the children achieve full growth by measuring height and weight velocities, growth, strength, and final stature. Body composition studies showed an overall decrease in the central deposition of fat and an increase in lead body mass with propranolol treatment. This decrease is likely to be related to the earlier findings of Morio and colleagues [16] and Herndon and colleagues [40] showing that peripheral lipolysis and subsequent development of hepatic steatosis are prevented with propranolol administration. By reducing peripheral lipolysis, the release of free fatty acids is decreased, leading to possible increases in insulin sensitivity. Lean body mass was increased in propranolol-treated patients. The low incidence of associated adverse events along with marked reduction in cardiac stress and the hypermetabolic response shows that propranolol can be safely administered to severely burned children.

Summary

In severely burned children, propagation of the catecholamine-induced hypermetabolic response can be reduced by propranolol administration. The degree of mitigation of the deleterious effects of burn injury depends on the dose of propranolol and duration of administration. Decreasing resting heart rate by 15% to 20% significantly reduces cardiac work over time. Proteolysis and lipolysis are similarly reduced, as a result of the decrease in resting energy expenditure and potentiation of catecholamine signaling. Instead of the typical net proteolysis that occurs after a severe burn injury, skeletal muscle protein synthesis is increased. These beneficial results (summarized in Table 3) were attained safely and largely without adverse events. The results of this study suggest that additional studies with a larger number of participants will show beneficial results in terms of growth, cardiac physiology, and the attenuation

Table 3
Results of β1 and β2 adrenergic receptor mediated signaling following a burn injury, without and with β blockade

Cardiac effects	Metabolism	Muscle protein	Fat metabolism
Burn Injury			
Increased HR	Increased REE	Degradation increased	Increased lipolysis
Increased hyperdynamic circulation		Synthesis decreased	Increased circulating triglycerides, free fatty acids
Increased cardiac work		Decreased lean body mass	Increased hepatic steatosis
Burn + Propranolol			
Decreased HR	Decreased REE	Degradation decreased	Decreased lipolysis
Decreased hyperdynamic circulation		Synthesis increased	Decreased circulating triglycerides, free fatty acids
Decreased cardiac work		Increased lean body mass	Decreased hepatic steatosis

of the metabolic syndrome. The authors are currently conducting 2 multicenter trials to test the administration of propranolol in severely burned children. The first is a multicenter study to determine the safety of acute administration of propranolol in severely burned adults. The second study is to confirm the results of a single study trial testing the safety and efficacy of propranolol administration for a full year after injury in severely burned children. We anticipate that the findings of our trial will be generalizable to patients with different types of surgical stress who are in similar hypermetabolic states.

METHODS

Administration and safety guidelines

Propranolol can be safely administered to patients in the ICU and in the outpatient setting with appropriate exclusion of ineligible patients, upward titration of the dose after initiation of therapy, and constant monitoring for adverse events.

Patients were excluded based on preexisting conditions that may complicate the evaluation of end points (including human immunodeficiency virus (HIV), AIDS, a 5-year history of malignancy, diabetes); those with conditions that may be worsened by β blockade (asthma); and those deemed clinically futile at admission because of the severity of their injuries.

Propranolol administration can begin within 24 to 72 hours after admission, after fluid levels are stabilized. Although earlier studies used intravenous administration of propranolol, we now give propranolol by nasogastric tube unless oral feeds cannot be tolerated. Propranolol is escalated from an initial dose of 1 mg/kg/d to ~4 mg/kg/d to achieve a decrease in resting heart rate of ~20% in the following manner. Propranolol is given at a dose of 0.3 to 1.0 mg/kg of bodyweight every 4 to 6 h to achieve a total dose of ~2 mg/kg/d. The dose is then titrated to achieve a decrease of 20% less than the average heart rate recorded for the patient during the 24 hours before propranolol administration. Monitoring of heart rate and blood pressure is continuous while the patient is in the ICU. A dose of propranolol is held, or decreased, when the mean blood pressure is less than 65 mm Hg. Therapy is reinitiated with incremental increases in propranolol doses until the study goal of an approximate decrease of 20% of basal heart rate is reestablished.

Kinetic studies of propranolol plasma drug concentrations in severely burned children have shown that peak concentrations were achieved in our patients within 30 minutes to 1 hour after administration [13]. Trough levels were attained by the second hour after administration. Propranolol's half-life is between 4 and 6 hours. We are currently determining whether this reduced half-life in pediatric burn patients is accompanied by retention of higher levels of metabolites in the circulation.

At discharge, patients older than 6 years of age were switched to the exentab formulation, enabling once-daily administration of propranolol. Children less than 6 years of age remained on liquid formulation given 4 times daily. At the time of discharge, patients were issued a blood pressure cuff and a diary for continued monitoring. After discharge, patients recorded their heart rate and blood pressure 4 times per day. When the heart rate was less than 60 bpm or blood pressure was less than the normal value for age, patients were instructed to contact their physician for instructions. Heart rate logs and pill audits were logged with each return to the clinic.

Potential side effects associated with propranolol administration include bradycardia, hypotension, cardiac arrhythmia, hypoglycemia, respiratory arrest, and death. Over the course of administering propranolol to more than 300 patients, we have recorded few adverse events. In all cases, administration of propranolol was halted and then reinitiated as described earlier.

Enrollment and ethics

Assessments were performed at admission, during the acute hospital stay, at the time of discharge, and at 3, 6, 9, and 12 months after burn injury. A written informed consent form, approved by the Institutional Review Board of the University of Texas Medical Branch (Galveston, TX), was signed by the legal guardian before enrollment in the study. In children older than 7 years of age, assent was obtained before the start of the study.

Standard burn care

The Galveston formula, a total of 5000 mL/m^2 TBSA burned + 2000 mL/m^2 TBSA lactated Ringer's solution, was used to determine the volume of fluid administered for fluid resuscitation during the first 24 hours. Within 48 hours of admission, all patients underwent burn wound excision and coverage with autograft or allograft. Bed rest for the first 4 days was followed by ambulation on each subsequent day until the following surgery. Patients underwent excision and grafting procedures every 6 to 7 days until 95% healing was achieved for all burned sites.

Enteral nutrition was administered to all patients via a nasogastric or nasoduodenal tube; Vivonex TEN enteral nutrition provides 6% fat, 15% protein, and 82% carbohydrate. Daily intake for the first week post-injury was calculated as 1500 kcal/m^2 TBSA + 1500 kcal/m^2 TBSA burned. From the first post-burn week until the time of discharge from the acute unit, daily intake was calculated as 1.4 times the resting energy expenditure measured weekly (see section on Indirect Calorimetry for more details). Retinol-binding protein, pre-albumin, and albumin measurements were performed on all hospitalized patients to check nutritional status. After hospital discharge, Boost (Nestle Health Care Nutrition, Nestlé SA, Vevey, Switzerland) was consumed 3 times daily to supplement the patients' dietary intake with 41 g of carbohydrate, 10 g of protein, and 4 g of fat per serving. Once the staff nutritionist confirmed that the patients' regular diet supplied 1.4 times the resting energy expenditure to meet the patient's caloric requirements, Boost was discontinued. Caretakers were interviewed to assess dietary intake daily when patients returned to the tub room, weekly while residing in the community, and at time points more than 6 months after burn injury when the patients returned for clinical care.

ASSESSMENTS

Cardiac and blood pressure measurements

Blood pressure and resting heart rate were measured and recorded using noninvasive cuff measurements or continuous arterial monitoring; measurements were continuous while the patients were in hospital. At all follow-up visits, measurements were recorded once. Patients and families were trained to use the blood pressure cuffs that were issued to them. Heart rate and blood pressure were then measured and recorded 4 times per day after discharge throughout the study. If the patient's heart rate was less than 60 bpm or the blood pressure was less than the normal value for age, patients and caretakers were instructed to call the study nurse or physician. The percent of predicted heart rate values were calculated by comparing burn patient heart rates and normograms from age-matched, healthy nonburned children [44,45]. The formula for calculating the percent of predicted heart rate used was actual heart rate/age-adjusted norm. The rate pressure product was calculated using the formula mean arterial pressure × heart rate [45].

A pediatrician reviewed the caretakers' heart rate and blood pressure diaries on a routine basis. The propranolol dose was titrated to achieve a systolic blood pressure and pulse within 15% of the mean values for the age-matched nonburned normal patient cohort. If a heart rate ranging from 70 bpm (teenagers) to 90 bpm (younger children) or systolic blood pressure from 90 mm Hg (teenagers) to 80 mm Hg (younger children) were recorded, then the next dose of propranolol was administered to the patients. If these parameters were not met, however, the propranolol dose was held and patients were assessed at the time when the next dose was to be administered. When administration of propranolol was missed several times within a week because of heart rate or blood pressure, the dose was then adjusted to ensure that the heart rate and blood pressure were in the correct range with treatment.

Indirect calorimetry

The resting energy expenditure was measured on resting patients between 12 AM and 5 AM on a weekly basis during the hospitalization period using a Sensor-Medics Vmax 29 metabolic cart (Yorba Linda, CA). Each minute, an analysis was performed on inspired and expired gas. When both oxygen consumption and carbon dioxide production reached and maintained a steady state for 5 min, the values were recorded. Normal values, predicted using the Harris-Benedict equation and body mass index, were compared with the measured values [26,48,49].

Body composition

Body composition was determined using dual-energy x-ray absorptiometry (DEXA) (QDR-4500W Hologic, Waltham, MA); PLBM, central fat, central mass, TLBMC, and TBMC, were measured. Daily calibrations using a spinal phantom in the single-beam, lateral, and anteroposterior modes were performed to minimize systemic deviations. Correct identification of bone, lean mass, air, and fat was ensured using a tissue bar phantom to calibrate the individual pixels in the image [27]. Before measurement, intravenous fluids and enteral feedings were discontinued for the duration of the examination and then reinitiated afterward. Results were expressed as percent change from patient baseline (determined within 3 ± 2 weeks after burn injury). At each time point, bone loss was calculated as the percent change from baseline. Patients were then stratified based on a loss of more than 5% in total body bone mineral content less the head per total body mass (TBMC/TBM) and TLBMC as determined by DEXA. The proportion of patients randomized to placebo or propranolol in each strata was recorded, and the likelihood (odds ratios ± 95% CI) of presenting a clinically significant bone loss of at least 5% in both of these parameters was estimated.

Measurement of hormones

Blood and urine were obtained at admission, during the acute hospitalization period at regular intervals, and at follow-up visits. Blood was collected using serum separator tubes and centrifuged (1320 rpm, 10 min). Serum was decanted and stored at −80°C for later analyses. High-performance liquid chromatography and enzyme-linked immunosorbent assay techniques were used to determine serum levels of parathyroid hormone, insulinlike growth factor (IGF) 1, IGF binding protein-3, osteocalcin, testosterone, albumin, and total protein, as described elsewhere [27,48,49]. Measurement of urinary catecholamine levels was performed as described elsewhere [27,48,49].

Stable isotope studies

Infusion of stable isotopes was performed by the Metabolic Core Facility at the Shriners Hospitals for Children – Galveston by previously published methods [4,10,12,16,20,41].

Gene expression studies

Messenger RNA was isolated from tissue biopsy samples and then sent to the Genomic Core at the University of Texas Medical Branch for processing. Gene expression was elucidated using Affymetrix Human Genome U95 microarrays. Data were analyzed as previously published [17,41].

Acknowledgments

The authors thank Deborah Benjamin, Wes Benjamin, Maria Cantu, Mario Celis, Tabatha Elliot, Kathryn Epperson, Eric Henry, Holly Goode, Kara Hougen, Joanna Huddleston, Mary Kelly, Xuyang Liang, Maria Magno, Liz Montemayor, Marc Nicolai, Sylvia Ojeda, Maricela Pantoja, Cathy Reed, Lisa Richardson, Lucile Robles, Pam Stevens, Sierra Tinney, Judith Underbrink, Becky Whitlock, the nutrition department, and the respiratory therapy team for their assistance in obtaining the study measurements. The authors thank Dr Kasie Cole for editing and proofreading the manuscript.

References

[1] Pereira CT, Murphy KD, Herndon DN. Altering metabolism. J Burn Care Rehabil 2005;26: 194–9.

[2] Jeschke MG, Gauglitz GG, Kulp GA, et al. Long-term persistance of the pathophysiologic response to severe burn injury. PLoS One 2011;6:e21245.
[3] Wilmore DW, Aulick LH. Metabolic changes in burned patients. Surg Clin North Am 1978;58:1173–87.
[4] Wolfe RR, Herndon DN, Peters EJ, et al. Regulation of lipolysis in severely burned children. Ann Surg 1987;206:214–21.
[5] Herndon DN, Tompkins RG. Support of the metabolic response to burn injury. Lancet 2004;363:1895–902.
[6] Reiss E, Pearson E, Artz CP. The metabolic response to burns. J Clin Invest 1956;35:62–77.
[7] Yurt RW, McManus AT, Mason AD Jr, et al. Increased susceptibility to infection related to extent of burn injury. Arch Surg 1984;119:183–8.
[8] Desborough JP. The stress response to trauma and surgery. Br J Anaesth 2000;85:109–17.
[9] Wilmore DW, Long JM, Mason AD Jr, et al. Catecholamines: mediator of the hypermetabolic response to thermal injury. Ann Surg 1974;180:653–69.
[10] Herndon DN, Barrow RE, Rutan TC, et al. Effect of propranolol administration on hemodynamic and metabolic responses of burned pediatric patients. Ann Surg 1988;208:484–92.
[11] Gore DC, Honeycutt D, Jahoor F, et al. Propranolol diminishes extremity blood flow in burned patients. Ann Surg 1991;213:568–73 [discussion: 573–4].
[12] Herndon DN, Hart DW, Wolf SE, et al. Reversal of catabolism by beta-blockade after severe burns. N Engl J Med 2001;345:1223–9.
[13] Williams FN, Herndon DN, Kulp GA, et al. Propranolol decreases cardiac work in a dose-dependent manner in severely burned children. Surgery 2011;149:231–9.
[14] Herndon DN, Rodriguez NA, Diaz EC, et al. Long-term propranolol use in severely burned pediatric patients: a randomized controlled study. Ann Surg 2012;256:402–11.
[15] Jeschke MG, Norbury WB, Finnerty CC, et al. Propranolol does not increase inflammation, sepsis, or infectious episodes in severely burned children. J Trauma 2007;62:676–81.
[16] Morio B, Irtun O, Herndon DN, et al. Propranolol decreases splanchnic triacylglycerol storage in burn patients receiving a high-carbohydrate diet. Ann Surg 2002;236:218–25.
[17] Barrow RE, Wolfe RR, Dasu MR, et al. The use of beta-adrenergic blockade in preventing trauma-induced hepatomegaly. Ann Surg 2006;243:115–20.
[18] Norbury WB, Jeschke MG, Herndon DN. Metabolism modulators in sepsis: propranolol. Crit Care Med 2007;35:S616–20.
[19] Baron PW, Barrow RE, Pierre EJ, et al. Prolonged use of propranolol safely decreases cardiac work in burned children. J Burn Care Rehabil 1997;18:223–7.
[20] Hart DW, Wolf SE, Mlcak R, et al. Persistence of muscle catabolism after severe burn. Surgery 2000;128:312–9.
[21] Selye H. Stress and the general adaptation syndrome. Br Med J 1950;1:1383–92.
[22] Kraft R, Herndon DN, Al-Mousawi AM, et al. Burn size and survival probability in paediatric patients in modern burn care: a prospective observational cohort study. Lancet 2012;379:1013–21.
[23] Finnerty CC, Herndon DN, Przkora R, et al. Cytokine expression profile over time in severely burned pediatric patients. Shock 2006;26:13–9.
[24] Jeschke MG, Chinkes DL, Finnerty CC, et al. Pathophysiologic response to severe burn injury. Ann Surg 2008;248:387–401.
[25] Jeschke MG, Finnerty CC, Herndon DN, et al. Severe injury is associated with insulin resistance, endoplasmic reticulum stress response, and unfolded protein response. Ann Surg 2012;255:370–8.
[26] Mlcak RP, Jeschke MG, Barrow RE, et al. The influence of age and gender on resting energy expenditure in severely burned children. Ann Surg 2006;244:121–30.
[27] Przkora R, Barrow RE, Jeschke MG, et al. Body composition changes with time in pediatric burn patients. J Trauma 2006;60:968–71.
[28] Williams FN, Herndon DN, Suman OE, et al. Changes in cardiac physiology after severe burn injury. J Burn Care Res 2011;32:269–74.

[29] Pereira CT, Herndon DN. The pharmacologic modulation of the hypermetabolic response to burns. Adv Surg 2005;39:245–61.
[30] Chang DW, DeSanti L, Demling RH. Anticatabolic and anabolic strategies in critical illness: a review of current treatment modalities. Shock 1998;10:155–60.
[31] Kinney JM, Long CL, Gump FE, et al. Tissue composition of weight loss in surgical patients. I. Elective operation. Ann Surg 1968;168:459–74.
[32] Rutan RL, Herndon DN. Growth delay in postburn pediatric patients. Arch Surg 1990;125: 392–5.
[33] Kulp GA, Herndon DN, Lee JO, et al. Extent and magnitude of catecholamine surge in pediatric burned patients. Shock 2010;33:369–74.
[34] Goodall M, Stone C, Haynes BW Jr. Urinary output of adrenaline and noradrenaline in severe thermal burns. Ann Surg 1957;145:479–87.
[35] Sutherland JA, Al Chekakie MO, Moran JF. Catecholamine-induced cardiomyopathy rapidly reversed with beta-blocker therapy. Congest Heart Fail 2009;15:193–5.
[36] Kassim TA, Clarke DD, Mai VQ, et al. Catecholamine-induced cardiomyopathy. Endocr Pract 2008;14:1137–49.
[37] Goldstein DS. Catecholamines and stress. Endocr Regul 2003;37:69–80.
[38] Carey JS, Mohr PA, Brown RS, et al. Cardiovascular function in hemorrhage, trauma and sepsis: determinants of cardiac output and cardiac work. Ann Surg 1969;170:910–21.
[39] Minifee PK, Barrow RE, Abston S, et al. Improved myocardial oxygen utilization following propranolol infusion in adolescents with postburn hypermetabolism. J Pediatr Surg 1989;24:806–10 [discussion: 810–1].
[40] Herndon DN, Nguyen TT, Wolfe RR, et al. Lipolysis in burned patients is stimulated by the beta 2-receptor for catecholamines. Arch Surg 1994;129:1301–4 [discussion: 1304–5].
[41] Herndon DN, Dasu MR, Wolfe RR, et al. Gene expression profiles and protein balance in skeletal muscle of burned children after beta-adrenergic blockade. Am J Physiol Endocrinol Metab 2003;285:E783–9.
[42] Oberbeck R. Therapeutic implications of immune-endocrine interactions in the critically ill patients. Curr Drug Targets Immune Endocr Metabol Disord 2004;4:129–39.
[43] Oberbeck R, Schmitz D, Wilsenack K, et al. Adrenergic modulation of survival and cellular immune functions during polymicrobial sepsis. Neuroimmunomodulation 2004;11: 214–23.
[44] Hazinski MF. Cardiovascular disorders. In: Hazinski MF, editor. Manual of pediatric critical care. St Louis, MO: Mosby; 1999. p. 84–288.
[45] Voors AW, Webber LS, Berenson GS. Resting heart rate and pressure-rate product of children in a total biracial community: the Bogalusa Heart Study. Am J Epidemiol 1982;116: 276–86.
[46] Harris JA, Benedict FG. A biometric study of basal metabolism in man. Washington, DC: Carnegie Institution of Washington; 1919.
[47] Porro LJ, Herndon DN, Rodriguez NA, et al. Five-year outcomes after oxandrolone administration in severely burned children: a randomized clinical trial of safety and efficacy. J Am Coll Surg 2012;214:489–502.
[48] Hart DW, Wolf SE, Herndon DN, et al. Energy expenditure and caloric balance after burn: increased feeding leads to fat rather than lean mass accretion. Ann Surg 2002;235: 152–61.
[49] Suman OE, Mlcak RP, Chinkes DL, et al. Resting energy expenditure in severely burned children: analysis of agreement between indirect calorimetry and prediction equations using the Bland-Altman method. Burns 2006;32:335–42.

Advances in Surgery 47 (2013) 199–211

ADVANCES IN SURGERY

What Is the Optimal Means of Staging Colon Cancer?

Elizabeth A. Arena, MD[a,b], Anton J. Bilchik, MD, PhD[a,b,c,*]

[a]Department of Surgical Oncology, John Wayne Cancer Institute, Saint John's Health Center, 2200 Santa Monica Boulevard, Santa Monica, CA 90404, USA; [b]Gastrointestinal Research Program, John Wayne Cancer Institute, Saint John's Health Center, 2200 Santa Monica Boulevard, Santa Monica, CA 90404, USA; [c]California Oncology Research Institute, Los Angeles, CA, USA

Keywords

• Colorectal cancer • Nonmetastatic • Locoregional • Staging

Key points

- Identifying lymph node metastases is essential for accurately staging patients with colon cancer.
- Adequate lymph node yield and removal of at least twelve lymph nodes is an important quality measure in colon cancer staging.
- Sentinel lymph node biopsy and molecular tumor cell identification are promising techniques to identify occult lymph node metastases and improve staging accuracy.

INTRODUCTION

Colorectal cancer remains the third most common cancer diagnosis in men and women in the United States, with an estimated 140,000 new cases and nearly 52,000 deaths expected during 2012 [1]. With advances in screening and treatment options, deaths from colorectal cancer have steadily declined over the last 2 decades [2]. Although surgical resection can be curative in patients whose disease is confined to the bowel wall, survival rates significantly decrease when disease spreads to regional lymph nodes. Adjuvant chemotherapy has been shown to improve survival of patients with locoregional and metastatic colon cancer [3–5]. In patients with nonmetastatic disease, cancer outcomes are primarily determined by regional lymph node involvement. However, up to one-quarter of

Supported by grant 2R01 CA90848-05A2 from the National Cancer Institute and by funding from the California Oncology Research Institute, Los Angeles, CA. The content is solely the responsibility of the authors and does not necessarily represent the official view of the National Cancer Institute or the National Institutes of Health.

*Corresponding author. John Wayne Cancer Institute, 2200 Santa Monica Boulevard, Santa Monica, CA 90404. *E-mail address:* bilchika@jwci.org

0065-3411/13/$ – see front matter
http://dx.doi.org/10.1016/j.yasu.2013.03.001

node-negative colon cancers will recur. Identifying patients with high-risk, node-negative colon cancer is an important challenge, as they may benefit from adjuvant chemotherapy if their disease is staged accurately [6].

Pathologic analysis of a limited sample of lymph nodes may miss a small metastasis and provide false-negative results. Quality measures promote analysis of a minimum number of lymph nodes to improve staging accuracy [7,8]. Furthermore, conventional pathologic analysis with single-level sectioning is subject to sampling error. New investigations into more focused analysis of lymph nodes, or "ultrastaging," by sentinel lymph node biopsy, immunohistochemistry (IHC), and reverse transcriptase polymerase chain reaction (RT-PCR) have shown promising results in upstaging colon cancer, predicting recurrence, and improving disease-free survival [9–12].

HISTORICAL STAGING

Staging for colorectal cancer has traditionally been anatomically based, as first characterized by the British pathologist Cuthbert Dukes in 1932 [13]. The Dukes classification is a simplified anatomic approach to staging colorectal cancer: Dukes A: tumor invasion into but confined to bowel wall; B: tumor invasion through the bowel wall but not involving lymph nodes; C: involvement of lymph nodes; and D: distant metastases. This classification was later modified by Astler and Coller in 1954 to further characterize the degree of invasion into the bowel wall [14]. Subsequently, in 1957 the American Joint Committee on Cancer (AJCC) adopted the tumor-node-metastasis (TNM) cancer staging system, and this has proven to be the most significant staging system (Fig. 1) we have to date. Several editions have been revised over the years, with the most recent 7th edition being initiated in 2010 [7,15]. Although TNM staging remains anatomically based, tumor biology also is important. Although currently not included in the staging model, AJCC recommendations are to note isolated tumor cells, tumor regression grade, the circumferential margin, microsatellite instability, perineural invasion, KRAS mutation status, and 18q loss of heterozygosity. These variables may have prognostic significance but require further study [7,15,16].

GENERAL CONSIDERATIONS FOR CURRENT STAGING OF COLON CANCER

The current recommendation for early detection of colorectal cancer is regular screening beginning at age 50, with fecal occult blood testing, sigmoidoscopy, or colonoscopy [16–18]. Patients who have a family history of colorectal cancer or polyps are encouraged to begin screening at a younger age. If biopsy specimen confirms invasive adenocarcinoma, laboratory tests should include a complete blood count, chemistry panel, and measurement of carcinoembryonic antigen. Baseline computed tomography of the chest, abdomen, and pelvis should be performed to evaluate for distant metastases. Positron emission tomography scan has limited utility in the initial staging workup of colon cancer [16–18]. Conventional TNM pathologic staging (Fig. 1) is then performed following oncologic resection of the involved segment of colon, which includes

ANATOMIC STAGE/PROGNOSTIC GROUPS

Stage	T	N	M	Dukes*	MAC*
0	Tis	N0	M0	–	–
I	T1	N0	M0	A	A
	T2	N0	M0	A	B1
IIA	T3	N0	M0	B	B2
IIB	T4a	N0	M0	B	B2
IIC	T4b	N0	M0	B	B3
IIIA	T1–T2	N1/N1c	M0	C	C1
	T1	N2a	M0	C	C1
IIIB	T3–T4a	N1/N1c	M0	C	C2
	T2–T3	N2a	M0	C	C1/C2
	T1–T2	N2b	M0	C	C1
IIIC	T4a	N2a	M0	C	C2
	T3–T4a	N2b	M0	C	C2
	T4b	N1–N2	M0	C	C3
IVA	Any T	Any N	M1a	–	–
IVB	Any T	Any N	M1b	–	–

NOTE: cTNM is the clinical classification, pTNM is the pathologic classification. The y prefix is used for those cancers that are classified after neoadjuvant pretreatment (for example, ypTNM). Patients who have a complete pathologic response are ypT0N0cM0 that may be similar to Stage Group 0 or I. The r prefix is to be used for those cancers that have recurred after a disease-free interval (rTNM).
* Dukes B is a composite of better (T3 N0 M0) and worse (T4 N0 M0) prognostic groups, as is Dukes C (any TN1 M0 and Any T N2 M0). MAC is the modified Astler-Coller classification.

Definitions

Primary Tumor (T)

- TX Primary tumor cannot be assessed
- T0 No evidence of primary tumor
- Tis Carcinoma in situ: intraepithelial or invasion of lamina propria[1]
- T1 Tumor invades submucosa
- T2 Tumor invades muscularis propria
- T3 Tumor invades through the muscularis propria into pericolorectal tissues
- T4a Tumor penetrates to the surface of the visceral peritoneum[2]
- T4b Tumor directly invades or is adherent to other organs or structures[2,3]

Regional Lymph Nodes (N)[4]

- NX Regional lymph nodes cannot be assessed
- N0 No regional lymph node metastasis
- N1 Metastasis in 1–3 regional lymph nodes
- N1a Metastasis in one regional lymph node
- N1b Metastasis in 2–3 regional lymph nodes
- N1c Tumor deposit(s) in the subserosa, mesentery, or nonperitonealized pericolic or perirectal tissues without regional nodal metastasis
- N2 Metastasis in 4 or more regional lymph nodes
- N2a Metastasis in 4–6 regional lymph nodes
- N2b Metastasis in 7 or more regional lymph nodes

Distant Metastasis (M)

- M0 No distant metastasis
- M1 Distant metastasis
- M1a Metastasis confined to one organ or site (for example, liver, lung, ovary, nonregional node)
- M1b Metastases in more than one organ/site or the peritoneum

[1] Tis includes cancer cells confined within the glandular basement membrane (intraepithelial) or mucosal lamina propria (intramucosal) with no extension through the muscularis mucosae into the submucosa.

[2] Direct invasion in T4 includes invasion of other organs or other segments of the colorectum as a result of direct extension through the serosa, as confirmed on microscopic examination (for example, invasion of the sigmoid colon by a carcinoma of the cecum) or, for cancers in a retroperitoneal or subperitoneal location, direct invasion of other organs or structures by virtue of extension beyond the muscularis propria (that is, a tumor on the posterior wall of the descending colon invading the left kidney or lateral abdominal wall; or a mid or distal rectal cancer with invasion of prostate, seminal vesicles, cervix, or vagina).

[3] Tumor that is adherent to other organs or structures, grossly, is classified cT4b. However, if no tumor is present in the adhesion, microscopically, the classification should be pT1-4a depending on the anatomical depth of wall invasion. The V and L classifications should be used to identify the presence or absence of vascular or lymphatic invasion, whereas the PN site-specific factor should be used for perineural invasion.

[4] A satellite peritumoral nodule in the pericolorectal adipose tissue of a primary carcinoma without histologic evidence of residual lymph node in the nodule may represent discontinuous spread, venous invasion with extravascular spread (V1/2), or a totally replaced lymph node (N1/2). Replaced nodes should be counted separately as positive nodes in the N category, whereas discontinuous spread or venous invasion should be classified and counted in the Site-Specific Factor category Tumor Deposits (TD).

Fig. 1. Current guidelines for the staging of colon cancer. (The original and primary source for this information is the *AJCC Cancer Staging Manual*, Seventh edition (2010), published by Springer-Verlag New York; used with the permission of the American Joint Committee on Cancer (AJCC), Chicago, Illinois.)

proximal ligation of the feeding vascular pedicle and en bloc lymphadenectomy of associated draining lymph nodes. The appropriate treatment plan is based on AJCC staging and incorporates select individual patient factors per the physician's discretion.

AJCC AND ITS LIMITATIONS

Although modifications to AJCC TNM staging over the years have improved its predictive ability, including the addition of adequate lymph node sampling as discussed later in this article, there remain serious limitations to the staging system. The current model cannot identify the 25% of high-risk node-negative patients who will develop recurrent colorectal cancer and may benefit from adjuvant therapy. Most importantly, the current model lacks a clear rank order by stage in predicting outcomes. For example, overall survival is worse in patients with stage IIA and IIB colon cancer than in patients with stage IIIA disease, whereas patients with stage IIC disease fare worse than patients with stage IIIB disease [19]. AJCC definitions of T, N, and M categories have become more complex, but the AJCC staging system remains limited in its prognostic accuracy. As a result, several modifications and additions have been proposed [9,11,19–25].

LYMPH NODE YIELD FOR IMPROVED STAGING

Over the last decade, the most significant evolution in staging colon cancer has been the recognition that adequate lymph node yield is necessary. With evidence mounting that removal of at least 12 lymph nodes is associated with improved survival, a consensus was reached by the International Union Against Cancer, the AJCC, the College of American Pathologists, and the National Cancer Institute that guidelines should include a 12-node minimum [26,27]. This consensus culminated in the National Quality Forum, which endorsed resection of a minimum of 12 lymph nodes for colon cancer and administration of adjuvant chemotherapy for patients with node-positive disease [8]. Regional lymphadenectomy in colon cancer can improve regional control of disease, staging accuracy, adjuvant treatment planning, and overall survival. The reported number of lymph nodes removed in a colectomy can vary based on surgical technique, extent of pathologic analysis, or patient factors. As early as 1989, Scott and Grace described a technique of fat clearance to increase the number of nodes identified [28]. Their study suggested that at least 13 nodes needed to be identified to stage Dukes B classified patients accurately [28]. Le Voyer and colleagues [29] reported a secondary survey of the Intergroup Trial INT-0089 and found, after controlling for number of nodes involved, survival increased as more nodes were analyzed. Even when no nodes were involved, overall and disease-specific survival was improved when more lymph nodes were analyzed. They concluded that the number of lymph nodes analyzed in colon cancer is itself a prognostic variable [29].

A large population-based study was reported in 2006 to explore the role of lymph node resection and survival further [30]. Investigators used the Surveillance, Epidemiology, and End Results (SEER) database from 1988 to 2000 to identify 82,896 patients with stage I to III colon cancer. Although a trend was noted for increased number of nodes removed during the study period, the median number of lymph nodes removed across all patients was only 9. For all stages examined, increased nodal sampling was associated with improved survival (Fig. 2) [30]. Importantly, multivariate regression found that mortality was significantly reduced when the number of removed lymph nodes was 15 versus 1 to 7.

A recent study identified a significant increase in lymph node yield over the last decade [31]. This retrospective analysis of 2 multicenter prospective trials examined 245 patients enrolled between 2001 and 2009. Lymph node yield was significantly higher from 2005 to 2008 (17 nodes) compared with 2001 to 2004 (15 nodes). Adherence to the 12-node minimum was only 70% in the earliest years and up to 94% in 2007 to 2008, showing a significant change through either improved surgical technique or improved pathologic identification of nodes. Interestingly, this study did not see a significant change in adjuvant therapy use over that time period, suggesting there may be a lag time for adjusting treatment plans [31].

LYMPH NODE RATIO

In addition to absolute number of lymph nodes removed, some investigators have reported that the ratio of positive nodes to total nodes may be a significant prognostic indicator in colon cancer [21,32,33]. Using the SEER database, Wang and colleagues [33] in 2008 created incremental subsets of lymph node ratios and found these ratios to be important prognostic indicators for patients with stage IIIB and IIIC disease. A smaller study by Lee and colleagues [21] examined 201 patients with stage III colon cancer and found lymph node ratios to be significant prognostic indictors for disease-free survival. Finally, a recent study examined lymph node ratio with or without adherence to the 12-node minimum [32]. This study found lymph node ratio to be an independently effective prognostic indicator for patients with stage III colon cancer, irrespective of number of nodes removed. Survival did seem greater in patients with 12 or more nodes examined. Large prospective studies remain necessary to determine if lymph node ratio should be added to the current cancer staging system.

ULTRASTAGING

The staging of colon cancer can be refined further by focused analysis of lymph nodes. Up to 20% to 30% of patients whose nodes are negative by conventional pathologic analysis will develop disease recurrence. Recurrence may be attributable to incomplete resection of tumor-bearing regional lymph nodes, aggressive tumor biology with occult residual disease spreading to extranodal sites, and/or occult nodal disease that has not been detected by standard pathologic analysis [11]. As many as 70% of tumor-positive lymph nodes contain tumor deposits less than 0.5 cm in diameter, which may easily be missed on standard analysis [9,34].

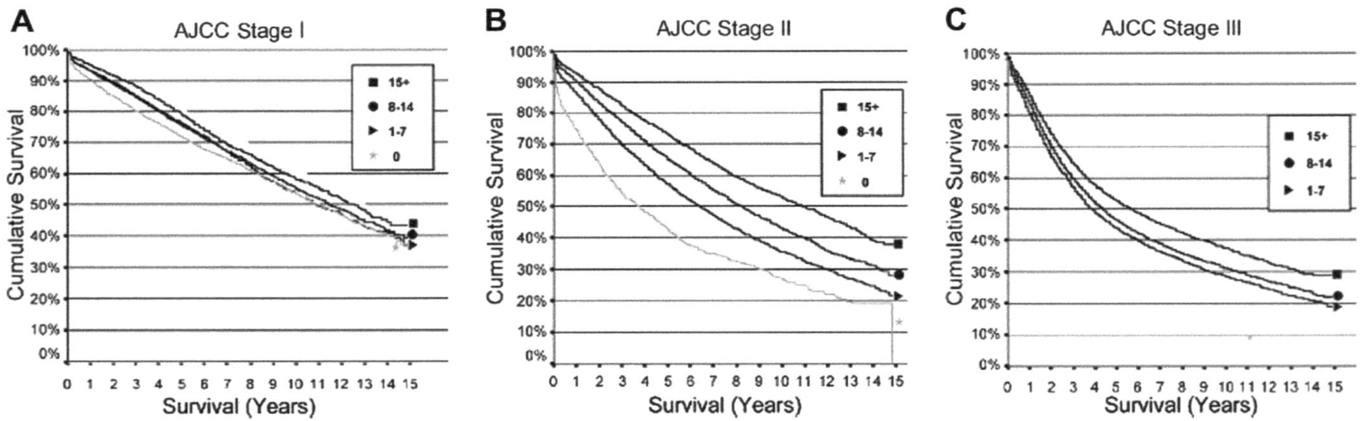

Fig. 2. Cumulative survival of patients with stage I, II, or III colon cancer increases with more extensive nodal examination. Survival was greatest when more than 15 lymph nodes were evaluated. (*Reprinted from* Chen SL, Bilchik AJ. More extensive nodal dissection improves survival for stages I to III of colon cancer: a population-based study. Ann Surg 2006;244:602–10; with permission.)

Conventional analysis of a 5-mm lymph node involves microscopic examination of 1 or 2 sections that are stained with hematoxylin and eosin (H&E). Standard methodology limits analysis to <1% of the lymph node and inability to detect small tumor cell aggregates [9,11]. Generally isolated tumor cells and micrometastases up to 2 mm in size require IHC staining to be identified. Serial sectioning and addition of specialized IHC stains or RT-PCR may improve nodal staging accuracy. Applying these techniques to all resected nodes would significantly increase the time and cost of analysis, but applying them to a selected sample of high-risk nodes could improve staging accuracy in a cost-efficient fashion.

SENTINEL LYMPH NODE BIOPSY

Lymphatic mapping with focused analysis of the sentinel lymph node was developed by Morton and colleagues [35] to identify nodal metastasis in patients with clinically localized cutaneous melanoma. It was subsequently adapted by Giuliano and colleagues [36] for staging breast cancer, and then by Bilchik and colleagues [37] for staging gastrointestinal malignancies [38]. The concept of sentinel lymph node biopsy is centered on the premise that lymphatic drainage from a primary tumor occurs in an orderly and progressive fashion, with the sentinel node representing the first draining node and the most likely site of metastasis when regional nodes become involved. In patients with melanoma and breast cancer, sentinel node biopsy can avoid unnecessary complete lymph node dissection with its associated risks of lymphedema and wound complications. In patients with colon cancer, lymphatic mapping with sentinel lymph node biopsy does not change the extent of lymph node resection because all patients undergo en bloc lymphadenectomy with segmental resection. However, lymphatic mapping and sentinel node biopsy can identify lymph nodes for focused pathologic analysis.

The feasibility of lymphatic mapping in gastrointestinal neoplasms was described in detail by Tsioulias and colleagues in 2000 [38]. This study examined 65 patients with gastrointestinal neoplasms, including 50 patients with large bowel adenocarcinoma. Lymphatic mapping was performed by injecting 0.5 to 1 mL of isosulfan blue dye circumferentially around the neoplasm. The draining lymphatic channel was visualized and the first 1 to 3 blue-stained nodes were marked in vivo. Standard en bloc resection was then performed and the specimen delivered to the pathology laboratory. Depending on the size of the node, each sentinel node was sectioned at 2-mm to 3-mm intervals. Focused analysis was performed with both H&E and IHC with a cytokeratin antibody cocktail. Nonsentinel nodes were analyzed with conventional pathologic sectioning and H&E staining. Sentinel nodes were successfully identified in 95% of the patients. The false-negative rate excluding rectal tumors was 4% (2/54). In 11 cases (17%), tumor deposits were identified by multiple sectioning or IHC only, resulting in upstaging through focused analysis [38]. A subsequent study by Wood and colleagues [39] further validated the use of lymphatic mapping in colorectal cancer, specifically the use of in vivo, ex vivo, and laparoscopic techniques. At least one sentinel node was identified in 96% of patients, and occult metastases were identified in 17% of patients [39].

Several other studies have reported a wide range in lymphatic mapping success rates from 58% to 100% [39–43]. Variations in accuracy and sensitivity may have reflected a lack of standardization of technique, retrospective analysis, and inexperience in the surgical and pathologic aspects of the technique. To examine the role of focused analysis of sentinel nodes in colon cancer further, a prospective multicenter trial was initiated [44]. One hundred thirty-two patients with stage I and II colorectal cancer were enrolled between 2001 and 2005 at 4 tertiary referral centers. Participating surgical and pathologic teams had performed lymphatic mapping at least 20 times before initiation of the trial. Sentinel nodes were identified in vivo as described earlier, or ex vivo immediately after resection if unable to determine in vivo (Fig. 3). Similar pathologic analysis with H&E and IHC staining was performed as described in the previous study, in addition to RT-PCR assay of sentinel nodes. Preliminary results were reported in 2006, with a success rate of 96% in identification of sentinel nodes. The sensitivity of lymphatic mapping and sentinel node analysis was 88%, and the false-negative rate was 7.4%. Upstaging occurred in 23.6% of patients. Interim analysis of this multicenter trial in 2007 [9] demonstrated successful identification of a sentinel node in 150 of 152 cases (99%). Possible upstaging with identification of macrometastases greater than 2 mm or micrometastases 0.2 to 2 mm in size occurred in 7 patients, and possible upstaging was seen in an additional 18 patients (22%), whose sentinel nodes contained small tumor clusters (<0.2 mm) identified by IHC or RT-PCR. At a mean follow-up of 25 months, 12 disease-specific recurrences occurred, 10 of which were in patients with a tumor-positive sentinel node. All patients with a negative sentinel node had no recurrence at that time, suggesting surgery alone may have been curative in these patients [9].

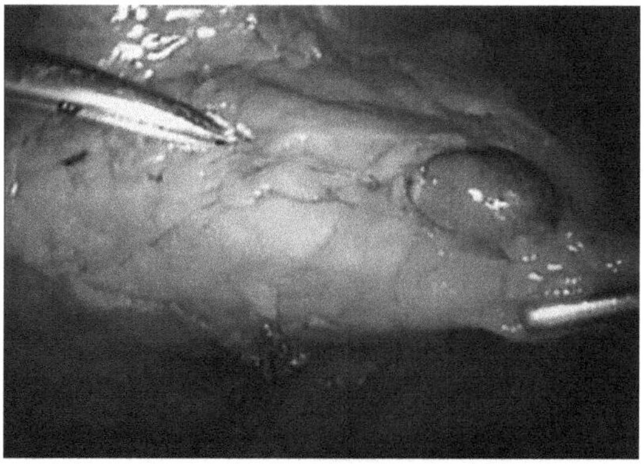

Fig. 3. Lymphatic mapping using isosulfan blue dye to identify a sentinel node in a patient with colon cancer. (*Reprinted from* Bilchik AJ, DiNome M, Saha S, et al. Prospective multicenter trial of staging adequacy in colon cancer: preliminary results. Arch Surg 2006;141:527–33 [discussion: 533–4]; with permission.)

A similar randomized multicenter controlled trial was undertaken by the United States Military Cancer Institute to help determine the clinical relevance of focused staging based on sentinel node analysis [11,45]. One hundred ninety-two patients with colon cancer were enrolled between 2002 and 2010 and randomized to standard nodal evaluation (control) or ultrastaging with ex vivo lymphatic mapping and sentinel node focused pathologic analysis with H&E/IHC. The rate of nodal positivity was 38.7% in the control group versus 57.3% in the ultrastaging group; the difference primarily reflected identification of small cell aggregates (<0.2 mm) in the sentinel node. Recent outcome analysis showed that median lymph node yield was 16 in the ultrastaging group versus 13 in the control group, and the 5-year disease-free survival rate in patients with node-negative disease was 86% in the ultrastaging group versus 71% in the control group (Fig. 4) [11]. This trial demonstrated that ultrastaging improved staging accuracy and disease-free survival in patients with early colon cancer.

ISOLATED TUMOR CELLS

Several studies have begun to demonstrate the unique prognostic significance of isolated tumor cells. A recent study by Mescoli and colleagues [22] highlighted the potential role for identifying patients with lymph nodes positive only for isolated tumor cells. The authors examined 312 patients who had stage I and II colorectal cancer and lymph nodes that were tumor-negative by conventional pathologic analysis. The high quality of lymph node resection in this study (mean number of resected nodes was 17 per patient) ensured adequate conventional pathologic analysis and helped determine the

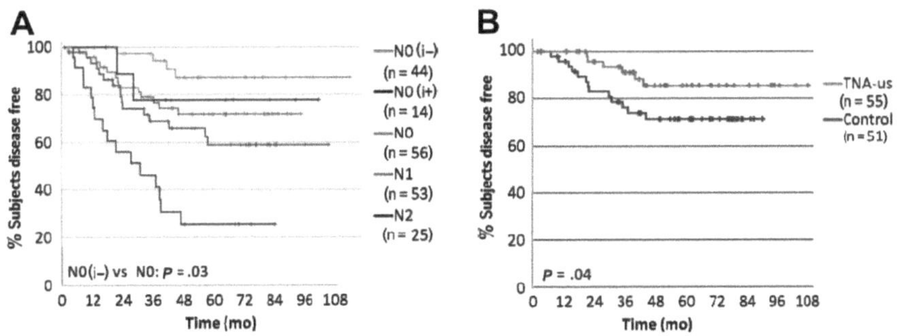

Fig. 4. Prognostic significance of ultrastaging in colon cancer. (*A*) Disease-free survival according to nodal disease volume in all patients. N0 (i+) and N0 (i−) represent patients whose nodes were positive or negative for isolated tumor cells or small clusters, respectively. (*B*) Disease-free survival of node-negative patients randomized to standard pathologic evaluation (Control) versus targeted nodal assessment and ultrastaging (TNA-us). (*Reprinted from* Nissan A, Protic M, Bilchik AJ, et al. United States Military Cancer Institute Clinical Trials Group (USMCI GI-01) randomized controlled trial comparing targeted nodal assessment and ultrastaging with standard pathologic evaluation for colon cancer. Ann Surg 2012;256:412–27; with permission.)

significance of isolated tumor cells, defined as single cells that appeared phenotypically malignant and stained positive with MFN116 anticytokeratin antibody [22]. Isolated tumor cells were significantly correlated with T value and stage. Recurrent colorectal cancer was found in 14% of patients with isolated tumor cells, compared with 4.7% of patients without isolated tumor cells. In univariate and multivariate analysis, the presence of isolated tumor cells was the only variable significantly associated with recurrence [22].

A meta-analysis of 39 studies [46] similarly showed the prognostic significance of isolated tumor cells for recurrent colorectal cancer in node-negative patients. In this study, a combination of IHC and RT-PCR techniques was used to identify isolated tumor cells and micrometastases. Over 4000 patients were included in the analysis, and results showed that molecular tumor cell detection was associated with lower rates of overall survival, disease-specific survival, and disease-free survival [46].

ALTERNATIVE MODELS

Some investigators have proposed innovative strategies to improve the prognostic accuracy of staging models in colon cancer [19,47,48]. By incorporating non-TNM factors, such as histologic grade, lymph node ratio, type of operation, and neoadjuvant and adjuvant treatment, Manilich and colleagues [47] identified the lymph node ratio as an important predictor for both colon and rectal cancer, whereas type of surgery was predictive for rectal cancer. Similarly, using the SEER database, Weiser and colleagues [19] incorporated additional demographic and tumor variables in the traditional TNM system and found inclusion of tumor grade, number of metastatic lymph nodes removed, age, and sex generated a more accurate predictive model for survival in colorectal cancer. These studies emphasize the need for further investigation into alternative models for colorectal cancer beyond the traditional AJCC staging.

SUMMARY

Although staging for colon cancer has become more complex over time, it is not clear that this complexity has improved prognostic assessment. Even with revisions in the 7th edition of the AJCC staging system, a clear rank order of prognosis from substage to substage has not been established. Improved staging models will need to be developed, and attempts at further identifying those high-risk patients within each stage may be clinically useful. Through improved quality measures with lymph node yield, advances in colon cancer staging accuracy have been made over the last decade. Determining how to incorporate ultrastaging and molecular techniques will be the challenge for future staging models.

References

[1] Siegel R, Naishadham D, Jemal A. Cancer statistics, 2012. CA Cancer J Clin 2012;62:10–29.

[2] Edwards BK, Ward E, Kohler BA, et al. Annual report to the nation on the status of cancer, 1975-2006, featuring colorectal cancer trends and impact of interventions (risk factors, screening, and treatment) to reduce future rates. Cancer 2010;116:544–73.
[3] Andre T, Boni C, Navarro M, et al. Improved overall survival with oxaliplatin, fluorouracil, and leucovorin as adjuvant treatment in stage II or III colon cancer in the MOSAIC trial. J Clin Oncol 2009;27:3109–16.
[4] Graham JS, Cassidy J. Adjuvant therapy in colon cancer. Expert Rev Anticancer Ther 2012;12:99–109.
[5] Kuebler JP, Wieand HS, O'Connell MJ, et al. Oxaliplatin combined with weekly bolus fluorouracil and leucovorin as surgical adjuvant chemotherapy for stage II and III colon cancer: results from NSABP C-07. J Clin Oncol 2007;25:2198–204.
[6] Baddi L, Benson A 3rd. Adjuvant therapy in stage II colon cancer: current approaches. Oncologist 2005;10:325–31.
[7] Edge SB, Compton CC. The American Joint Committee on Cancer: the 7th edition of the AJCC cancer staging manual and the future of TNM. Ann Surg Oncol 2010;17: 1471–4.
[8] National Quality Forum Endorses Consense Standards for Diagnosis and Treatment of Breast and Colorectal Cancer: National Quality Forum; first posted April 12, 2007, Web Based Press Release. Available at: http://www.facs.org/cancer/qualitymeasures.html. Accessed November 2, 2012.
[9] Bilchik AJ, Hoon DS, Saha S, et al. Prognostic impact of micrometastases in colon cancer: interim results of a prospective multicenter trial. Ann Surg 2007;246:568–75 [discussion: 575–7].
[10] Iddings D, Ahmad A, Elashoff D, et al. The prognostic effect of micrometastases in previously staged lymph node negative (N0) colorectal carcinoma: a meta-analysis. Ann Surg Oncol 2006;13:1386–92.
[11] Nissan A, Protic M, Bilchik AJ, et al. United States Military Cancer Institute Clinical Trials Group (USMCI GI-01) randomized controlled trial comparing targeted nodal assessment and ultrastaging with standard pathological evaluation for colon cancer. Ann Surg 2012;256:412–27.
[12] Wasif N, Faries MB, Saha S, et al. Predictors of occult nodal metastasis in colon cancer: results from a prospective multicenter trial. Surgery 2010;147:352–7.
[13] Dukes CE. The classification of cancer of the rectum. J Pathol 1932;35:323–32.
[14] Astler VB, Coller FA. The prognostic significance of direct extension of carcinoma of the colon and rectum. Ann Surg 1954;139:846–52.
[15] Edge SB, Byrd DR, Compton CC, et al, editors. AJCC cancer staging manual. 7th edition. New York: Springer; 2010.
[16] National Comprehensive Cancer Network. Colon Cancer v.2.2013. Available at: http://www.nccn.org/professionals/physician_gls/pdf/colon.pdf. Accessed November 2, 2012.
[17] U.S. Preventive Services Task Force. Screening for colorectal cancer: U.S. Preventive Services Task Force recommendation statement. Ann Intern Med 2008;149:627–37.
[18] Qaseem A, Denberg TD, Hopkins RH Jr, et al. Screening for colorectal cancer: a guidance statement from the American College of Physicians. Ann Intern Med 2012;156: 378–86.
[19] Weiser MR, Gonen M, Chou JF, et al. Predicting survival after curative colectomy for cancer: individualizing colon cancer staging. J Clin Oncol 2011;29:4796–802.
[20] Bilchik A, Stojadinovic A. Is it time to move beyond lymph node evaluation in the staging of colon cancer? Arch Surg 2010;145:830–1.
[21] Lee HY, Choi HJ, Park KJ, et al. Prognostic significance of metastatic lymph node ratio in node-positive colon carcinoma. Ann Surg Oncol 2007;14:1712–7.
[22] Mescoli C, Albertoni L, Pucciarelli S, et al. Isolated tumor cells in regional lymph nodes as relapse predictors in stage I and II colorectal cancer. J Clin Oncol 2012;30:965–71.

[23] Poston GJ, Figueras J, Giuliante F, et al. Urgent need for a new staging system in advanced colorectal cancer. J Clin Oncol 2008;26:4828–33.
[24] Sinicrope FA, Shi Q. Combining molecular markers with the TNM staging system to improve prognostication in stage II and III colon cancer: are we ready yet? J Natl Cancer Inst 2012;104:1616–8.
[25] Telian SH, Bilchik AJ. Significance of the lymph node ratio in stage III colon cancer. Ann Surg Oncol 2008;15:1557–8.
[26] Compton CC, Fielding LP, Burgart LJ, et al. Prognostic factors in colorectal cancer. College of American Pathologists Consensus Statement 1999. Arch Pathol Lab Med 2000;124: 979–94.
[27] Goldstein NS, Sanford W, Coffey M, et al. Lymph node recovery from colorectal resection specimens removed for adenocarcinoma. Trends over time and a recommendation for a minimum number of lymph nodes to be recovered. Am J Clin Pathol 1996;106: 209–16.
[28] Scott KW, Grace RH. Detection of lymph node metastases in colorectal carcinoma before and after fat clearance. Br J Surg 1989;76:1165–7.
[29] Le Voyer TE, Sigurdson ER, Hanlon AL, et al. Colon cancer survival is associated with increasing number of lymph nodes analyzed: a secondary survey of intergroup trial INT-0089. J Clin Oncol 2003;21:2912–9.
[30] Chen SL, Bilchik AJ. More extensive nodal dissection improves survival for stages I to III of colon cancer: a population-based study. Ann Surg 2006;244:602–10.
[31] Stojadinovic A, Nissan A, Wainberg Z, et al. Time-dependent trends in lymph node yield and impact on adjuvant therapy decisions in colon cancer surgery: an international multi-institutional study. Ann Surg Oncol 2012;19(13):4178–85.
[32] Chen SL, Steele SR, Eberhardt J, et al. Lymph node ratio as a quality and prognostic indicator in stage III colon cancer. Ann Surg 2011;253:82–7.
[33] Wang J, Hassett JM, Dayton MT, et al. Lymph node ratio: role in the staging of node-positive colon cancer. Ann Surg Oncol 2008;15:1600–8.
[34] Rodriguez-Bigas MA, Maamoun S, Weber TK, et al. Clinical significance of colorectal cancer: metastases in lymph nodes <5 mm in size. Ann Surg Oncol 1996;3:124–30.
[35] Morton DL, Wen DR, Wong JH, et al. Technical details of intraoperative lymphatic mapping for early stage melanoma. Arch Surg 1992;127:392–9.
[36] Giuliano AE, Kirgan DM, Guenther JM, et al. Lymphatic mapping and sentinel lymphadenectomy for breast cancer. Ann Surg 1994;220:391–8 [discussion: 398–401].
[37] Bilchik AJ, Giuliano A, Essner R, et al. Universal application of intraoperative lymphatic mapping and sentinel lymphadenectomy in solid neoplasms. Cancer J Sci Am 1998;4: 351–8.
[38] Tsioulias GJ, Wood TF, Morton DL, et al. Lymphatic mapping and focused analysis of sentinel lymph nodes upstage gastrointestinal neoplasms. Arch Surg 2000;135:926–32.
[39] Wood TF, Saha S, Morton DL, et al. Validation of lymphatic mapping in colorectal cancer: in vivo, ex vivo, and laparoscopic techniques. Ann Surg Oncol 2001;8:150–7.
[40] Bembenek AE, Rosenberg R, Wagler E, et al. Sentinel lymph node biopsy in colon cancer: a prospective multicenter trial. Ann Surg 2007;245:858–63.
[41] Evangelista W, Satolli MA, Malossi A, et al. Sentinel lymph node mapping in colorectal cancer: a feasibility study. Tumori 2002;88:37–40.
[42] Joosten JJ, Strobbe LJ, Wauters CA, et al. Intraoperative lymphatic mapping and the sentinel node concept in colorectal carcinoma. Br J Surg 1999;86:482–6.
[43] Kitagawa Y, Fujii H, Mukai M, et al. The role of the sentinel lymph node in gastrointestinal cancer. Surg Clin North Am 2000;80:1799–809.
[44] Bilchik AJ, DiNome M, Saha S, et al. Prospective multicenter trial of staging adequacy in colon cancer: preliminary results. Arch Surg 2006;141:527–33 [discussion: 533–4].
[45] Stojadinovic A, Nissan A, Protic M, et al. Prospective randomized study comparing sentinel lymph node evaluation with standard pathologic evaluation for the staging of colon

carcinoma: results from the United States Military Cancer Institute Clinical Trials Group Study GI-01. Ann Surg 2007;245:846–57.
[46] Rahbari NN, Bork U, Motschall E, et al. Molecular detection of tumor cells in regional lymph nodes is associated with disease recurrence and poor survival in node-negative colorectal cancer: a systematic review and meta-analysis. J Clin Oncol 2012;30:60–70.
[47] Manilich EA, Kiran RP, Radivoyevitch T, et al. A novel data-driven prognostic model for staging of colorectal cancer. J Am Coll Surg 2011;213:579–88, 588.e1–2.
[48] Roth AD, Delorenzi M, Tejpar S, et al. Integrated Analysis of molecular and clinical prognostic factors in stage II/III colon cancer. J Natl Cancer Inst 2012;104:1635–46.

Advances in Surgery 47 (2013) 213–225

ADVANCES IN SURGERY

The Effect of Do-Not-Resuscitate Status on Postoperative Mortality in the Elderly Following Emergency Surgery

John E. Scarborough, MD[a,*], Theodore N. Pappas, MD[b]

[a]Department of Surgery, Duke University School of Medicine, DUMC 2837, Durham, NC 27710, USA; [b]General and Advanced Gastrointestinal Surgery, Department of Surgery, Duke University School of Medicine, DUMC 3479, Durham, NC 27710, USA

Keywords

• Do-not-resuscitate orders • Elderly • Emergency surgery

Key points

- General surgeons are likely to treat an increasing number of elderly patients with preexisting DNR orders or other advanced directives.
- Surgical patients with preexisting DNR orders are generally more acutely and chronically ill than patients without such orders.
- DNR patients are more likely to die after emergency general surgery than non-DNR patients, even after adjustment for acute and chronic comorbidity.
- A primary reason for the excess postoperative mortality experienced by DNR patients is their decreased willingness (relative to non-DNR patients) to undergo aggressive management of major postoperative complications.
- Further research is warranted to investigate the contribution of "failure-to-pursue-rescue" to surgical mortality in elderly patients.

INCIDENCE OF PREOPERATIVE DO-NOT-RESUSCITATE ORDERS AMONG ELDERLY EMERGENCY GENERAL SURGERY PATIENTS

The use of do-not-resuscitate (DNR) orders and other advanced directives is increasingly common among medical and surgical patients in the United States [1,2]. In a study of Medicare patients hospitalized for a variety of medical indications, Wenger and colleagues [2] found that 13% of patients from 1985 to 1986 carried DNR orders compared with only 10% of patients from 1981 to 1982. This temporal trend was statistically significant even after adjustment

*Corresponding author. *E-mail address*: scarb005@mc.duke.edu

0065-3411/13/$ – see front matter
http://dx.doi.org/10.1016/j.yasu.2013.04.001

for the degree of sickness at hospital admission and other patient-related factors. The same study demonstrated that DNR orders were generally written earlier during hospitalization in the later time period, which the authors attributed to an increasing recognition among physicians and patients of the importance of discussions about end-of-life issues. Further evidence of the increasing use of DNR orders derives from studies of the intensive care unit population in the United States. Jayes and colleagues [3] analyzed the use of DNR orders among a consecutive sample of 17,440 intensive care unit admissions from 40 hospitals across the country from 1988 to 1990. The authors found the prevalence of DNR orders during this time period to be 9%, which was significantly greater than the 5.4% prevalence demonstrated during a similar study conducted approximately one decade earlier. Again, the authors found a temporal trend toward DNR orders being written earlier after a patient's admission in the latter time period.

The increasing use of DNR orders is not confined to patients with medical conditions or to nonsurgical intensive care units. Meissner and colleagues [4] found a 1.6% prevalence of DNR orders among patients admitted to a 50-bed surgical intensive care unit between 2002 and 2006, with one-third of those patients having their DNR order in place before actually being admitted to the surgical intensive care unit. Nathens and colleagues [5] used data from the multicenter, prospective National Study on the Costs and Outcomes of Trauma data source to determine the frequency of DNR use among patients requiring intensive care unit admission secondary to trauma. Among the 69 US trauma centers included in that study, the incidence of DNR orders among severely injured patients was 7%. Eachempati and colleagues [6] performed a prospective study of all patients requiring surgical intensive care unit admission after emergency surgery at a tertiary care hospital between 2000 and 2004. Of the 723 patients included in that analysis, 12.7% were made DNR at some point during their admission. Finally, data from American College of Surgeons National Surgical Quality Improvement (ACS-NSQIP; a nationally validated, risk-adjusted, outcomes-based program that includes information about DNR status) demonstrate that 0.5% to 4.2% of patients undergoing surgical procedures carry preexisting DNR orders, with the incidence of having a DNR order depending on the acuity of the operative intervention, the age of the patient, and the types of procedures being performed [7,8]. Thus, the increasing use of advanced directives and the aging of the United States will most likely mean that general surgeons will attend to an increasing number of elderly patients with DNR orders who develop emergency general surgery conditions [9,10].

CHARACTERISTICS OF ELDERLY EMERGENCY GENERAL SURGERY PATIENTS WITH PREEXISTING DNR ORDERS

In general, patients who carry DNR orders tend to be older and more acutely ill than patients without such orders. For example, DNR patients from the previously cited analysis by Jayes and colleagues [3] had an average age of 68.5 ± 0.4 years, compared with 58.5 ± 0.2 years for patients without DNR orders. DNR patients in that study were also more acutely ill than non-DNR patients, as evidenced by their higher Acute Physiology and Chronic Health Evaluation III score at intensive care unit admission (91.9 ± 0.2 for DNR patients vs 45.8 ± 0.2 for non-DNR patients; $P<.001$). DNR patients are also more likely than non-DNR patients to carry certain chronic comorbid diagnoses. For example, 86% of DNR patients from the Jayes study exhibited one or more chronic medical conditions compared with only 59.8% of non-DNR patients.

Patients with preexisting DNR orders who subsequently consent to operation are also generally more ill than patients without such orders. This is demonstrated definitively by the analysis by Saager and colleagues [7] of 576,745 surgical patients from the 2005 to 2008 ACS-NSQIP database. The authors' study sample included all adult surgical patients from that data source excepting those who required mechanical ventilation preoperatively, displayed evidence of systemic inflammatory response syndrome or systemic sepsis, or who were in a comatose state at the time of their index operation. A total of 2687 (0.47%) of patients from that sample possessed DNR orders before their index procedure, with the mean age of DNR patients being 75 ± 15 years compared with 55 ± 17 years for non-DNR patients. In addition to being older, DNR patients in the ACS-NSQIP database were also more likely than non-DNR patients to have comorbid conditions, such as cerebrovascular disease hypertension, and to display evidence of acute physiologic deterioration as demonstrated by a higher American Society of Anesthesiologists preoperative physical status classification (mean 3.1 ± 0.7 for DNR patients vs 2.4 ± 0.7 for non-DNR patients) [7].

The discrepancy in the general health of DNR versus non-DNR patients is evident even when considering only elderly patients with emergency general surgical conditions. Such patients with a preoperative DNR order have been shown to have a higher incidence of chronic diseases, such as chronic obstructive pulmonary disease, bleeding disorders (including the use of oral anticoagulant medications, such as warfarin or clopidogrel), and chronic kidney disease when compared with non-DNR elderly patients [8]. Elderly emergency general surgery patients with preexisting DNR orders are also more likely than similar patients without such orders to have a nonindependent functional status (31.6% vs 8.2% of non-DNR patients; $P<.0001$); an acute alteration in mental status (12.3% for DNR patients vs 5.2% for non-DNR patient; $P<.0001$); or preoperative malnutrition (as measured by a 59% vs 35% incidence of preoperative hypoalbuminemia; $P<.0001$). Finally, elderly DNR surgical patients are more likely than non-DNR patients to carry a diagnosis of cancer (8.3% vs 4.6%; $P<.0001$). It is therefore clear that elderly emergency general surgery patients who have preexisting DNR orders are, in general, more acutely and chronically ill than patients who do not have such orders.

WHY DO ELDERLY PATIENTS WITH DNR ORDERS CONSENT TO EMERGENCY OPERATION?

Given their generally high levels of acute and chronic illness, why do elderly DNR patients consent to an emergency general surgery procedure? It is important to note that DNR orders technically and legally apply only to situations in which cardiopulmonary resuscitation is required to prevent death, and can never be assumed to extend to other forms of aggressive medical treatment. That being said, it is also generally the case that DNR patients be less inclined than non-DNR patients to accept aggressive medical interventions that fall short of cardiopulmonary resuscitation [5].

Unfortunately, there is no published study in the surgical literature that explicitly surveys elderly surgical patients with preexisting DNR orders about their rationale for accepting emergency operation. However, reasonable inference can be drawn from surveys of nonsurgical patients that have been published in the geriatric and palliative care literature. For example, Clemency and Thompson reported the results of their in-depth semistructured interviews of 18 patients who had terminal illness (eg, AIDS or cancer) and a documented DNR order [11]. Each patient was asked about the intentions behind their DNR orders, and was then presented with various theoretical scenarios designed to assess their willingness to accept either palliative or nonpalliative medical and surgical interventions. All but three of the patients interviewed stated that they would consent to an operation despite their terminal condition and DNR status. These patients stated that they would willingly undergo procedures that were needed for palliation of pain or discomfort related to the patient's terminal illness, and procedures that were unrelated to the terminal illness but which if successful would enable the patient to return to their present quality of life.

Members of the Study to Understand Prognoses and Preferences for Outcomes and Risks of Treatments (SUPPORT) investigator group conducted a survey analysis of 917 adults hospitalized with Stage III or IV non–small cell lung cancer or metastatic colon cancer to determine the relative importance to those patients of life-extending versus palliative therapeutic interventions [12]. The investigators found that patients were more likely to accept life-extending (and potentially pain-producing) therapy as opposed to palliation only if they believed that such therapy would leave them with a high probability of living for at least 6 additional months. Conversely, patients who perceived their probability of living at least 6 more months as a result of life-extending therapy were more likely to opt for palliative "comfort care." The SUPPORT investigators found discordance between patients' and physicians' estimates of the likelihood of success of life-extending therapy, with the physicians' less optimistic estimates ultimately proving to be more accurate.

Extrapolating from these studies of the treatment preferences of terminally ill patients, it becomes evident that elderly patients may readily consent to emergency general surgery even if they have preexisting DNR orders. The potential reasons for providing such consent may include a desire to alleviate pain that is associated with the emergency surgical condition, a hope that successful treatment of the condition will allow the patient to return to their baseline quality of life after resolution of incisional pain or discomfort, and a willingness to accept aggressive intervention for conditions that are not immediately related to the patient's primary medical illness. Given the high probability of severe systemic illness or death that would result from nonoperative management of most emergency general surgical conditions, it is not surprising that elderly patients consent to surgical intervention even when they are otherwise averse to aggressive medical intervention.

OUTCOMES ASSOCIATED WITH EMERGENCY OPERATION AMONG ELDERLY PATIENTS WITH PREEXISTING DNR ORDERS

Only two published studies have specifically described the postoperative outcomes of emergency general surgery patients who have preexisting DNR orders [8,13,14]. Because both of these studies involve the analysis of data from the ACS-NSQIP Program Participant User Files, a brief review of that data source is warranted. ACS-NSQIP is a nationally validated, risk-adjusted, outcomes-based program developed for the purpose of measuring and improving the quality of surgical care in private-sector academic and community hospitals [15]. Participation in the program is voluntary, and as of 2010 reached 258 US hospitals [16]. ACS-NSQIP collects patient-specific data on 135 variables, including acute and chronic comorbid conditions, procedure characteristics, and 30-day postoperative mortality and morbidity. The data are prospectively collected at each institution by an on-site ACS-trained surgical clinical reviewer, and are subject to frequent auditing to ensure accuracy and reliability [15]. Included among the comprehensive list of patient-related variables captured by the program is preoperative DNR status. Patients are defined by ACS-NSQIP as having such an order only if it is located in the patient's hospital chart in the 30 days before their index procedure and contains a signature or cosignature by an attending physician [16]. Patients whose DNR order was rescinded immediately before index operation are classified as being DNR by ACS-NSQIP reviewers. Conversely, patients with whom DNR status was discussed but not formalized are not considered by ACS-NSQIP reviewers to be DNR.

Our group's first analysis of emergency general surgery patients with DNR orders used data from the 2005 to 2009 ACS-NSQIP participant user files to determine the specific outcomes after emergency general surgery for bowel obstruction [13]. The mean age of the 242 DNR patients that were included in this analysis was 81 $\pm$ 11 years. A total of 24% of these patients were admitted from a chronic care facility, and 21.5% were classified as having a nonindependent preoperative functional status. The procedures performed in these patients included adhesiolysis only in 27.3%; small bowel resection or bypass in 29.8%; and colon resection (with or without anastomosis) in 30%. The 30-day postoperative mortality rate for these patients was 29.8% and the overall 30-day postoperative morbidity rate was 47.1%. The most common postoperative complications sustained included prolonged mechanical ventilation (defined as >48 hours, with a 19% incidence); sepsis or septic shock (18.6%); pneumonia (13.2%); urinary tract infection (7%); superficial surgical site infection (5.8%); and unplanned reintubation (5.4%). The mortality rate of patients who sustained one or more postoperative complications was 41.2%, an incidence that was significantly higher than in patients with no identifiable postoperative complications (19.5%). After adjustment for comorbid illness and procedure characteristics, the odds of dying associated with occurrence of a postoperative complications was 3.19 (95% confidence interval [CI], 1.70–5.99; $P<.0001$). We concluded from these findings that DNR patients who consent to emergency surgery for bowel obstruction have a high incidence of postoperative mortality and mortality, and that their risk of death is substantially increased if they experience a postoperative complication.

To assess the independent effect of preoperative DNR status on outcomes after emergency surgery for bowel obstruction, we then used propensity score matching methods to create a cohort of non-DNR patients who were statistically similar to the DNR patients from our sample with respect to incidence of chronic comorbid illness, physical status at the time of operation, and procedure characteristics [13]. Comparing the postoperative outcomes of this matched cohort revealed a significantly higher 30-day mortality rate for DNR patients (30.4% DNR vs 21.4% non-DNR; odds ratio [OR], 1.54; 95% CI, 1.01–2.35; $P = .04$) that persisted even after adjusting for the presence or absence of a postoperative complication. We concluded from this finding that the presence of a preoperative DNR order is an independent risk factor for postoperative mortality in patients undergoing emergency surgery for bowel obstruction.

Our group has more recently performed a larger study of ACS-NSQIP data to determine whether the association between DNR status and mortality after emergency surgery for bowel obstruction extends to all types of emergency general surgical procedures [8]. In this later study, we included all patients from the 2005 to 2010 ACS-NSQIP participant user files who were aged 65 years or older and who underwent emergency surgery for 1 of 10 common diagnoses. A total of 25,558 patients (24,497 without and 1061 with preexisting DNR orders) were included for analysis. In general, DNR patients exhibited a higher acuity of illness preoperatively and were more likely to carry chronic comorbid diagnoses. Diagnosis-specific 30-day postoperative outcomes for this cohort of elderly emergency general surgery patients with preexisting DNR orders are shown in Fig. 1 [8].

Given the significant baseline differences observed between DNR and non-DNR patients, we then developed a propensity matching algorithm to draw from the non-DNR population those patients who were most similar to the DNR patients with respect to acute and chronic severity of illness [8]. Our propensity matching algorithm also included markers of nutritional and functional status, indication for operation, and markers of procedure complexity, such as operative time and total work relative value units associated with index

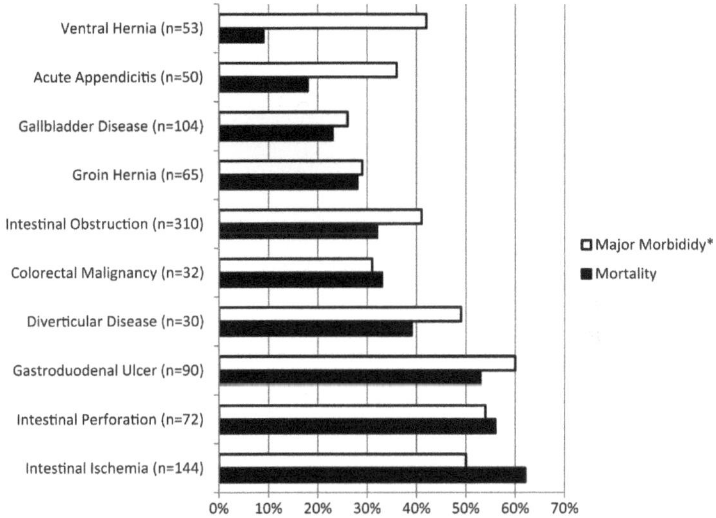

Fig. 1. Diagnosis-specific 30-day postoperative outcomes for elderly patients with preexisting DNR orders who undergo emergency general surgery. *Patients were considered to have sustained major postoperative morbidity if they developed one or more of the following complications: organ/space surgical site infection, wound dehiscence, pneumonia, pulmonary embolism, mechanical ventilation requirement greater than 48 hours, unplanned reintubation, cardiac arrest requiring cardiopulmonary resuscitation, myocardial infarction, progressive renal insufficiency, acute renal failure requiring dialysis, stroke, comatose state greater than 24 hours in duration, failure of graft/prosthesis requiring intervention, bleeding requiring more than 3 units packed red blood cells within 72 hours after index operation, systemic sepsis, or septic shock.

operation (Table 1) [17]. Using this algorithm, we were able to create a cohort of 1053 non-DNR patients who were well matched for all patient- and procedure-related variables. We then compared the early postoperative outcomes of this well-matched cohort. We found that DNR patients were significantly more likely than non-DNR patients to die within 30 days of their procedure (36.9% vs 22.3%; OR, 2.07; 95% CI, 1.69–2.55; $P<.0001$), but were not significantly more likely to experience major postoperative complications (42.1% vs 40.2%; OR, 1.08; 95% CI, 0.91–1.29; $P = .38$). Thus, preoperative DNR status is a significant predictor of mortality but not major morbidity for elderly patients who receive an emergency general surgical procedure.

Other studies have also used data from ACS-NSQIP to investigate the impact of DNR status on postoperative outcomes, although these are not confined to elderly patients or to emergency procedures. Kazaure and colleagues [17] performed a retrospective cohort study of 4128 surgical patients with and 4128 patients without preoperative DNR orders drawn from the 2005 to 2008 ACS-NSQIP Participant User Files. The DNR and non-DNR patients in this study were matched by age and by type of index procedure (which included colectomy, lower extremity amputation, cholecystectomy,

Table 1
Patient- and procedure-related variables available in ACS-NSQIP that were used to match DNR and non-DNR patients undergoing emergency general surgery

Type of variable	Variable
Demographic characteristics	Age
	Gender
	Body mass index
	Preoperative admission status
	Intraoperative surgical trainee participation
Chronic comorbid conditions	Preoperative functional status
	Physical mobility
	Diabetes mellitus
	Chronic obstructive pulmonary disease
	Congestive heart failure
	Coronary artery disease
	Renal dysfunction
	Chronic steroid use
	Bleeding disorder
	Known malignancy
	Cerebrovascular disease
Acute physiologic characteristics	Acute alteration in level of consciousness
	American Society of Anesthesiologists Physical Status Classification
	Preoperative mechanical ventilation
	Preoperative infected wound
	Preoperative transfusion
	Prior operation in preceding 30 d
	Preoperative serum albumin
	Preoperative sepsis classification
Intraoperative characteristics	Emergency surgical diagnosis
	Operative time
	Incisional wound classification
	Intraoperative transfusion
	Total work relative value units

Data from Scarborough JE, Pappas TN, Bennett KM, et al. Failure-to-pursue rescue: explaining excess mortality in elderly emergency general surgical patients with preexisting "do-not-resuscitate" orders. Ann Surg 2012;256:453–61.

small bowel procedure, exploratory laparotomy, femur fracture repair, or appendectomy). The authors included emergency and elective procedures in their analysis, with DNR patients from the matched cohort being more likely than non-DNR patients to receive operation in an emergency setting (34.6% vs 24.1%; $P<.001$). The authors found that overall mortality in DNR patients was 23.1%, compared with only 8.4% for non-DNR patients. Of the seven procedures included for analysis, mortality rates between the two groups were comparable only for femur fracture repair and appendectomy. Because there was a significant difference in the baseline characteristics of the DNR and non-DNR patients in their study sample, the authors used conditional logistic regression analysis to compare mortality rates after adjustment for comorbid disease burden and acuity of illness at presentation. After such adjustment, preoperative DNR status retained significance as a predictor of 30-day postoperative mortality (adjusted odds ratio of mortality associated with a preoperative order 2.2; 95% CI, 1.8–2.8; $P<.0001$). Unlike the findings from our study, Kazaure and colleagues found DNR patients to have a higher rate of major postoperative complications (26.2% vs 20.3%; $P<.0001$), although the authors did not subject this comparison to any type of risk adjustment.

Further evidence of the independent effect of preoperative DNR status on postoperative outcomes comes from the previously cited study by Saager and colleagues [7]. From their overall study sample of 576,745 surgical patients from the 2005 to 2008 ACS-NSQIP data source, the authors used a 1:3 propensity-matching algorithm to match DNR and non-DNR patients for demographic and preoperative comorbid characteristics. To match for the type of operation performed, the authors used software from the Agency for Health care Research and Quality to classify each patient's procedure (as determined by their primary Current Procedure Terminology code) into 1 of 244 clinically meaningful categories. The result of this algorithm was the creation of a cohort of 2199 DNR patients and 6002 non-DNR patients who were well-matched for most demographic and comorbid characteristics. Using complex statistical methods, the authors then compared the primary outcomes of the matched cohort of DNR and non-DNR patients [7]. The authors found that DNR status did not influence the incidence of major postoperative morbidity (15.5% for DNR patients vs 15% for non-DNR patients; hazard ratio [HR] for DNR status, 0.97; 95% CI, 0.86–1.10; $P = .65$), and that the presence of a preoperative DNR order was actually associated with a significantly lower incidence of minor postoperative morbidity (10.4% vs 11.9%; HR, 0.84; 95% CI, 0.72–0.97; $P = .02$). Secondary analysis of specific postoperative complications demonstrated that DNR patients were significantly less likely than non-DNR patients to sustain superficial surgical site infection, organ/space surgical site infection, unplanned reintubation, and prolonged mechanical ventilation. Although not more likely to sustain complications, DNR patients from the matched cohort were significantly more likely than their non-DNR counterparts to die within 30 days of operation, with a mortality rate of 12.5% observed among DNR patients compared with only 5.2% among non-DNR patients (HR, 2.3 for DNR status; 95% CI, 1.9–2.7; $P<.001$).

Thus, there is clear evidence patients with preoperative DNR orders have significantly higher postoperative mortality rates when compared with patients without such orders, but similar rates of major postoperative morbidity. The incidence of mortality and morbidity seem to be highest among elderly patients who consent to emergency operation.

EXPLAINING THE EXCESS MORTALITY OF ELDERLY EMERGENCY GENERAL SURGERY PATIENTS WITH PREEXISTING DNR ORDERS

An important finding from our analysis of elderly emergency general surgery patients may help to explain why the presence of a preoperative DNR order represents an independent risk factor for postoperative mortality [8]. Specifically, we found that patients from our propensity-matched cohort who suffered one or more major postoperative complications were significantly more likely to die if they had a preoperative DNR order. This outcome (death in the setting of a major postoperative complication) has been commonly referred to as "failure-to-rescue" [18,19]. The failure-to-rescue rate for DNR patients from our propensity-matched cohort was 56.7%, compared with 41.4% for non-DNR patients (OR, 2.07; 95% CI, 1.30–3.38; $P = .001$). The specific major complications that were associated with higher mortality in DNR patients compared with non-DNR patients included renal insufficiency, myocardial infarction, organ/space surgical site infection, pneumonia, prolonged mechanical ventilation, and septic shock.

Because the two groups in our propensity-matched cohort were so well-matched for patient- and procedure-related factors, we did not believe that the increased failure-to-rescue rate among DNR patients can be attributed to their being more sick than non-DNR patients. Instead, we interpreted our findings to mean that patients with DNR orders were more likely than patients without such orders to succumb to major complications for reasons unrelated to their physiologic condition. Crucial to this interpretation was our finding that DNR patients were significantly less likely than non-DNR patients to undergo reoperation within 30 days of their index procedure (reoperation rate 8.3% for DNR patients vs 12% for non-DNR patients; OR, 0.67; 95% CI, 0.50–0.90; $P = .006$). Because the two groups were well-matched patient- and procedure-related factors, and because they exhibited a similar incidence of major postoperative morbidity, there is no reason to believe that DNR patients would be less likely to need reoperation. Using reoperation as a marker of aggressiveness of postoperative care, we concluded from our findings that DNR patients are therefore less likely than non-DNR patients to receive aggressive management of major postoperative complications, and are therefore more likely to die when such complications occur. In general, there are two potential reasons patients with preoperative DNR orders might be treated less aggressively in the postoperative period compared with patients without preoperative DNR orders: either the physicians caring for DNR patients are less likely to offer aggressive intervention for major complications, or the patients themselves are less likely to accept such intervention.

There is some evidence from the medical literature of physician bias against aggressive treatment of DNR patients. Wenger and colleagues [20] studied the outcomes of a nationally representative sample of Medicare patients hospitalized with congestive heart failure, acute myocardial infarction, pneumonia, stroke, or hip fracture. After adjustment for differences in sickness at admission and other patient- and hospital-related factors, the authors found that in-hospital mortality was higher for DNR patients than non-DNR patients (40% vs 9%; $P < .001$), and attributed this difference to potential differences in the aggressiveness of physician management of these illnesses. Holtzman and colleagues [21] reviewed the nursing home charts of a random sample of 1605 Medicaid beneficiaries from one county in Minnesota and found that nursing home patients with DNR orders received less aggressive medical care than patients without such orders, and that in many cases patients with DNR orders but no other advanced directives had care limited beyond the withholding of cardiopulmonary resuscitation. These and other studies make clear the possibility of an unintentional bias among physicians against treating medically ill patients who have DNR orders with appropriate aggressiveness [22].

Importantly, there is no evidence within the surgical literature to suggest surgeon-driven undertreatment of DNR patients who have consented to undergo operation. For example, in their propensity-matched analysis of adult DNR and non-DNR patients undergoing both elective and emergency general surgical procedures, Saager and colleagues [7] found no difference in the duration of operation or in the use of intraoperative blood transfusion. Similarly, in our analysis of elderly patients undergoing emergency general surgery procedures, we found the procedures received by DNR patients to be generally of the same duration and complexity as those received by non-DNR patients [8]. Thus, there is no indication from the available evidence that surgical patients with preexisting DNR orders are treated any less aggressively than non-DNR patients by their surgeons, with further evidence provided by the similar postoperative complication rates observed for the two groups both in our analysis and that of Saager and colleagues.

Thus, the excess mortality observed among elderly emergency general surgery patients who have preexisting DNR orders can best be explained by their decreased willingness relative to non-DNR patients to accept aggressive management of major postoperative complications when such complications occur. Although this decision may seem paradoxic in light of the fact that these patients initially consented to emergency operation, the anecdotal observations of any surgical intensivist clearly support the concept of "failure-to-pursue-rescue" as a primary reason for the excess mortality witnessed among surgical patients with preexisting DNR orders. Such patients typically have only a limited amount of time in which to decide whether or not to consent to surgical management of their emergency condition. Given that the alternative to such management is likely death or severe systemic illness, and given that most emergency general surgical conditions are associated with significant physical discomfort and duress, it is not surprising that even elderly patients with a predilection against aggressive medical intervention would decide to accept emergency surgery. Understandably, such patients may hold out the hope that their postoperative course will be uneventful and that they may have some chance of returning to their presurgical quality of life. When events, such as major postoperative complications, conspire to obfuscate these hopes, patients might then reasonably decide that further aggressive intervention (eg, dialysis, coronary catheterization, or reoperation) is no longer consistent with their goals of care [23].

SUMMARY

Elderly patients who have preexisting DNR orders experience a high incidence of mortality and major morbidity within 30 days after emergency general surgery. Although not a risk factor for major morbidity, preoperative DNR status does represent an independent risk factor for mortality after emergency general surgery. The most plausible reason for the excess mortality in DNR patients is their decreased willingness to undergo aggressive treatment of major postoperative complications. Whether patient-driven failure-to-pursue-rescue also explains to some extent the high mortality of non-DNR elderly emergency general surgery patients deserves further investigation.

References

[1] Silveira MJ, Kim SY, Langa KM. Advance directives and outcomes of surrogate decision making before death. N Engl J Med 2010;362:1211–8.
[2] Wenger NS, Pearson ML, Desmond KA, et al. Changes over time in the use of do not resuscitate orders and the outcomes of patients receiving them. Med Care 1997;35:311–9.
[3] Jayes RL, Zimmerman JE, Wagner DP, et al. Do-not-resuscitate orders in intensive care units: current practices and recent changes. J Am Med Assoc 1993;270:2213–7.
[4] Meissner A, Genga KR, Studart FS, et al. Epidemiology of and factors associated with end-of-life decisions in a surgical intensive care unit. Crit Care Med 2010;38:1060–8.
[5] Nathens AB, Rivara FP, Wang J, et al. Variation in the rates of do not resuscitate orders after major trauma and the impact of intensive care unit environment. J Trauma 2008;64:81–91.
[6] Eachempati SR, Hydo L, Shou J, et al. Sex differences in creation of do-not-resuscitate orders for critically ill elderly patients following emergency surgery. J Trauma 2006;60:193–8.
[7] Saager L, Kurz A, Deogaonkar A, et al. Pre-existing do-not-resuscitate orders are not associated with increased postoperative morbidity at 30 days in surgical patients. Crit Care Med 2011;39:1036–41.
[8] Scarborough JE, Pappas TN, Bennett KM, et al. Failure-to-pursue rescue: explaining excess mortality in elderly emergency general surgical patients with preexisting "do-not-resuscitate" orders. Ann Surg 2012;256:453–61.
[9] Spencer G. Projections of the population of the United States age, sex, and race: 1988-2080. Washington, DC: US Bureau of the Census; 1989.
[10] Cherniak EP. Increasing use of DNR orders in the elderly worldwide: whose choice is it? J Med Ethics 2002;28(5):303–7.
[11] Clemency MV, Thompson NJ. Do not resuscitate orders in the perioperative period: patient perspectives. Anesth Analg 1997;84:859–64.
[12] Weeks JC, Cook F, O'Day SJ, et al. Relationship between cancer patients predictions of prognosis and their treatment preferences. J Am Med Assoc 1998;279(21):1709–14.
[13] Speicher PJ, Lagoo-Deenadayalan SA, Galanos AN, et al. Expectations and outcomes in geriatric patients with do-not-resuscitate orders undergoing emergent surgical management of bowel obstruction. Arch Surg 2013;148(1):23–8.
[14] Turrentine FE, Wang H, Simpson VB, et al. Surgical risk factors, morbidity, and mortality in elderly patients. J Am Coll Surg 2006;203:865–77.
[15] Ingraham AM, Richards KE, Hall BL, et al. Quality improvement in surgery: the American College of Surgeons National Surgical Quality Improvement Program approach. Adv Surg 2010;44:251–67.
[16] American College of Surgeons National Surgical Quality Improvement Program. User guide for the 2010 participant user file. 2011. Available at: http://site.acsnsqip.org/participant-use-data-file?. Accessed September 23, 2012.
[17] Kazaure H, Roman S, Sosa JA. High mortality in surgical patients with do-not-resuscitate orders. Arch Surg 2011;146(8):922–8.

[18] Ghaferi AA, Birkmeyer JD, Dimick JB. Complications, failure to rescue, and mortality with major inpatient surgery in Medicare patients. Ann Surg 2009;250:1029–34.
[19] Ghaferi AA, Birkmeyer JD, Dimick JB. Variation in hospital mortality associated with inpatient surgery. N Engl J Med 2009;361:1368–75.
[20] Wenger NS, Pearson ML, Desmond KA, et al. Outcomes of patients with do-not-resuscitate orders. Toward an understanding of what do-not-resuscitate orders mean and how they affect patients. Arch Intern Med 1995;155(19):2063–8.
[21] Holtzman J, Pheley AM, Lurie N. Changes in orders limiting care and the use of less aggressive care in a nursing home population. J Am Geriatr Soc 1994;42(3):275–9.
[22] Chen JT, Sosnov J, Lessard D, et al. Impact of do-not-resuscitate orders on quality of care performance measures in patients hospitalized with acute heart failure. Am Heart J 2008;156(1):78–84.
[23] Kaldijian LC, Broderick A. Developing a policy for do not resuscitate orders within a framework of goals of care. Jt Comm J Qual Patient Saf 2011;37:11–9.

Advances in Surgery 47 (2013) 227–249

ADVANCES IN SURGERY

Incidental Gall Bladder Cancer

Anu Behari, MS, Vinay K. Kapoor, FRCS*

Department of Surgical Gastroenterology, Sanjay Gandhi Post-Graduate Institute of Medical Sciences (SGPGIMS), Raibareli Road, Lucknow 226014, Uttar Pradesh, India

Keywords

• Cholecystectomy • Completion extended cholecystectomy
• Extended cholecystectomy • Gall bladder cancer • Gall stone disease
• Laparoscopic cholecystectomy

Key points

- Gall bladder cancer (GBC) is termed incidental GBC when the diagnosis of GBC is made for the first time on histologic examination of the gall bladder specimen after simple cholecystectomy for presumed gall stone disease.
- Most patients with incidental GBC, except those with T1a (mucosal) disease, for which simple cholecystectomy alone is enough, and those with distant metastases, need reoperation.
- Work up before the reoperation includes ultrasonography, computed tomography, positron emission tomography, and staging laparoscopy, mainly to exclude distant metastases.
- The surgical procedure for incidental GBC is completion extended cholecystectomy, which includes resection of a 2-cm wedge of liver in the gall bladder bed and lymphadenectomy.
- Incidental GBC is usually early and potentially resectable; early and appropriate management can achieve long-term survival, and even cure, in a disease with an otherwise dismal outlook.

INTRODUCTION

Gall stone disease (GSD) is common worldwide. Cholecystectomy is the treatment of choice for symptomatic GSD and is one of the most common abdominal operations performed. There is a strong association between GSD and gall bladder cancer (GBC). Incidental GBC (IGBC, also variously called inapparent, occult, subclinical, or unsuspected GBC) (ie, GBC detected for the first time on histologic examination of a gall bladder [GB] removed for

*Corresponding author. *E-mail address:* vkkapoor.india@gmail.com

0065-3411/13/$ – see front matter
http://dx.doi.org/10.1016/j.yasu.2013.04.003

presumed GSD), is an unpleasant shock for the patient as well as the surgeon. The diagnosis of IGBC raises several management issues: does the patient require reoperation? What should be the preoperative workup before the second surgery? What procedure is required? [1]. But at the same time, considering the generally dismal prognosis of GBC (mainly because of the advanced stage in most cases when it is diagnosed preoperatively or at operation), fortuitous discovery of an IGBC, which is early GBC (usually limited to the mucosa or muscle), and its appropriate management, may offer a chance of long-term survival and even cure. Most cholecystectomies are now performed laparoscopically. Laparoscopic cholecystectomy (LC) carries a potential risk of perforation of the GB and bile spill, resulting in an increased risk of peritoneal dissemination and wound (port site) metastases. This situation can, theoretically at least, vitiate the results of the second surgical procedure and make even early and potentially curable IGBC incurable. This review provides an overview of the issues and controversies in the management of IGBC.

DEFINITIONS

Various investigators use the term incidental GBC to describe several different clinical scenarios leading to considerable confusion. It is important to have a uniformity of nomenclature, both for formulation of treatment guidelines as well as for comparison of results. We have proposed that the following terms should be used depending on the presentation and timing of diagnosis of GBC.

Obvious: diagnosis of GBC is apparent on clinical examination (surgical obstructive jaundice [SOJ], GB lump Fig. 1) or radiologic investigations (ultrasonography [US] [Fig. 2] and computed tomography [CT] [Fig. 3] showing GB mass).

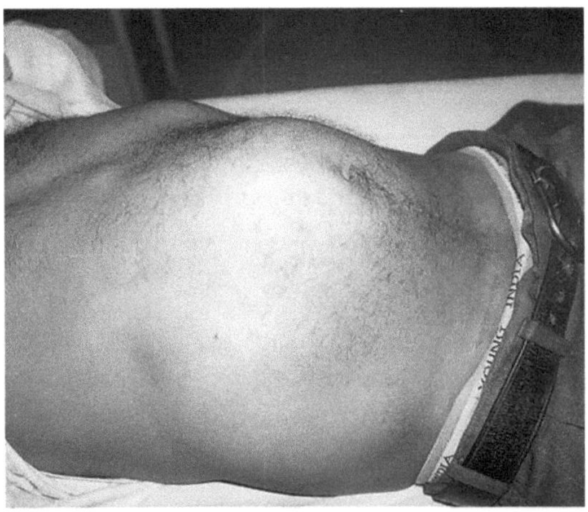

Fig. 1. Large clinically obvious GB lump.

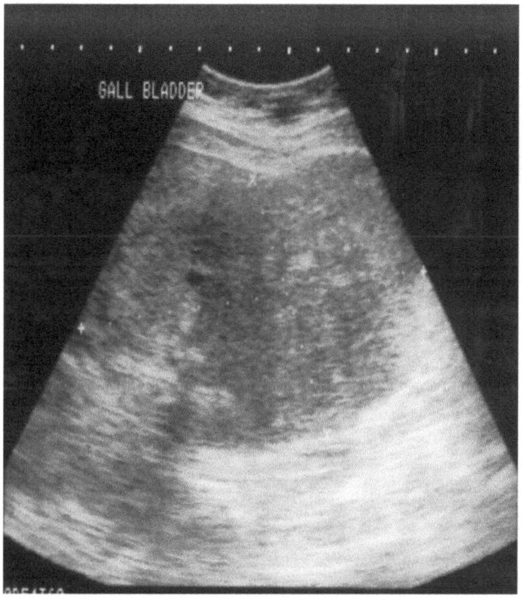

Fig. 2. Ultrasonographic image showing a GB mass.

Suspected: US and CT show focal irregular GB wall thickening (Fig. 4) (diffuse regular GB wall thickening suggests chronic cholecystitis or xanthogranuolomatous cholecystitis [XGC] [Fig. 5], porcelain GB [Fig. 6], or single large sessile polyp [Fig. 7]).

Unsuspected (unexpected): there is no clinical or radiologic suspicion of GBC; GBC is suspected during operation for presumed GSD, for example, densely adherent omentum (Fig. 8), contracted thick-walled GB, obliterated

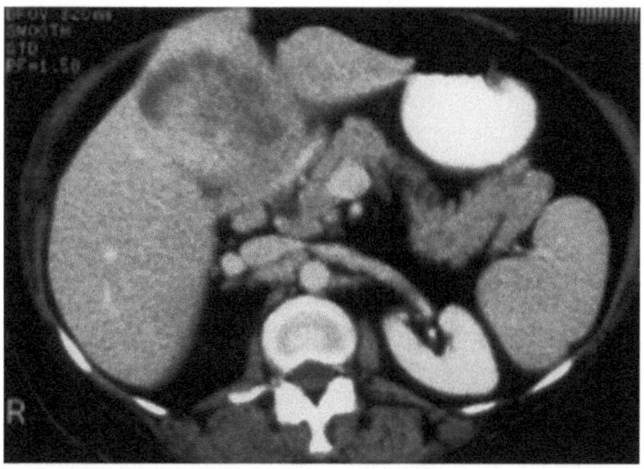

Fig. 3. GB mass filling the lumen of the GB as seen on contrast-enhanced CT of the abdomen: radiologically obvious GBC.

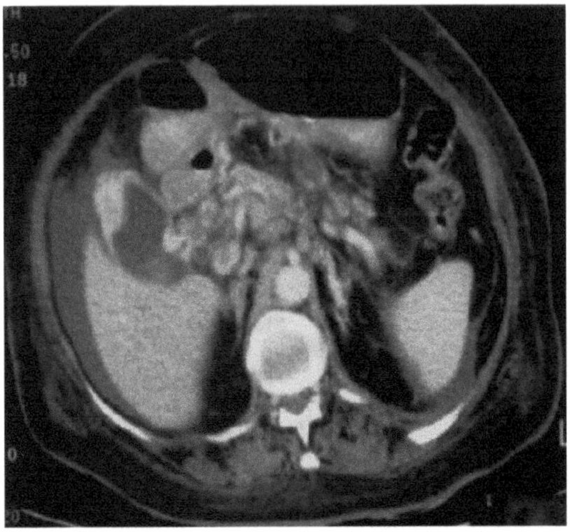

Fig. 4. Contrast-enhanced CT showing focal thickening of GB wall: suspicious GBC.

Calot triangle (Fig. 9), difficult GB bed (although all these findings can be present in chronic inflammation also); ulcer (Fig. 10), nodule, or focal GB wall thickening is discovered on gross examination of the opened specimen.

Incidental: GBC is not suspected at operation or even on gross examination of the GB specimen; it is detected for the first time on histologic examination of the GB only. This is true IGBC and is the one that is discussed in this review.

Missed: routine histologic examination of the GB did not reveal GBC but patient develops recurrence within few months (an early GBC was missed even on routine histology of the GB).

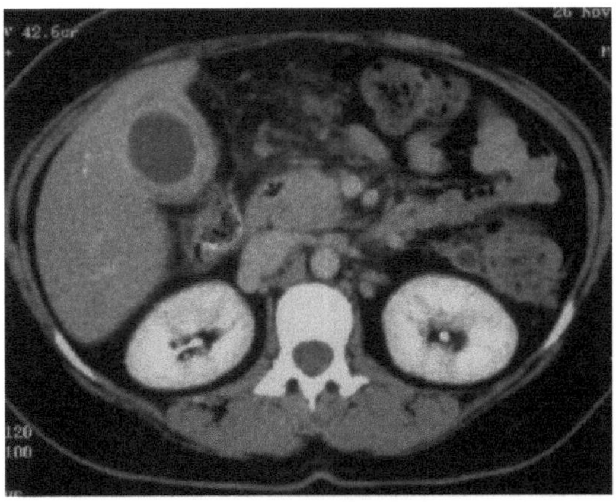

Fig. 5. Diffusely thickened GB wall, suggestive of inflammation.

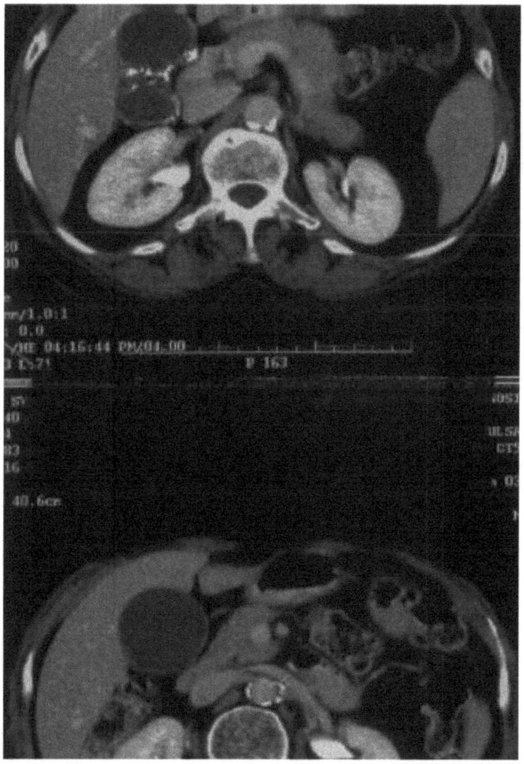

Fig. 6. Contrast-enhanced CT abdomen showing focal GB wall calcification: porcelain GB.

INCIDENCE

IGBC may be encountered in approximately 1% of all cholecystectomies. Recent reports [2,3] of IGBC after LC report rates ranging from 0.5% to 2.1%. With the increasing number of LCs being performed for GSD, the number of IGBCs is expected to increase [4]. Even with an expected incidence of 1%, as many as 5000 incidental GBCs are diagnosed in more than 500,000 cholecystectomies performed in the United States every year. Rates of IGBC may be higher for some subgroups of patients with GSD (eg, elderly patients, those with acute cholecystitis/empyema GB [5], Mirizzi syndrome [6,7], porcelain GB [8], and single large sessile GB polyp [9]).

MANAGEMENT

Rationale

Treatment of IGBC is based on the following considerations:

- Simple cholecystectomy in presence of GBC is likely to transgress tumor-bearing tissue planes. This situation is most likely when the tumor has spread

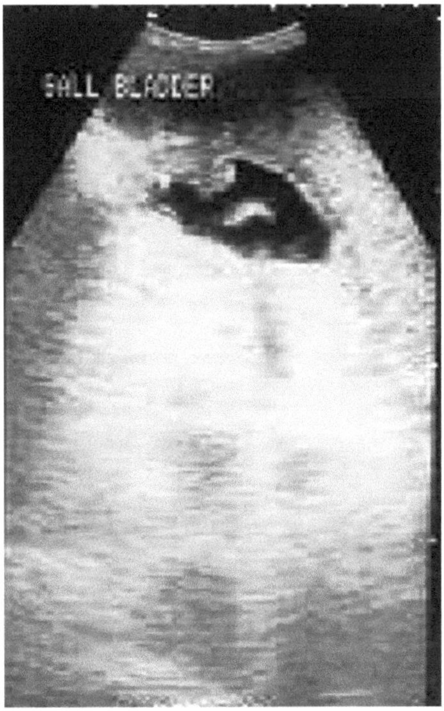

Fig. 7. Single, sessile polypoidal lesion of the GB on US: suspicious GBC.

beyond the muscle into the perimuscular/subserosal plane (the plane of dissection during simple cholecystectomy).

- There is a high chance of residual disease, either in the GB bed in the liver or in the draining lymph nodes (LNs) after a simple cholecystectomy in the presence

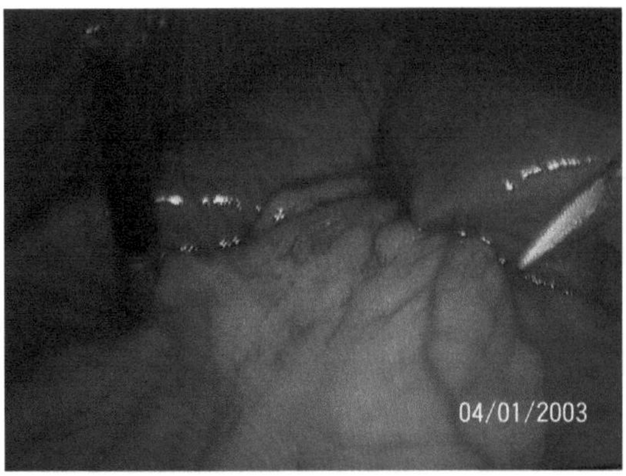

Fig. 8. Omentum found densely adherent to GB during LC, unsuspected GBC.

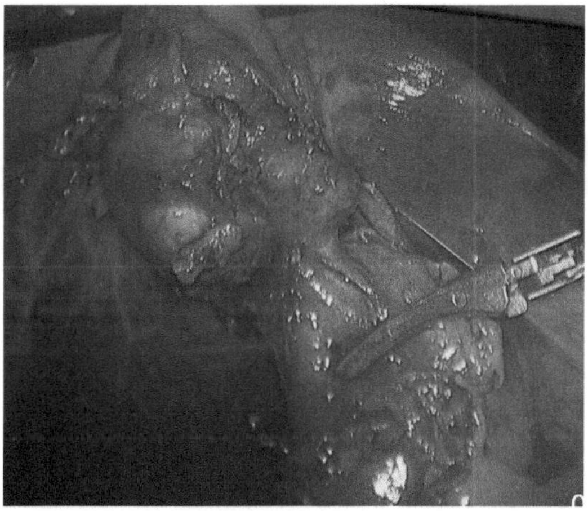

Fig. 9. Obliterated Calot triangle during LC: unsuspected GBC.

of an IGBC. The likelihood of this residual disease increases with increasing depth of tumor (T stage). A recent retrospective analysis of 435 GBC cases referred to the Memorial Sloan Kettering Cancer Center (MSKCC), New York over a 10-year period reported that 47% were discovered incidentally on LC; 100 (74%) of the 146 patients who were reexplored were found to have residual disease [10].

- Looking specifically into the incidence of finding residual disease at the time of re-resection, Pawlik and colleagues [11] found that the re-resected specimen contained residual/additional disease in 46.4% of patients: 0%, 10.4%, and 36.4% of patients with T1, T2, and T3 disease, respectively were found to have residual disease in the liver and LN metastases were found in 12.5%, 31.3%, and 45.5% of patients with T1, T2, and T3 tumors, respectively.
- LN involvement in GBC increases with increasing transmural spread and varies from 0% for T1a, up to 11% for T1b, 46% to 62% for T2, and 79% to 83% for

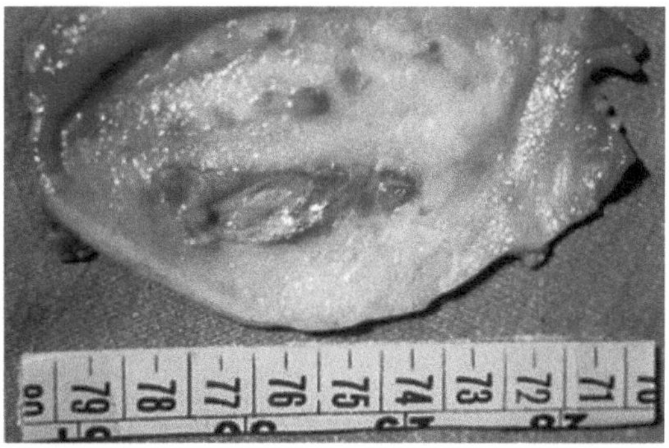

Fig. 10. Ulcer in the GB specimen cut open after LC: unsuspected GBC.

T3 and T4 tumors [12–15]. In tumors close to the GB neck, the cystic duct margin or even the common bile duct (CBD) may have microscopic residual disease.

- Because the cystic LN may or may not be removed along with the GB in a simple cholecystectomy, complete information about the stage (LN status) of the disease is not available. Moreover, cystic LN is not a sentinel LN for GB, and other LNs may be involved even if the cystic LN is negative. Involvement of draining LNs is one of the most important predictors of poor prognosis in GBC.
- Completion extended cholecystectomy (CEC) (ie, re-resection with removal of the GB bed in liver and LN dissection) may not only allow complete staging of the disease but may also provide survival benefit depending on the stage of the disease (see later discussion).
- If the cholecystectomy had been performed laparoscopically, there may be seeding of the port sites (especially the port of GB extraction) and also tumor dissemination; this possibility becomes even more likely if there is perforation of the GB with bile spill during cholecystectomy.
- Most often, the cholecystectomy is performed at a center other than the referral center. There may be delay in referral, allowing time for tumor spread; also, complete operative details (eg, about bile spill, use of a bag for GB extraction, which port was used for GB extraction) may not be available.
- Although some patients with IGBC may be at a very early (Tis or T1a) stage and, therefore, no further management other than the simple cholecystectomy, which has already been performed, may be required, many are likely to have early (T1b and T2) disease, in which further therapy with re-resection is likely to make a significant positive difference in prognosis. T2 tumors (the ones most likely to benefit from re-resection) constituted 59% (43/73), 49% (48/98), and 46% (13/28) of IGBC reported by Wakai and colleagues, Shirai and colleagues, and Toyonaga and colleagues, respectively, from Japan [16–18]. Similar figures have been reported by other investigators [2,3,19]. In our series of 44 IGBCs, the T stage distribution was T1a in 4, T1b in 16, T2 in 15, and T3 in 9 patients (Behari and Kapoor, unpublished data, 2013).

For Tis (in situ) and T1a (mucosal) tumors, simple cholecystectomy alone is enough and no further treatment is required. The reported incidence of LN metastases is about 1.8%, and low (1.1%) recurrence rates have been reported, 50% of these being in CBD [12]. If, therefore, the cystic duct margin is positive, CBD resection is required. Numerous series report excellent long-term survival for T1a tumors with simple cholecystectomy (see section on results of surgery).

For T1b (muscularis propria) tumors, controversy still persists. Although according to some reports, simple cholecystectomy alone is enough, others recommend reoperation with excision of the GB bed in liver and lymphadenectomy because of the high incidence of residual disease and chances of recurrence after simple cholecystectomy alone. The reported rates of LN metastases (11%) as well as recurrence (9%) are higher than those for T1a tumors. A higher recurrence rate of 12.5% has been reported after simple cholecystectomy compared with a 2.7% after extended cholecystectomy for T1b tumors [12]. However, based on our experience, we continue to perform (and advocate) reoperation for CEC for T1b tumors.

For T2 (perimuscular/subserosal) tumors, there is a high chance of presence of residual disease in the GB bed as well as in the draining LNs, and there is plenty of literature support for reoperation with liver resection (most often a 2-cm nonanatomic wedge or segment IVb+V) and lymphadenectomy (see section on results of surgery).

For T3 (perimuscular/subserosal) tumors, although the chances of residual disease are high, improvement in survival with re-resection has not been reported consistently; there are some reports of improvement in survival with re-resection, whereas others have reported no such benefit. However, we advocate that, in the absence of distant metastases, even T3 tumors should be offered the benefit, albeit small, of reoperation for CEC.

TIMING OF SURGERY

Although most surgeons would like to reoperate soon after a diagnosis of IGBC has been made, there are no clear guidelines as to what is the upper limit of the time interval before which re-resection should be performed to have a beneficial effect. However, the longer the time interval, the higher the risk of spread and dissemination, precluding reoperation for re-resection with intent to cure [20]. In a small experience of 11 patients with T2 tumors that were re-resected, Muratore and colleagues [21] reported that the survival was significantly better (median 46.7 months, 5-year 100%) for the group of patients operated sooner (mean cholecystectomy, resection interval of 2.2 months) than those who were operated late (mean cholecystectomy, resection interval of 11.3 months); all patients in the latter group died within 25 months. However, every patient with IGBC, irrespective of the time interval after simple cholecystectomy, should receive the benefit of reoperation for re-resection, the only contraindication being the presence of distant spread.

WORKUP BEFORE REOPERATION

Despite an incidental diagnosis and a higher chance of having localized disease amenable to cure after appropriate re-resection, many patients with IGBC have nonlocalized disease for which even re-resection does not have any impact on survival. The aim of the preoperative workup is to identify distant spread and avoid an unnecessary laparotomy in patients with disseminated disease.

Details of the index simple cholecystectomy, especially with regards to bile spill, use of a bag for GB extraction, and port used for GB extraction, should be obtained, if possible. Also, the specimen, paraffin blocks, and slides of the removed GB should be obtained for a review for the site (fundus, body, or neck/cystic duct), type (papillary or otherwise), T status, N status (if cystic LN was included in the specimen), cystic duct margin, lymphovascular and perineural invasion, grade and differentiation of the tumor.

After a detailed clinical examination to rule out obvious distant metastases (eg, liver nodules, ascites, pelvic deposits, left supraclavicular LN, umbilical nodule), the sequence of investigations includes US of the abdomen, chest radiography (better still, chest CT), CT of the abdomen, positron emission tomography (PET) scan (optional), and staging laparoscopy, mainly to look for any distant metastasis, which is then confirmed by fine-needle aspiration cytology (FNAC), because presence of distant spread rules out a reoperation. We consider even distant (celiac, superior mesenteric and aortocaval) LNs as distant spread [22]. If these LNs are seen on CT, they are targeted for FNAC; if not, they are biopsied during laparotomy (Fig. 11). Presence of a mass in the GB fossa on preoperative CT has been reported to be associated with a poor prognosis even after an attempted second curative resection [21]. In the context of IGBC, CT suffers from the limitations of not being able to identify very small lesions and in not being able to distinguish residual/recurrent tumor from inflammatory or postsurgical scarring.

The role of PET in the context of IGBC is still evolving. PET has been postulated to have a role complementary to CT in the preoperative staging algorithm of patients with IGBC. Shukla and colleagues [23] studied 80 patients with IGBC with PET-CT. Fifty-five (70%) of these patients had disseminated disease, and 24 (30%) patients had local and potentially resectable disease. Twenty-one of these patients could be resected, and in 7 (33%) of them, there was residual disease. The sensitivity and positive predictive values of PET-CT for residual disease were 29% and 20%, respectively. Butte and colleagues [24], with their experience of 32 patients with IGBC, concluded that for patients presenting with stage T1b or greater IGBC, the use of PET-CT helps reduce the number of patients undergoing nontherapeutic reexploration and thus might be a useful tool for the selection of patients for potentially curative treatment. In their study, PET-CT identified 10 (31%) patients with disseminated disease and changed surgical management in 8 (25%) of them. More prospective studies are needed to put the role of PET-CT in preoperative staging workup for IGBC in proper prospective.

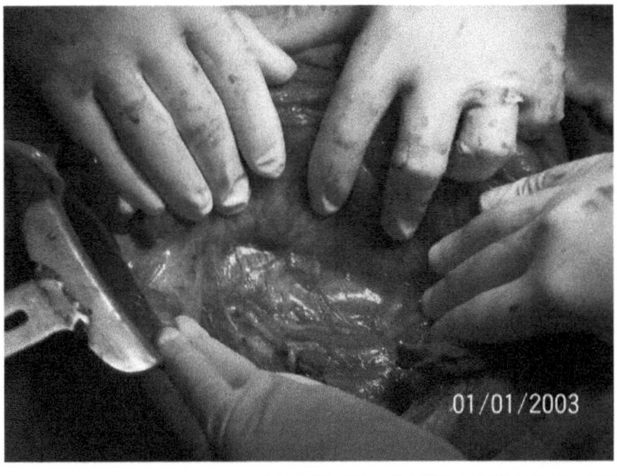

Fig. 11. Biopsy of para-aortic LNs after full Kocherization of duodenum at laparotomy.

STAGING LAPAROSCOPY

For a planned radical resection for preoperatively diagnosed GBC, staging laparoscopy is advised in all patients, because it picks up small, superficial, surface hepatic (Fig. 12), omental and peritoneal metastases undetected on preoperative imaging and may avoid an unnecessary laparotomy in as many as one-third of cases [25]. For patients with IGBC undergoing re-resection, Butte and colleagues [26] reported that the chances of having disseminated disease is related to the T stage, positive resection margin, and poor differentiation, and staging laparoscopy is more likely to have a high yield in this subgroup of patients. In these investigators' experience, the overall yield of staging laparoscopy was low in patients with IGBC undergoing reexploration for curative surgery. Of the 138 patients who underwent reexploration, 19 had dissemination. Staging laparoscopy was performed in 46 patients and picked up dissemination in only 2 of the 10 patients with dissemination. Because most cholecystectomies are performed laparoscopically and LC is associated with a significant risk of bile spill, which in turn increases the likelihood of tumor dissemination even in early tumors [27], in our opinion, staging laparoscopy should remain a part of the algorithm of management of IGBC until further studies are available. Like most other surgeons managing GBC, we have encountered disseminated disease after cholecystectomy even for T1 lesions and continue to perform (and advocate) staging laparoscopy before re-resection in patients with IGBC also.

SURGERY FOR IGBC

If preliminary laparoscopy followed by laparotomy does not reveal metastatic disease or distant (celiac, superior mesenteric or aortocaval) LN spread, one can proceed with CEC, including a 2-cm nonanatomic wedge (Fig. 13)/segment IVb+V liver resection along with standard LN dissection in which cystic (12c), pericholedochal (12b), hilar (12h), proper hepatic artery (12a), periportal (12p),

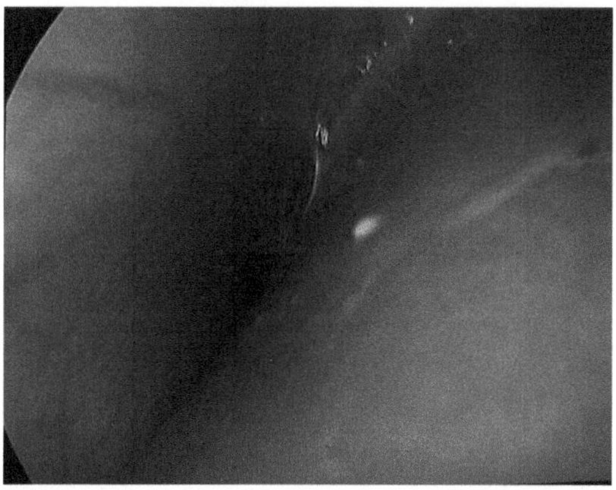

Fig. 12. Metastatic deposit on the liver surface during staging laparoscopy.

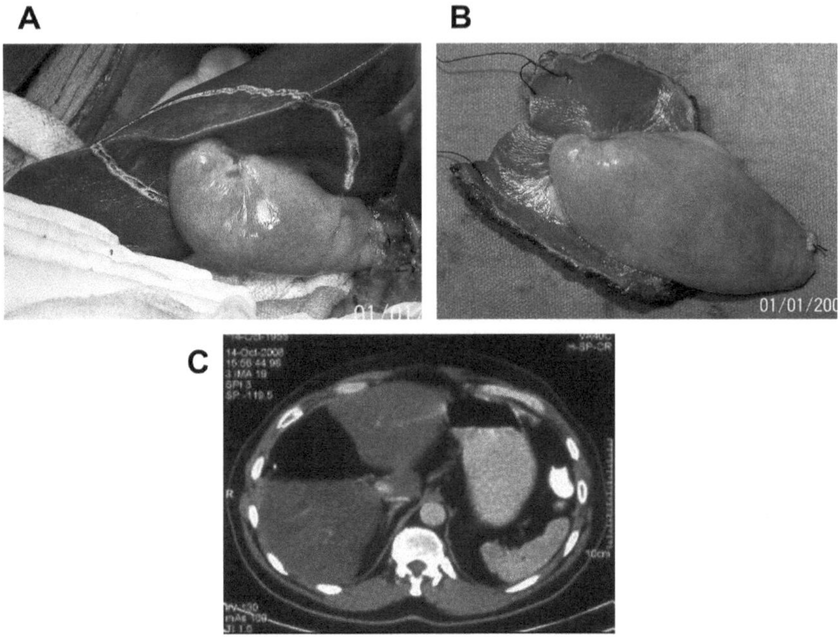

Fig. 13. (A) 2 cm wedge of liver marked in preparation for resection. (B) Extended cholecystectomy specimen containing gall bladder and 2 cm wedge of liver. (C) CT scan in a patient who had undergone extended cholecystectomy.

posterosuperior pancreaticoduodenal (13a), and common hepatic artery LNs are removed with skeletonization of hepatic artery, portal vein, and the bile duct in the hepatoduodenal ligament (Fig. 14). There are no randomized comparisons between wedge resection and segment IVb+V resection, but

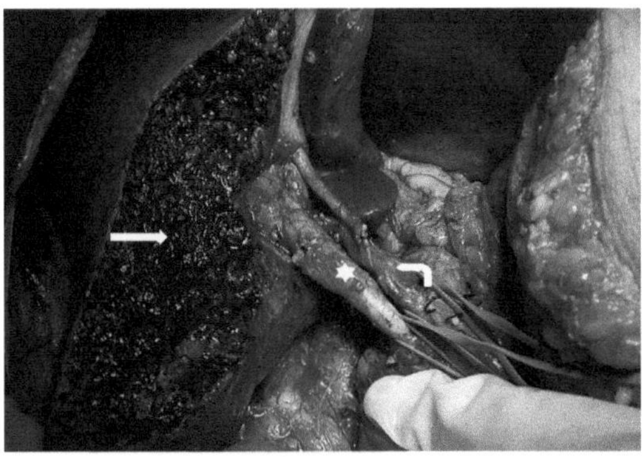

Fig. 14. Operative field after extended cholecystectomy: liver bed after wedge resection (*straight arrow*) and hepatoduodenal ligament after LN dissection. Star: Common bile duct. Curved line: Hepatic artery.

data from the German Cancer Registry suggest that for T1 lesions, wedge excision is sufficient and that for T2 tumors segment IVb+V resection offers survival advantage [28]. Routine excision of the CBD is not warranted because it has been shown to increase the morbidity without providing any survival benefit. In a report that analyzed collated data from a French multicenter database on experience with IGBC, Fuks and colleagues [29] reported that resection of CBD increased postoperative complications (60% vs 23%, $P = .0001$); it increased neither R0 resection nor overall survival (OS). However, if the cystic duct margin of the cholecystectomy specimen shows malignant cells, a CBD excision needs to be added. Some surgeons advocate locating the cystic duct margin, re-resecting it for frozen section examination, and performing a CBD excision if this margin is positive [30].

The issue of port site excision during reoperation remains controversial. There is no consensus regarding the questions whether port sites should be excised at all, whether all ports or only the port of extraction should be excised, whether presence of tumor cells in the excised port sites indicates disseminated disease, and whether port site excision provides only staging and prognostic information and not survival benefit.

Port site recurrence rates for GBC after LC have been reported to range from 0% to 40%, and higher rates are associated with GB perforation and bile spill during cholecystectomy. Results of an international survey that included Swiss, German, and Austrian surgeons, who reported a total of 117,840 LCs, revealed 479 IGBCs and 70 patients had port site metastases. In as many as 52 patients with port site metastases, the tumor was confined to the GB wall (T0–13, T1–13 and T2–36), port site metastasis was seen in the port of GB extraction in 49 and in other ports in 37 patients [31].

In a recent study of 113 patients with IGBC from the MSKCC, 69 of whom underwent port site excision and 44 of whom did not undergo port site excision, 13 (19%) were found to have port site metastases. Port site metastases were seen only in patients with T2 or T3 tumors and correlated with the development of peritoneal metastases ($P = .01$). Median survival of patients with T2/T3 disease without port site metastasis was 42 months compared with 17 months in patients with port site metastases ($P = .005$). When only patients with R0 resections were compared and adjusted for T and N stage, port site resection was not associated with better overall ($P = .23$) or recurrence-free survival ($P = .69$) and led the investigators to conclude that port site excision was not associated with less disease recurrence or improved survival and should not be considered mandatory during definitive surgical treatment of IGBC [32]. The retrospective nature of the study and the fact that port site excision was dependent on the surgeon's choice and was not a definitive protocol limit the validity of these conclusions. Occasionally, a solitary port site deposit is the only site of disease, indicating that it is a local recurrence rather than dissemination and is amenable to resection for cure. We continue to perform (and advocate) full-thickness (skin to peritoneum) excision (Fig. 15) of all 4 port sites during CEC for IGBC.

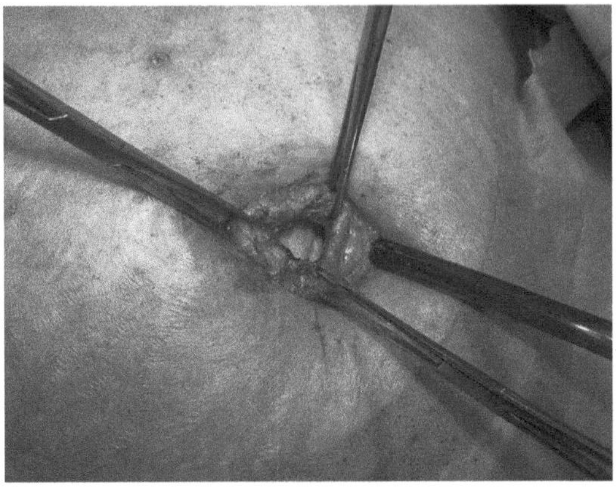

Fig. 15. Full-thickness excision of port site during CEC.

INDICATIONS/CONTRAINDICATIONS FOR REOPERATION

Decision recommendations for reoperation are based primarily on T stage (the information that is available most often). The effect of other factors related to tumor biology (eg, tumor differentiation, presence of unfavorable histologic markers such as perineural or lymphovascular invasion) on chances of improvement in survival after reoperation should also be taken into consideration. As an example, not all T2 tumors have the 5-year survival greater than 90% reported by some investigators; the reported figures vary from 60% to more than 90%. Also, a subgroup of patients with T2 tumors does not have significant survival benefit after reoperation.

The management algorithm of patients with IGBC is summarized in Fig. 16.

ADJUVANT THERAPY

The role of chemoradiotherapy as an alternative to surgery or as an adjuvant after surgery for IGBC is far from clear. This is not surprising because this issue remains unsettled even for GBC in general. A recent systematic review and meta-analysis of adjuvant therapy (chemotherapy, radiotherapy [RT] or both) in biliary tract cancers (BTC) including GBC reported a nonsignificant improvement in OS with any adjuvant treatment compared with surgery alone (pooled odds ratio [OR], 0.74; $P = .06$). There was no difference between GBC and bile duct cancers. Those receiving chemotherapy or chemotherapy -RT derived statistically greater benefit than RT alone (OR, 0.39, 0.61, and 0.98, respectively; $P = .02$). The greatest benefit was seen for LN-positive disease (OR, 0.49; $P = .004$) and after R1 resection (OR, 0.36, $P = .002$) [33]. Another pooled analysis of 104 chemotherapy trials involving 1368 patients with BTC conducted during 1999 to 2006 suggested differences in clinical behavior and responsiveness to chemotherapy between GBC and other BTCs [34]). Among all patients, the median time to progression (TTP) and OS were 4.1 months

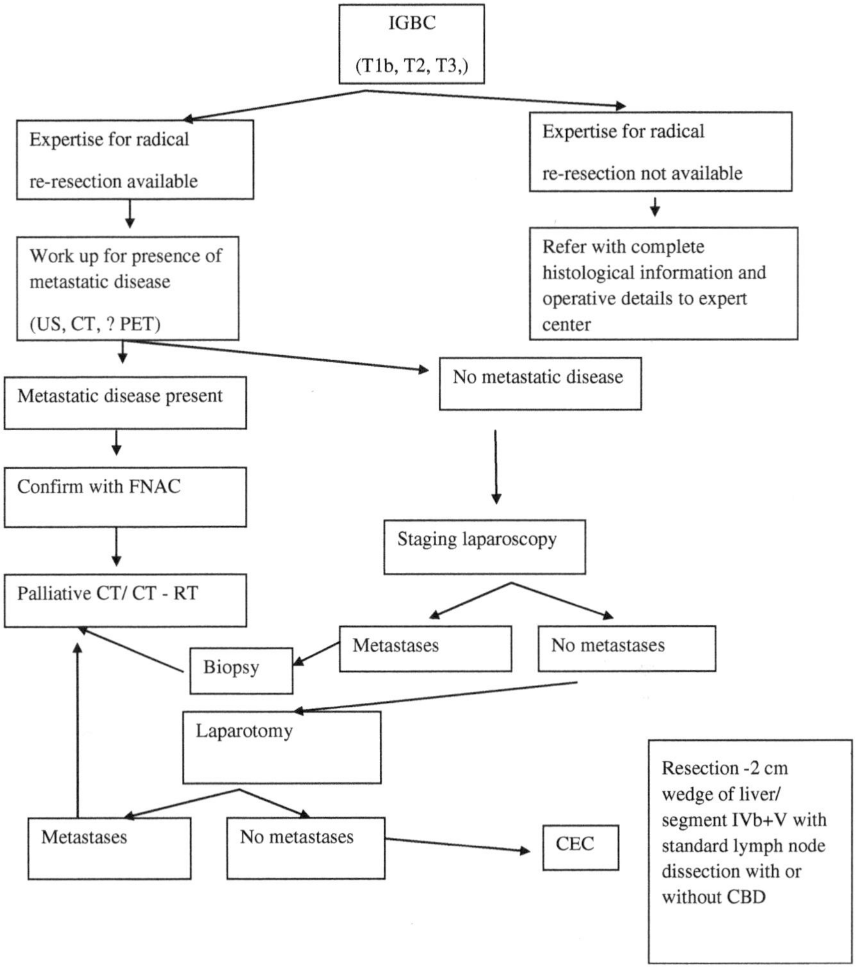

Fig. 16. Management algorithm for IGBC. CT, chemotherapy; RT, radiotherapy.

and 8.2 months, respectively. A subgroup analysis of GBC versus cholangiocarcinoma (CC), however, showed a significantly higher response rate (RR) of 36% in GBC versus 18% in CC, whereas the median OS was longer in patients with CC (9.3 months) than that for GBC (7.2 months). This study showed that gemcitabine-containing and platinum-containing regimens led to consistently greater RRs and TTP than other therapies.

Extrapolating evidence from these reports to IGBC, adjuvant therapy should probably be given to:

1. Patients with T2 or more, node-positive and margin-positive disease (patients with these features have been predicted to obtain a survival benefit with addition of

adjuvant therapy from a nomogram built from a parametric survival model from the SEER [Surveillance Epidemiology and End Results]-Medicare database) [35]
2. Patients with histologic markers of aggressive behavior (eg, lymphovascular and perineural invasion and poorly differentiated tumors)
3. Patients who had bile spill during the index cholecystectomy

In addition, patients who cannot undergo or refuse reoperation for CEC should receive chemoradiotherapy as the second best option.

RESULTS OF SURGERY FOR IGBC

GBC is one of the most aggressive cancers of the gastrointestinal tract (probably even more aggressive than those of the pancreas, liver, and stomach). Overall prognosis is poor, but patients with IGBC who usually have early stages of the disease and are managed appropriately are potentially curable.

In a report from the MSKCC [10], best results (median survival 72 months) were obtained in patients who were found to have no residual disease at reoperation followed by those who had residual disease but underwent R0 resection (19 months); those who underwent R1/R2 resection had a median survival of 13 months only.

For T1a tumors, 5-year survival greater than 90% after simple cholecystectomy has been reported by several investigators [36–38]; no survival advantage is provided by re-resection [39]. For patients with T1b lesions, although some groups report excellent survival with simple cholecystectomy alone, with no significant improvement in survival after extended cholecystectomy [18,36–38,40,41], others recommend addition of resection of GB bed and LN dissection, based on reported incidences of locoregional failure after simple cholecystectomy and improved survival after extended cholecystectomy (Table 1) [39,42–45]. However, a recent systematic review [12] concluded that there was no evidence to suggest superiority of extended cholecystectomy over simple cholecystectomy for T1b tumors.

Survival results for T2 GBC show a consistent improvement in survival with extended cholecystectomy (Table 2). Although 5-year survival after simple

Table 1
Results of surgery for T1b GBC after simple cholecystectomy and extended cholecystectomy

	No. of patients		5-year survival		
Series	SC	EC	SC	EC	*P* value
Goetze & Paolucci [39], 2008	49	23	42	79	.03
Cangemi et al [44], 2006	08	03	37.5	100	<.01
Yildirim et al [41], 2005	05	03	50	100	NS
Kim et al [40], 2002	06	03	100	100	NS
Wakai et al [37], 2001	13	12	100	75	NS
Ouchi et al [42], 1994	05	02	42	100	<.05

Abbreviations: EC, extended cholecystectomy; NS, not significant; SC simple cholecystectomy.

Table 2
Results of simple and extended cholecystectomy for T2 GBC

Series	No. of patients	Procedure (number of patients)	5-y survival (%)
Shirai et al [17], 1992	45	SC (35) EC (10)	40.5 90
Yamaguchi & Tsuneyoshi [48], 1992	25	SC	36
Oertli et al [49], 1993	17	SC	24
Matsumoto et al [52], 1992	09	EC	100
Bartlett et al [51], 1996	08	EC	88
Paquet [50], 1998	05	EC	80
de Aretxabala et al [47], 1997	38	SC (18) EC (20)	20 70
Fong et al [20], 2000	53	SC (16) EC (37)	19 61
Muratore et al [21], 2003	11	EC	100% for 8 patients with no preoperative disease All patients with preoperative disease died within 25 mo
Wise et al [53], 2001	10	SC (5) EC (5)	80% died between 6.5 and 21 mo All alive at 15–83 mo
Aramaki et al [54], 2004	22	SC (1) EC (21)	88.9% vs 31.3% for those with and without lymphatic invasion, respectively

Abbreviations: EC, extended cholecystectomy; SC simple cholecystectomy.

cholecystectomy has been reported to range from 19% to 40% [17,46–49], the figures after extended cholecystectomy range from 70% to 100% [17,20,21,47,50–54].

Some reports of improvement in survival after re-resection are available for T3 tumors [20,29,55]. However, the German Cancer Registry experience reported no survival benefit for 32 of the 85 patients with T3 GBC who underwent extended resection [56].

A recent report of IGBC after LC reported that prognostic factors for poorer survival were male gender ($P = .026$), age older than 65 years ($P = .013$), presence of inflammation ($P = .009$), nonpolypoidal gross type ($P = .003$), pT stage ($P = .001$), and moderately or poorly differentiated tumor ($P = .001$). Tumor differentiation was a significantly independent predictor of poor prognosis [19].

Despite a significant survival advantage for patients with T1b/T2 GBC who undergo radical resection, this treatment has been reported to be significantly underused. Jensen and colleagues [57] in an analysis of data from the SEER Registry from 1988 to 2004, reported that of the 4631 patients who underwent surgery for early-stage GBC, 90% underwent cholecystectomy alone and only 10% of patients underwent radical surgery.

Specifically discussing the 382 patients with T2 tumors, identified from the SEER database between 1988 and 2002, Wright and colleagues [58] reported that 238 (62%) underwent cholecystectomy alone, 76 (19.8%) underwent cholecystectomy with LN dissection, and only 14 (4%) patients underwent an appropriate radical procedure, thus confirming that most patients with T2 GBC in the United States were not managed according to the national recommendations.

On similar lines, an analysis of SEER data from 1998 to 2003 of 2835 patients with GBC (T1–T3) showed that most patients with GBC received inappropriate treatment: 91% underwent simple (not extended) cholecystectomy and 95% had an inadequate lymphadenectomy [59]).

EFFECT OF OPEN VERSUS LC

LC has a high likelihood of GB perforation, bile spill, and tumor seeding of the peritoneal cavity, which is likely to vitiate the results of attempted curative resection later. Exploring the association between GB perforation during LC and port site/peritoneal recurrence, Wakai and colleagues [16], in a study of 28 patients, reported that the incidence of port site/peritoneal recurrence was higher in patients with GB perforation (3/7, 43%) than in those without GB perforation (0/21, 0%) ($P = .011$). The outcome after LC was worse in the 7 patients with GB perforation (cumulative 5-year survival of 43%) than in those without (cumulative 5-year survival of 100%) ($P < .001$).

In a recent study looking at the effect of bile spill on subsequent curative surgery and survival in GBC, Lee and colleagues [60] reported a higher incidence of R1 and R2 resections and a significantly diminished OS (25.8 months vs 72.6 months, $P = .014$) and disease-free survival (20.9 months vs 71.4 months $P = .028$) in patients with GBC who had bile spill during LC compared with those with no bile spill. All patients with bile spill and recurrent disease had metastatic disease. Another study [61] looking at the effect of LC found similarly distressing results, and investigators reviewing the Western literature on early GBC initially removed by LC and their own series found 21 patients with T1 and 42 patients with T2 disease. One-year Kaplan-Meier survival (T1, 89%; T2, 71%) and 3-year survival (T1, 47%; T2, 40%) of these patients was worse than previous reports for open cholecystectomy indicating that an initial LC with its potential for bile spill can convert potentially curable early GBC to incurable disease. Patients with preoperative findings suspicious for GBC should undergo open exploration with intent to perform a radical cancer operation as the primary procedure if the diagnosis is then confirmed intraoperatively. According to the German Cancer Registry data [62], intraoperative GB perforation results in significant ($P = .047$) prognostic disadvantage. In the event of perforation, even the use of retrieval bags does not protect against this disadvantage. Reports of poorer results for IGBC in patients with acute cholecystitis and empyema GB also associate it with the higher possibility of GB perforation and bile spill because of difficulty in handling the inflamed GB [19].

However, many other reports [63–65] of IGBC diagnosed after LC do not report any disadvantage of the laparoscopic approach and contend that although the surgical approach might be associated with a different pattern of recurrence, the long-term survival is determined by the disease stage only.

FOLLOW-UP

Follow-up after resection for IGBC includes clinical evaluation, US, CT, and PET [66], but whether regular proactive follow-up is of any benefit to the patient is debatable, because recurrences in GBC are hardly ever resectable for cure and can be palliated only, for which follow-up of self-referral of symptoms is also good enough.

PREVENTION

Every effort should be made to avoid GB perforation and bile spill during cholecystectomy because recurrence rates are higher with intraoperative GB perforation than without (38.4% vs 27.2%) [63].

If technically possible, cystic LN should be included in the GB specimen; it is easier for the pathologist to detect a metastasis in the LN than an early primary lesion in the GB. All GBs (at least in geographic areas and ethnic populations in which GBC is common) should be removed in a bag to prevent port site contamination with tumor cells (Fig. 17). However, use of a bag does not prevent dissemination if the GB was opened during cholecystectomy, resulting in bile spill.

Risk of IGBC is higher in older patients, and especially those with acute cholecystitis, empyema GB, Mirizzi syndrome, history of previous or coexisting CBD stones, and thick-walled GB. Special precautions to prevent bile spill need to be taken during cholecystectomy for such indications.

All removed GBs must be opened (Fig. 18) and carefully examined by the surgeon in the operating room to look for any abnormality (eg, ulcer, nodule,

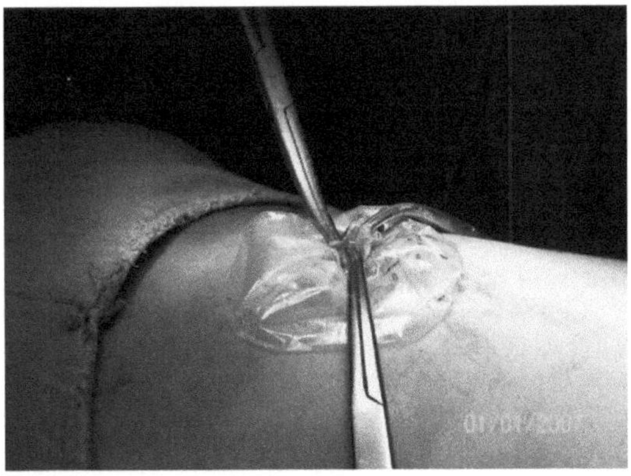

Fig. 17. GB being extracted in a bag to prevent contamination of port site.

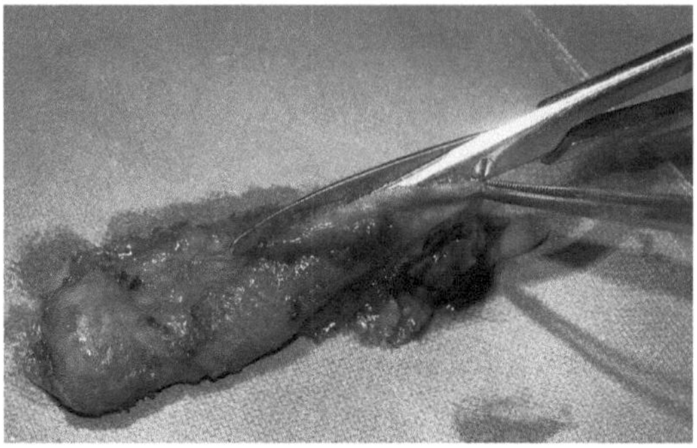

Fig. 18. GB being cut open after removal for examination for any findings suspicious of GBC.

thickening) that suggests GBC; if present, it should be subjected to frozen section examination (if facilities and expertise for frozen section are not available, the suspicious area can be touched on a glass slide and subjected to imprint cytology), which, if positive, should lead to conversion to laparotomy for completion of extended cholecystectomy then and there. Although recommended and mandatory, this system is not routinely practiced, even in Japan [67].

All GBs, even if they look normal on gross examination, should be subjected to histologic examination so as to detect an IGBC. Preferably, multiple serial sections should be taken. There are some reports [68–70] that suggest that a grossly normal GB need not be sent for histologic examination, but we do not agree with this approach, because the cost of histologic examination of the GB is small (compared with the total cost of cholecystectomy) but the price the patient pays for a 'missed', early, resectable, and potentially curable GBC resulting in inevitable recurrence, which is usually advanced and invariably unresectable, for cure is high [71].

References

[1] Kapoor VK. Incidental gall bladder cancer. Am J Gastroenterol 2001;96:627–9.

[2] Yamamoto H, Hayakawa N, Kitagawa Y, et al. Unsuspected gallbladder carcinoma after laparoscopic cholecystectomy. J Hepatobiliary Pancreat Surg 2005;12(5):391–8.

[3] Kwon AH, Imamura A, Kitade H, et al. Unsuspected gallbladder cancer diagnosed during or after laparoscopic cholecystectomy. J Surg Oncol 2008;97(3):241–5.

[4] Shih SP, Schulick RD, Cameron JL, et al. Gallbladder cancer: the role of laparoscopy and radical resection. Ann Surg 2007;245(6):893–901.

[5] Lohsiriwat V, Vongjirad A, Lohsiriwat D. Value of routine histopathologic examination of three common surgical specimens: appendix, gallbladder, and hemorrhoid. World J Surg 2009;33(10):2189–93.

[6] Redaelli CA, Büchler MW, Schilling MK, et al. High coincidence of Mirizzi syndrome and gallbladder carcinoma. Surgery 1997;121(1):58–63.

[7] Prasad TL, Kumar A, Sikora SS, et al. Mirizzi syndrome and gallbladder cancer. J Hepatobiliary Pancreat Surg 2006;13(4):323–6.

[8] Stephen AE, Berger DL. Carcinoma in the porcelain gallbladder: a relationship revisited. Surgery 2001;129(6):699–703.

[9] Kwon W, Jang JY, Lee SE, et al. Clinicopathologic features of polypoid lesions of the gallbladder and risk factors of gallbladder cancer. J Korean Med Sci 2009;24(3):481–7.
[10] Duffy A, Capanu M, Abou-Alfa GK, et al. Gallbladder cancer (GBC): 10-year experience at Memorial Sloan-Kettering Cancer Centre (MSKCC). J Surg Oncol 2008;98(7):485–9.
[11] Pawlik TM, Gleisner AL, Vigano L, et al. Incidence of finding residual disease for incidental gallbladder carcinoma: implications for re-resection. J Gastrointest Surg 2007;11(11): 1478–86 [discussion: 1486–7].
[12] Lee SE, Jang JY, Lim CS, et al. Systematic review on the surgical treatment for T1 gallbladder cancer. World J Gastroenterol 2011;17(2):174–80.
[13] Kondo S, Nimura Y, Kamiya J, et al. Mode of tumor spread and surgical strategy in gallbladder carcinoma. Langenbecks Arch Surg 2002;387(5–6):222–8.
[14] Shimada H, Endo I, Fujii Y, et al. Appraisal of surgical resection of gallbladder cancer with special reference to lymph node dissection. Langenbecks Arch Surg 2000;385(8): 509–14.
[15] Tsukada K, Kurosaki I, Uchida K, et al. Lymph node spread from carcinoma of the gallbladder. Cancer 1997;80(4):661–7.
[16] Wakai T, Shirai Y, Hatakeyama K. Radical second resection provides survival benefit for patients with T2 gallbladder carcinoma first discovered after laparoscopic cholecystectomy. World J Surg 2002;26(7):867–71.
[17] Shirai Y, Yoshida K, Tsukada K, et al. Inapparent carcinoma of the gallbladder. An appraisal of a radical second operation after simple cholecystectomy. Ann Surg 1992;215(4):326–31.
[18] Toyonaga T, Chijiiwa K, Nakano K, et al. Completion radical surgery after cholecystectomy for accidentally undiagnosed gallbladder carcinoma. World J Surg 2003;27(3): 266–71.
[19] Choi SB, Han HJ, Kim CY, et al. Incidental gallbladder cancer diagnosed following laparoscopic cholecystectomy. World J Surg 2009;33(12):2657–63.
[20] Fong Y, Jarnagin W, Blumgart LH. Gallbladder cancer: comparison of patients presenting initially for definitive operation with those presenting after prior noncurative intervention. Ann Surg 2000;232(4):557–69.
[21] Muratore A, Amisano M, Viganò L, et al. Gallbladder cancer invading the perimuscular connective tissue: results of reresection after prior non-curative operation. J Surg Oncol 2003;83(4):212–5.
[22] Kapoor VK, Sonawane RN, Haribhakti SP, et al. Gall bladder cancer: proposal for a modification of the TNM classification. Eur J Surg Oncol 1998;24:487–91.
[23] Shukla PJ, Barreto SG, Arya S, et al. Does PET-CT scan have a role prior to radical re-resection for incidental gallbladder cancer? HPB (Oxford) 2008;10(6):439–45.
[24] Butte JM, Redondo F, Waugh E, et al. The role of PET-CT in patients with incidental gallbladder cancer. HPB (Oxford) 2009;11(7):585–91.
[25] Agrawal S, Sonawane RN, Behari A, et al. Laparoscopic staging in gallbladder cancer. Dig Surg 2005;22(6):440–5.
[26] Butte JM, Gönen M, Allen PJ, et al. The role of laparoscopic staging in patients with incidental gallbladder cancer. HPB (Oxford) 2011;13(7):463–72.
[27] Wibbenmeyer LA, Wade TP, Chen RC, et al. Laparoscopic cholecystectomy can disseminate in situ carcinoma of the gallbladder. J Am Coll Surg 1995;181(6):504–10.
[28] Goetze TO, Paolucci V. Adequate extent in radical re-resection of incidental gallbladder carcinoma: analysis of the German Registry. Surg Endosc 2010;24(9):2156–64.
[29] Fuks D, Regimbeau JM, Le Treut YP, et al. Incidental gallbladder cancer by the AFC-GBC-2009 Study Group. World J Surg 2011;35(8):1887–97.
[30] Zhu AX, Hong TS, Hezel AF, et al. Current management of gallbladder carcinoma. Oncologist 2010;15(2):168–81.
[31] Paolucci V, Schaeff B, Schneider M, et al. Tumor seeding following laparoscopy: international survey. World J Surg 1999;23(10):989–95 [discussion: 996–7].

[32] Maker AV, Butte JM, Oxenberg J, et al. Is port site resection necessary in the surgical management of gallbladder cancer? Ann Surg Oncol 2012;19(2):409–17.
[33] Horgan AM, Amir E, Walter T, et al. Adjuvant therapy in the treatment of biliary tract cancer: a systematic review and meta-analysis. J Clin Oncol 2012;30(16):1934–40.
[34] Eckel F, Schmid RM. Chemotherapy in advanced biliary tract carcinoma: a pooled analysis of clinical trials. Br J Cancer 2007;96(6):896–902.
[35] Wang SJ, Lemieux A, Kalpathy-Cramer J, et al. Nomogram for predicting the benefit of adjuvant chemoradiotherapy for resected gallbladder cancer. J Clin Oncol 2011;29(35):4627–32.
[36] Shirai Y, Yoshida K, Tsukada K, et al. Early carcinoma of the gallbladder. Eur J Surg 1992;158(10):545–8.
[37] Wakai T, Shirai Y, Yokoyama N, et al. Early gallbladder carcinoma does not warrant radical resection. Br J Surg 2001;88:675–8.
[38] de Aretxabala X, Roa I, Hepp J, et al. Early gallbladder cancer: is further treatment necessary? J Surg Oncol 2009;100(7):589–93.
[39] Goetze TO, Paolucci V. Immediate re-resection of T1 incidental gallbladder carcinomas: a survival analysis of the German Registry. Surg Endosc 2008;22:2462–5.
[40] Kim EK, Lee SK, Kim WW. Does laparoscopic surgery have a role in the treatment of gallbladder cancer? J Hepatobiliary Pancreat Surg 2002;9:559–63.
[41] Yildirim E, Celen O, Gulben K, et al. The surgical management of incidental gallbladder carcinoma. Eur J Surg Oncol 2005;31:45–52.
[42] Ouchi K, Suzuki M, Tominaga T, et al. Survival after surgery for cancer of the gallbladder. Br J Surg 1994;81:1655–7.
[43] Wagholikar GD, Behari A, Krishnani N, et al. Early gallbladder cancer. J Am Coll Surg 2002;194(2):137–41.
[44] Cangemi V, Fiori E, Picchi C, et al. Early gallbladder carcinoma: a single-center experience. Tumori 2006;92:487–90.
[45] Shukla PJ, Barreto G, Kakade A, et al. Revision surgery for incidental gallbladder cancer: factors influencing operability and further evidence for T1b tumours. HPB (Oxford) 2008;10(1):43–7.
[46] Fong Y, Heffernan N, Blumgart LH. Gallbladder carcinoma discovered during laparoscopic cholecystectomy: aggressive reresection is beneficial. Cancer 1998;83(3):423–7.
[47] de Aretxabala XA, Roa IS, Burgos LA, et al. Curative resection in potentially resectable tumours of the gallbladder. Eur J Surg 1997;163(6):419–26.
[48] Yamaguchi K, Tsuneyoshi M. Subclinical gallbladder carcinoma. Am J Surg 1992;163(4): 382–6.
[49] Oertli D, Herzog U, Tondelli P. Primary carcinoma of the gallbladder: operative experience during a 16 year period. Eur J Surg 1993;159(8):415–20.
[50] Paquet KJ. Appraisal of surgical resection of gallbladder carcinoma with special reference to hepatic resection. J Hepatobiliary Pancreat Surg 1998;5(2):200–6.
[51] Bartlett DL, Fong Y, Fortner JG, et al. Long-term results after resection for gallbladder cancer. Implications for staging and management. Ann Surg 1996;224(5):639–46.
[52] Matsumoto Y, Fujii H, Aoyama H, et al. Surgical treatment of primary carcinoma of the gallbladder based on the histologic analysis of 48 surgical specimens. Am J Surg 1992;163(2):239–45.
[53] Wise PE, Shi YY, Washington MK, et al. Radical resection improves survival for patients with pT2 gallbladder carcinoma. Am Surg 2001;67(11):1041–7.
[54] Aramaki M, Matsumoto T, Shibata K, et al. Factors influencing recurrence after surgical treatment for T2 gallbladder carcinoma. Hepatogastroenterology 2004;51(60):1609–11.
[55] Foster JM, Hoshi H, Gibbs JF, et al. Gallbladder cancer: defining the indications for primary radical resection and radical re-resection. Ann Surg Oncol 2007;14(2):833–40.
[56] Goetze TO, Paolucci V. Benefits of reoperation of T2 and more advanced incidental gallbladder carcinoma: analysis of the German registry. Ann Surg 2008;247(1):104–8.

[57] Jensen EH, Abraham A, Habermann EB, et al. A critical analysis of the surgical management of early-stage gallbladder cancer in the United States. J Gastrointest Surg 2009;13(4):722–7.
[58] Wright BE, Lee CC, Iddings DM, et al. Management of T2 gallbladder cancer: are practice patterns consistent with national recommendations? Am J Surg 2007;194(6):820–5 [discussion: 825–6].
[59] Coburn NG, Cleary SP, Tan JC, et al. Surgery for gallbladder cancer: a population-based analysis. J Am Coll Surg 2008;207(3):371–82.
[60] Lee JM, Kim BW, Kim WH, et al. Clinical implication of bile spillage in patients undergoing laparoscopic cholecystectomy for gallbladder cancer. Am Surg 2011;77(6):697–701.
[61] Weiland ST, Mahvi DM, Niederhuber JE, et al. Should suspected early gallbladder cancer be treated laparoscopically? J Gastrointest Surg 2002;6(1):50–6 [discussion: 56–7].
[62] Goetze TO, Paolucci V. Use of retrieval bags in incidental gallbladder cancer cases. World J Surg 2009;33(10):2161–5.
[63] Cucinotta E, Lorenzini C, Melita G, et al. Incidental gall bladder carcinoma: does the surgical approach influence the outcome? ANZ J Surg 2005;75:795–8.
[64] Chan KM, Yeh TS, Jan YY, et al. Laparoscopic cholecystectomy for early gallbladder carcinoma: long-term outcome in comparison with conventional open cholecystectomy. Surg Endosc 2006;20(12):1867–71.
[65] Whalen GF, Bird I, Tanski W, et al. Laparoscopic cholecystectomy does not demonstrably decrease survival of patients with serendipitously treated gallbladder cancer. J Am Coll Surg 2001;192(2):189–95.
[66] Kumar R, Sharma P, Kumari A, et al. Role of 18F-FDG PET/CT in detecting recurrent gallbladder carcinoma. Clin Nucl Med 2012;37(5):431–5.
[67] Akatsu T, Ueda M, Shimazu M, et al. Long-term survival of patients with gallbladder cancer detected during or after laparoscopic cholecystectomy. World J Surg 2005;29(9):1106–9 [discussion: 1110].
[68] Taylor HW, Huang JK. 'Routine' pathological examination of the gallbladder is a futile exercise. Br J Surg 1998;85(2):208.
[69] Bazoua G, Hamza N, Lazim T. Do we need histology for a normal-looking gallbladder? J Hepatobiliary Pancreat Surg 2007;14(6):564–8.
[70] Mittal R, Jesudason MR, Nayak S. Selective histopathology in cholecystectomy for gallstone disease. Indian J Gastroenterol 2010;29(1):26–30.
[71] Behari A, Kapoor VK. Does gall bladder cancer divide India? Indian J Gastroenterol 2010;29(1):3–7.

Advances in Surgery 47 (2013) 251–270

ADVANCES IN SURGERY

General Surgery Residency Training Issues

Mary E. Klingensmith, MD[a], Frank R. Lewis, MD[b,*]

[a]Department of Surgery, Washington University School of Medicine, 4566 Scott Avenue, St Louis, MO, USA; [b]American Board of Surgery, 1617 JFK Boulevard, Suite 860, Philadelphia, PA 19103, USA

Keywords

- General surgery residency • General surgery training
- American Board of Surgery oral examination
- Environmental and technological change • 80-hour workweek

Key points

- The changes in general surgery that have occurred have been disruptive to residency training, and to date there has been inadequate compensation for these.
- Evidence is now emerging of significant issues in the overall performance of recent graduates from at least 3 sources: the evaluation of external agents who incorporate these graduates into their practice or group, the opinions of the residents themselves, and the performance of graduates on the oral examination of the American Board of Surgery during the past 8 years.
- The environmental and technological causes of the present situation represent improvements in care for patients, and are clearly irreversible. Hence, solutions to the problems must be sought in other areas.
- To address the issues effectively, greater recognition and engagement are needed by the surgical community so that effective solutions can be crafted.
- These will need to include improvements in the efficiency of teaching, with the assumption of greater individual resident responsibility for their knowledge, the establishment of more defined standards for knowledge and skills acquisition by level of residency training, with flexible self-assessment available online, greater focus of the curriculum on current rather than historical practice, increased use of structured assessments (including those in a simulated environment), and modifications to the overall structure of the traditional 5-year residency.

Disclaimer: The comments presented in this article are the personal observations and opinions of the authors and do not reflect any actions, opinions, policies, or positions of the American Board of Surgery.

*Corresponding author. *E-mail address:* flewis@absurgery.org

0065-3411/13/$ – see front matter
http://dx.doi.org/10.1016/j.yasu.2013.05.001

INTRODUCTION

Many operations done by general surgeons, and the way in which they are done, have undergone radical change during the past 2 decades, yet the impacts on residency training have not been generally recognized. The change has come about because of 2 principal factors: evolutionary and technological change. Change has occurred in the treatment of several common diseases, and the conversion of a major proportion of abdominal surgery from an open to a laparoscopic approach.

In addition to the change in the nature of the surgery done, the impact of the 80-hour workweek on resident experience with urgent and emergent conditions has also been significant. The impact of this on the professional maturation of residents and the development of resident independence and autonomy has not been adequately recognized or analyzed.

This article describes qualitatively the nature of the changes, the negative impacts on resident training, and some proposed measures to mitigate the impact.

ENVIRONMENTAL AND TECHNOLOGICAL CHANGE IN DISEASE MANAGEMENT

Four common disease categories that involve intra-abdominal pathology have undergone major technological change in management during the past 20 years.

Benign peptic ulcer disease

Benign gastric and duodenal ulcer disease has been a staple of general surgical management for decades, for treatment of the complications of bleeding, perforation, and intractability. Three advances in medical treatment have markedly altered the incidence of these complications, and the consequent need for surgical intervention: H2 receptor blockers, proton pump inhibitors, and treatment of *Helicobacter pylori* gastric infection. As a result of medical management with these 3 modalities, intractability of ulcer disease has virtually disappeared, and perforation and hemorrhage have been markedly reduced. As a result, surgery is infrequently necessary today for treatment of peptic ulcer complications and resident experience with gastric surgery is largely limited to malignancy and bariatric surgery. Interestingly, the increase in laparoscopic bariatric surgery has provided the bulk of a typical resident experience in gastric surgery in recent years, but exposure to these procedures is highly variable, and residents are rarely the operating surgeon in these complex technical procedures.

Biliary tree stone disease

Common duct stone disease is a frequently occurring problem, typically causing ductal obstruction or pancreatitis, which in the past often required surgical intervention for stone removal. Today, the technological innovations possible with flexible endoscopy and endoscopic retrograde cholangiopancreatography have allowed most stones to be extracted endoscopically; these have markedly reduced the need for common duct exploration and stone removal. The consequence of this on resident training has been so dramatic that most graduating surgical residents today have done no common duct explorations, which was previously a common part of abdominal surgical experience.

Abdominal vascular surgery

Intra-abdominal aorto-iliac occlusive and aneurysmal disease have been treated by both general surgeons and vascular surgeons since the 1950s, when synthetic vascular graft replacements first became available. These diseases were typically treated with aorto-iliac and aorto-femoral graft replacement via open abdominal procedures. Two changes, both technological, occurred in the 1990s that altered this scenario: endovascular manipulation of occlusive disease became feasible and effective, allowing the dilatation and stenting of most aorto-iliac lesions; and intraluminal endovascular graft insertion, a remarkable technological achievement, was developed for the treatment of aneurysmal disease, with markedly reduced patient morbidity from the treatment. Both of these procedures are technologically complex, and competence in the performance of such procedures became possible only with the additional training that occurred with vascular fellowship after general surgical training. General surgical residents were unable to get sufficient experience with these procedures to become proficient, effectively removing aorto-iliac vascular disease from the conditions that they could treat.

Trauma

Injuries have constituted a significant portion of general surgical experience for decades, and continue to do so, but the nature of traumatic injuries, and their management, has changed significantly. Three specific events account for this: the incidence of abdominal penetrating trauma, which requires surgical intervention in 80% to 90% of cases, decreased markedly in the United States between 1992 and 2002. Overall, the incidence of penetrating trauma decreased by approximately 60% to 70% during this decade in all geographic regions, both urban and rural, and has remained low to the present time. Despite the dramatic nature of this decline, it has largely escaped public notice and the attention of criminologists, and no generally accepted explanation has been advanced as to causation. One recent analysis [1] identified 4 factors as potentially responsible for the decline in violent injuries: increases in the intensity of urban policing, the rising prison population, the receding crack epidemic, and the legalization of abortion. Surprisingly, factors such as gun control laws and tougher policing strategies do not appear important in explaining the decline. Whatever the reason, the decrease caused a marked reduction in the need for abdominal surgery in most urban centers, as penetrating trauma has always been the injury requiring the largest proportion of open surgical intervention.

In addition to the decline in penetrating trauma, the incidence of blunt trauma, due largely to automobile trauma, declined by about 20% between 1980 and 2010, as seat belts and airbags came into universal usage. Although blunt trauma is mostly managed nonoperatively and requires surgery only 10% to 20% of the time, this caused a further decrease in the operative experience of residents and trauma surgeons.

Last, from the mid 1980s to 2000, the advent of computerized tomographic (CT) scanning, and the steady increase in resolution of that modality, made it possible to diagnose in greater detail the intra-abdominal pathology that was present with most blunt trauma and with some penetrating trauma. The increased diagnostic accuracy often allowed the anatomic details of intra-abdominal pathology to be more fully defined and therefore reduced the need for exploratory laparotomy, which was often nontherapeutic when the pathology was relatively minor. The efficacy and resolution of CT scanning was great enough that it led to an entirely new genre of nonoperative trauma management for blunt trauma affecting the liver, spleen, pancreas, and kidney, when ongoing bleeding was not a problem.

The 3 changes detailed in the preceding paragraphs led to a decline of 70% to 80% in the incidence of abdominal exploration necessary for trauma management in trauma centers today. Whereas previously surgical residents would commonly document 40 to 50 trauma cases requiring abdominal exploration by completion of training, today the Residency Review Committee for Surgery has lowered the required threshold to 10.

All of these changes in disease management have been beneficial to patients, and have reduced the magnitude of treatment and the physiologic disruption that were previously present with these disease processes and their treatment. At the same time, they have markedly reduced the experience of surgical residents in performing open abdominal surgery, and decreased their breadth of experience.

IMPACT OF LAPAROSCOPIC SURGERY

The last and most significant technological change that has occurred is the development of laparoscopic surgery for intra-abdominal surgical management, replacing open surgery and the large abdominal incision that was previously necessary. Laparoscopic surgery arrived on the US scene about 1990, and has expanded steadily since that time, as laparoscopic surgical capabilities and instrumentation have improved. Initially, laparoscopic surgery was largely limited to simple procedures, such as cholecystectomy, which did not require significant amounts of intra-abdominal suturing or performance of intestinal anastomoses. With increasing experience, the range and complexity of procedures has progressively expanded, and today more complex procedures involving intestinal anastomoses, such as laparoscopic colectomy and laparoscopic gastric bypass, are routinely performed with low morbidity.

When laparoscopic surgery was introduced to the United States in the 1990s, the academic community was slow to awaken to the revolution it represented, slow to adopt laparoscopic surgery in most academic centers, and slow to develop significant numbers of faculty who were proficient in its performance. As a result, it advanced more rapidly in the private practice community, often accompanied by a significant entrepreneurial element. Surgical faculty in academic centers were often late in acquiring laparoscopic surgery expertise, and as a result, most residents in the early years of its development did not get a robust experience because they had insufficient faculty to act as role models, teachers, and advocates.

The private practice community early on developed private community hospital fellowships, which were not located at academic centers, and began training fellows who had already completed surgical training, but were in need of further training in laparoscopy. Such fellowships were outside the Accreditation Council for Graduate Medical Education (ACGME) accreditation system, and did not entail certification in a subspecialty defined by the American Board of Medical Specialties (ABMS). Increases in the numbers of these fellowships was encouraged by funding from device manufacturers who sold the equipment needed for laparoscopic surgery, and who saw the benefit of expanding the fellowships that would train surgeons to use the equipment they manufactured. Funding was generally provided by the manufacturers to pay the salary of the fellows during their training, and often for other costs of establishing and operating the fellowships. The availability of such funding continues to the present time, and operates outside any regulatory framework related to surgical education.

Because of the slower development of laparoscopic surgery in the academic community, the paucity of academic faculty who were proficient in laparoscopic surgery in its early years, and the development of private community fellowships in laparoscopic surgery, the training of surgery residents in laparoscopic surgery advanced more slowly than it might have. Although the Residency Review Committee (RRC) for Surgery has been steadily increasing the requirements for surgical resident training, it is still the rule that the most complex laparoscopic surgery is reserved for fellows in postresidency fellowships and not for residents during surgical training, although there is no reason this should be the case.

A recent review of the laparoscopic experience of graduating surgical residents in 2010–2011 compared with 2005 showed that the median laparoscopic experience had increased from 170 to 253 operations per resident, but the number of complex laparoscopic cases during 5 years of residency increased only from 49 to 82 during the same period [2].

In summary, the principal change in surgical residency training of the past 20 years has been the loss of many areas of open abdominal surgery, but at the same time this has not been replaced by a comparable volume of the same surgery done by complex laparoscopic techniques. Moving this laparoscopic experience back into surgical residency would be possible today, as the deficiency in faculty who are proficient in laparoscopic surgery has been fully corrected, but the laparoscopic surgery fellowships that are in competition with residents for cases are already in existence and are maintained in part by external funding unrelated to hospital or educational budgets. Because this entire funding mechanism operates outside any regulatory framework, neither the ACGME nor the ABMS have any control over these fellowships or their impact on resident training.

IMPACT OF THE 80-HOUR WORKWEEK

The imposition of the 80-hour workweek by the ACGME in 2003 produced a dramatic change in the scheduling of most resident rotations and the hours spent by residents in the hospital. Research before 2003, although not extensive or rigorous in most cases, indicated that surgical residents on average spent 90 to 100 hours per week in the hospital, if their time on night call was included. If a resident spends an average of 100 hours in the hospital for 48 weeks yearly for 5 years, then he or she has spent approximately 24,000 hours in the hospital during residency. If one does the same calculation for 90-hour workweeks, the time in hospital is 21,600 hours, and if 80 hours, it is 19,200 hours. If a resident decreases from 100-hour weeks to 80-hour weeks, therefore, the reduction in total hours over 5 years is 4800 hours, and if from 90 hours to 80 hours, it is 2400 hours. The first figure is equal to 1 year of 100-hour weeks, and the second to 6 months of 100-hour weeks. Thus, the impact of the 80-hour week on surgical residents is that it has effectively reduced in-hospital time by 6 to 12 months in most programs, a 10% to 20% overall reduction in clinical time.

The time that residents spend on daytime activity Monday to Friday has been minimally affected by the 80-hour week, and constitutes the bulk of their clinical experience. One can estimate this daytime weekday commitment as 5 days per week $\times$ 12 hours per day $=$ 60 hours per week. The balance of their time is spent in night and weekend duty. If they were previously working 100-hour weeks, approximately 40 hours per week was spent in night and weekend responsibilities. If 90 hours per week, 30 hours per week was devoted to night/weekend activity, and with an 80-hour week, 20 hours are so devoted, assuming the daytime weekday responsibilities are invariant. These "back-of-the-napkin" calculations show that the transition from a 100-hour week to an 80-hour week reduces night and weekend experience by 50%, and a 90-hour to 80-hour transition by 33%.

Elective surgical experience doing scheduled nonemergent cases in the operating room has been minimally impacted by the 80-hour week, which is why the numbers quoted in the literature regarding resident experience seem to show little change [2]. However, the overall in-hospital experience, and particularly the opportunity to see and participate in the management of urgent and emergent conditions, and to have a greater degree of independence, autonomy, and indirect supervision, has been dramatically reduced, on the order of 33% to 50%, as noted. The effect of this on resident professional maturation, self-reliance, clinical judgment, and independent functioning has not been previously recognized or studied, but almost certainly has had major adverse impact.

Other effects of the 80-hour workweek on residents' attitudes toward their ethical responsibilities to patients are more difficult to quantitate, but may have more long-term effects and greater negative impact on patient care. These effects are not a direct result of the 80-hour workweek itself, but of the rigidity and highly prescriptive nature of the rules by which it has been implemented. Three such effects will be described.

The rigidity of the work rules that limit the length of resident shifts have necessitated residents' departure from the hospital despite any consideration of the patient care process in which they are engaged. Residents who have admitted and carefully worked up a patient during the night will be arbitrarily sent home the next morning and excluded from often critical evaluation or treatment, including urgent and emergent operations, which will be "handed off" to someone else. Such requirements abrogate the essentials of continuity of care that residents should learn, a critical element of optimal patient care. In essence, 2000 years of evolved medical ethics, which have dictated that the doctor's welfare should always be subordinated to that of the patient, have been overturned and replaced by teaching and concrete example in which the resident's work hours and sleep history trump anything related to the care of the patient. This attitudinal change will not end with the completion of residency, but will be carried forward in postresidency fellowships and practice by current generations of residents, and is fundamentally changing the perceived ethical obligations of physicians toward their patients. The long-term effects are already being reflected by a global change in attitude toward taking emergency calls after entering practice, with less willingness to be on-call for urgent and emergent problems. This is currently one of the most pressing national problems hospitals face in providing 24/7 access to care across all specialties.

The second effect of the work hours requirements is that there are multiple shifts and teams of doctors who provide care over a period of time, whereas previously such care was usually by a single team of doctors who provided care on a 24/7 basis. This change has necessitated "handoffs," in which clinical responsibility is transferred from one group of doctors to another, but such handoffs nearly always create discontinuities in the full transfer of clinical information. There have been dozens of articles in the literature looking for better systems by which handoff information may be transferred, but no one has recognized the fundamental issue that much of the essential clinical information, which is important in critically ill patients, is qualitative and subjective, and not subject to objective quantitation. The degree and location of abdominal tenderness and guarding, the perfusion and temperature of an extremity, or the overall appearance, mental status, and demeanour of a patient, are all important observations for an experienced clinician in following and evaluating critically ill patients. None of these can be verbally transferred to another physician with any real appreciation of the subtleties involved. As a result, handoffs always result in decrements in the quality of care because the information transfer is incomplete, and the greatest impact will occur in the most critically ill patients.

It is noteworthy that the ACGME, which oversees graduate medical education, has just completed a comprehensive meta-analysis of the literature evaluating the effect of the work hours on patient quality of care, and has concluded that overall there has been a significant negative effect on surgical patients [3]. This reinforces what most clinicians have been observing since 2003.

The third significant effect of the work hours is that it has fostered resident dishonesty in reporting their work hours. Most residents feel a strong moral responsibility toward their patients, and recognize that the specifics of the work hours requirements are often detrimental to patient care, continuity of care, and resident learning. Because they want to do the right thing for patients in virtually all cases, the only way they can accomplish this is to sometimes lie about their duty hours so as to protect themselves and their residency program from sanctions; such behavior has been extensively documented by the ACGME. A policy that forces dishonest behavior so as to deliver optimal patient care is clearly inappropriate if not immoral.

VARIABLE QUALITY OF RESIDENCY PROGRAMS

In an effort to control quality and ensure compliance with training standards, residency programs in general surgery undergo periodic review by the RRC for Surgery of the ACGME. When a program is reviewed, the success of trainees in achieving a passing score on the qualifying (written) and certifying (oral) examinations of the ABS the first time they are taken (based on 5-year average results) are objective measures of teaching effectiveness of the program; achieving a success rate of 65% on both examinations is a minimum standard for RRC accreditation. Fig. 1 is a scatter plot showing success rate in first-time passage on the qualifying and certifying examinations for individual training programs. Ideally, all training programs would have uniform success in trainee performance, with 100% of trainees passing both examinations on the first attempt. The reality is that there is great variability in overall program performance, and approximately 18% of programs fall below the 65% thresholds for either the qualifying or certifying examination.

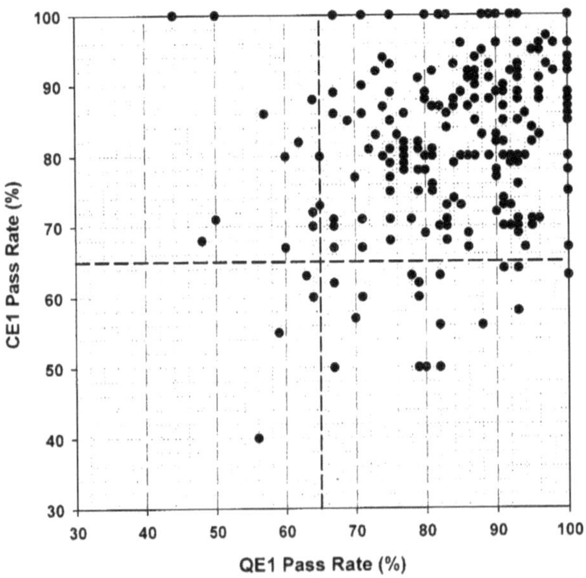

Fig. 1. Five-year first-time pass rate: All residency programs 2010 to 2011.

A further analysis of these data by program size is shown in Fig. 2, in which the first-time pass rates on both examinations are examined as a function of program size. The 6 pairs of bars correspond respectively to programs graduating 2, 3, 4, 5, 6, and more than 6 residents per year. It can be seen that for the qualifying examination there is a strong dependence on program size, with more than a 10% spread from the smallest to the largest programs in 5-year success rates. For the certifying examination there is a similar trend, but it does not reach statistical significance.

An analysis by Fuhrman and colleagues [4] of these data concluded that the larger programs have greater success because of greater resources for the support of resident training, ranging from dedicated paid faculty to more numerous learning aids and resources. The breadth and variety of surgery done at larger institutions may also play a role. It is also possible that the differences might be a result of the greater attractiveness of larger programs, and the greater competitiveness of residents who apply to, and are selected by them.

RESIDENT OPINION

The fraction of residents finishing general surgical residency who continue their training in a postresidency specialty or subspecialty fellowship has been steadily increasing for the past 3 decades, and at the present time exceeds 80%. The reasons for this are multiple, but among others is their belief that they are not ready for independent practice and require further training to

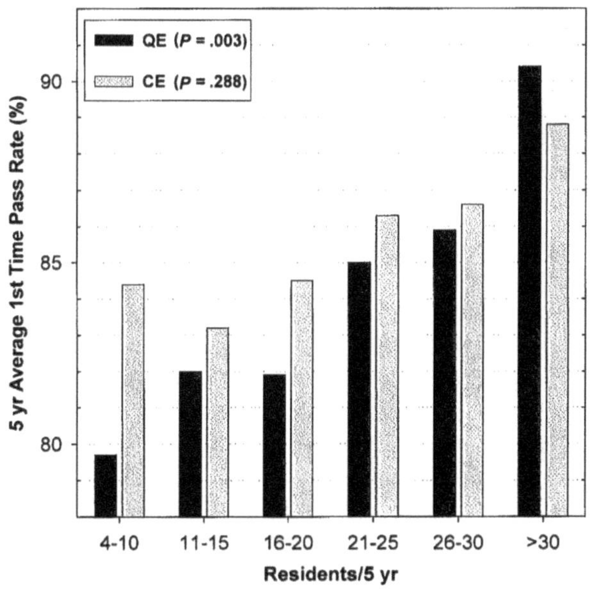

Fig. 2. Effect of program size on Qualifying Examination and Certifying Examination first-time pass rates.

be competent or competitive in a specific area. Most of these fellowships are of 1-year duration, but many extend to 2 or 3 years beyond the 5 years of surgical training.

An extensive survey of resident opinion regarding surgical training was completed by Heather Yeo and colleagues in 2009 [5], and is the most authoritative such survey ever conducted. They obtained input from 4402 surgical residents at all levels of seniority, representing 82% of all categorical residents at the time, from 248 of 249 surgical programs.

Several questions were asked with regard to postresidency specialty training, as follows:

When presented with the statement "General surgeons must become specialty trained to be successful," 55% of residents agreed and 26% disagreed (the remainder were neutral).

For the statement "I must complete specialty training to be competitive in the market," 64% agreed and 21% disagreed.

For the statement "If I complete specialty training I'll have a better lifestyle," 63% agreed and 12% disagreed.

For the statement "If I complete specialty training I'll have a better income," 78% agreed and 7% disagreed.

From these responses it seems clear that residents feel training beyond residency is necessary if they are to be successful in practice and competitive in the marketplace. Because the job market for general surgeons per se is stronger today than the market for most surgical specialists, these impressions relative to competitiveness and practice success are in fact incorrect, although the conclusions about lifestyle and income may be accurate.

In any case, it is clear that 4 of 5 finishing general surgery residents, for whatever reason, undertake further training before they enter practice. Thus, for practical purposes, the length of surgical training for more than 80% of surgical residents is 6 to 7 years, not 5 years.

AMERICAN BOARD OF SURGERY EXAMINATION PERFORMANCE

The American Board of Surgery conducts a written examination after completion of residency primarily focused on the testing of objective knowledge across the breadth of general surgical subjects. On successful completion, a subsequent oral examination is conducted by 6 independent examiners who are all experienced practicing surgeons, to evaluate clinical management, safety of clinical decision making, clinical judgment in difficult surgical situations, and management of common complications. The method of conducting this examination and the grading standards have not changed over an extended period of time.

Failure rates on the written and oral examinations are shown in Fig. 3 for the past 20 years. It can be seen that performance on the written examination has been consistent during this time, with no evidence of major change. The oral

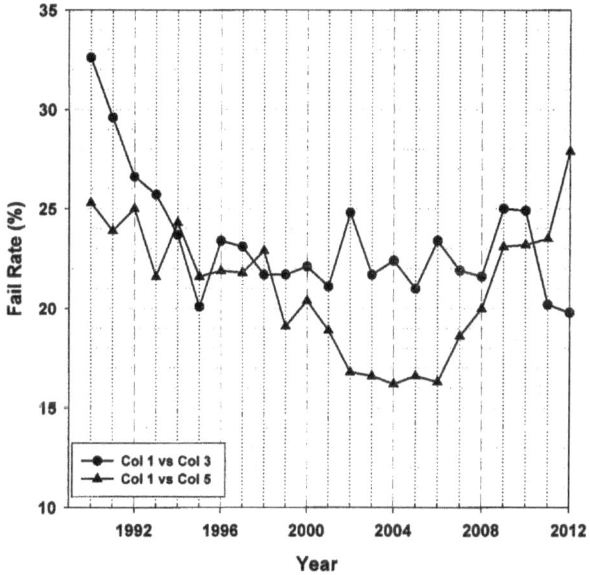

Fig. 3. American Board of Surgery examination fail rates by year.

examination, on the other hand, showed the lowest failure rate during a plateau phase from 2002 to 2006, then began a steady rise to the present time, with an overall increase in the failure rate from 16% to 28% during the past 6 years.

Although this change correlates with the implementation of the 80-hour workweek following 2003, and with successive yearly cohorts of residents working within this rubric, it also corresponds to other changes in the surgical environment already described, in particular the increasing role of laparoscopic surgery, the loss of several areas of open abdominal surgical experience, and a reduction in independence and autonomy for senior residents. Thus, causation cannot be determined for the increase in the oral examination failure rate with any degree of confidence, but it does appear that there has been a decline in residents' perceived abilities in clinical care decision making and management, although their factual knowledge of surgical subjects as tested by the written examination has not changed.

GRADED RESPONSIBILITY, AUTONOMY, AND INDEPENDENT FUNCTIONING IN RESIDENCY

The legal strictures relative to residency training have a logical inconsistency that has never been adequately addressed. For the duration of residency, until the last day of the fifth year of training, residents are not considered capable of independent or autonomous functioning and the treatments they render to patients are always considered to be dependent on the oversight of a responsible attending surgeon who provides direct or indirect supervision as necessary, and is legally responsible for the resident's actions. One day later, after completing residency, the same resident is legally considered to be "board eligible" and is subsequently "board certified," and in both instances is considered to possess sufficient competence to function independently and to manage the full gamut of surgical conditions in all patients without supervision or oversight by anyone else. That such a dramatic enhancement of competence can occur overnight is obviously illogical and fallacious.

What actually occurs, and what is the signal accomplishment of residency training in the United States since the model defined by William Halsted in the 1890s, is that surgical residents improve their knowledge and surgical capabilities continually throughout 5 years of residency and become progressively more able to manage complex conditions with increasing time.

A successful model has evolved in which the hierarchy of residency and faculty oversight, beginning with the attending surgeon who is in charge and extending downward through different levels of resident supervision of other residents, allows the development of progressively more detailed knowledge and skills with residents functioning at progressively increasing levels of responsibility. Attendings and more senior residents initially teach and oversee more junior residents in the performance of the dozens of skills necessary for diagnostic evaluation and patient management; as junior residents become competent in these, they begin to function with a degree of independence and no longer need direct supervision.

During the early years of residency, competence is initially gained in basic skills and simple operations. With increasing experience, diagnostic skills increase and the ability to evaluate and manage more complex diseases evolves. Manual skills in performance of operations increases in parallel with this, and the ability to perform more complex technical procedures similarly evolves, but it is universally accepted in surgical training that it is much more difficult to acquire the diagnostic acumen and surgical judgment needed for independent practice than it is to acquire the manual skills.

Residents may initially learn how to do operations by watching others, but ultimately they must manage patients themselves and do operations themselves if they are to become competent and capable of independent practice. The American system of resident education is unique in that residency training allows residents to do so while being directly overseen and supervised by attendings who are already competent in the management of patients and performance of operations and who allow residents to manage patients and perform operations while being directly observed and overseen to prevent errors from occurring. The ability of residents to do this in progressively more complex situations is a hallmark of increasing years of experience, and in the ideal residency environment they reach the point in which they can do the full spectrum of operations by the completion of residency training.

This system has been negatively impacted by the 80-hour workweek as stated previously, but additionally by the decline in opportunities for assisting at operations in most training programs, where the opportunity to watch, before doing, is gained. Longitudinal experience with patients, from preoperative admissions through prolonged postoperative stays has been markedly reduced by the transition from inpatient to outpatient treatment for large numbers of surgical operations. Hernia repair, breast surgery, and cholecystectomy, 3 staples of general surgical experience, are all managed primarily as outpatients today, and residents have minimal opportunity to evaluate these patients before surgery or to follow them afterward to observe their clinical course. It was through more prolonged in-hospital stays that residents were exposed to many of the conversations about and with patients, where matters instilling judgment, issues around palliation, and provision of ethical and compassionate care took place. By reductions in work hours and changes in the "typical" inpatient, the opportunities for mentoring and apprenticeships are reduced, a formerly central component to the training process.

ADDRESSING THE ISSUES

The environmental and technological changes described previously are irreversible and have fundamentally altered the types of disease that require surgical treatment as well as the way in which the treatment is done. Such change will undoubtedly continue, and the directions in which surgery will evolve in the future are not predictable. The most effective way to address the current issues is therefore to look at the things that can be changed in resident training, the many areas in which improvements in resident teaching are possible, and the areas in which residents' capabilities could be productively expanded.

Defining and continually updating the curriculum

The starting point for making change in residency is to recognize that much of what is being taught is obsolete, and addresses diseases that are no longer a significant problem, or those for which surgical treatment is rarely needed. Teaching and testing the extensive amount of information that exists with regard to gastric physiology, for example, is of little value to current residents who will rarely see a complication of benign peptic ulcer disease. The subjects taught in the curriculum should be continually updated to correspond to medical problems that are currently seen and treated, and new areas of technological development should be rapidly incorporated so that residents are kept abreast of current information. Bariatric surgery currently represents the most common operation that is performed in many hospitals, yet residents generally have limited knowledge of the subjects related to the causes of obesity, the physiologic changes that occur following bariatric surgery, or the technical details of the various operations performed. In most residencies they have almost no direct operative experience in developing competence in performing the procedures themselves.

There should be a continuous process by which the medical conditions that are currently being treated and the surgical treatments administered are tracked and used to modify the teaching curriculum so as to keep residents knowledgeable regarding the current diseases they will be treating. Knowledge related to diseases that are no longer a significant problem, although it may be intellectually fascinating, should be pruned from the active curriculum.

Improving the efficiency of learning

The general process of teaching residents has changed little in several decades, and is still primarily based on a preceptorship model in which the resident learns about whatever happens to walk through the door of the hospital that day, rather than through a comprehensive curriculum that covers all relevant subjects in a defined period of time, with competency testing at regular intervals to evaluate comprehension and understanding. The principles of education that are widely known and applied elsewhere are not central to residency teaching. This in large part is because the service demands placed on residents keep them continually responding to the next significant patient care problem throughout the day and prevent structured time from being set aside for didactic teaching. Realistically, the patient care needs that residents provide will never be eliminated because the service they provide carries teaching benefit as well as generating diverse experience with the management of all types of patient conditions; extensive experience in dealing with these diverse situations is essential to making them competent practitioners.

As a result, residency teaching cannot be a didactic classroom experience, as it is in graduate schools. What could occur, however, is the delivery of a more defined and comprehensive curriculum to residents at an individual level through the multiplicity of handheld devices and small computers that are available today, usable in any environment. Teaching of residents needs to evolve to a system in which the learning primarily occurs at the individual resident level, rather than via classroom or other group experience, but it should be governed by a structured and defined curriculum that the resident can access in his or her own time frame and in any environment in which he or she finds time available for learning. Numerous studies have shown that the 80-hour workweek has not resulted in increased time reading and studying by trainees. If we wish to change this, the expectations must be more explicitly defined via a curriculum that outlines specific levels of achievement by year of residency, and provides low-stakes online methods of self-assessment. Setting, measuring, and tracking achievement of these standards can help offset concerns over training program variability, as all trainees will meet the same thresholds of performance, irrespective of training environment.

The variety of on-line and sophisticated resources for learning, including annotated operative videos, the SCORE portal and curriculum, and other resources make self-directed learning more efficient now than it has ever been. Teaching material can be delivered easily in discrete increments, and can be accompanied by self-assessment on completion that provides comparative performance data relative to one's peers, or to an absolute standard. The enormous success and rapid growth of the Khan Academy teaching modules [6] has demonstrated in the past few years just how dynamic such a model can be, as well as how effective and attractive it is to users. An almost identical model could be developed for resident learning.

Similarly, maximal learning needs to occur in all available clinical opportunities. This can be achieved in 2 ways. First, to the extent feasible, physician extenders (physician assistants and nurse practitioners) should assume the "service" components of resident work so that maximal time for clinical assessments and therapeutic decision making can be left for the residents, as well as maximal time for participation in the operating room. Second, the teaching faculty in training programs need to understand how to teach more effectively and deliberately. We need to be cognizant of the changes to the case mix that has occurred over the past few decades and train residents deliberately in focused areas. For instance, given the urgent but rare nature of perforated peptic ulcer, residents need to be trained on the principles of gastric surgery on the cases they are seeing in elective situations, such as bariatric surgery. Teaching faculty need to be deliberate in their goals for each operation they do with trainees, with specific teaching done in every case. The laparotomy being performed for a cancer resection could and should also include a brief description and demonstration of how one might obtain vascular control of traumatic injuries to any number of intra-abdominal organs. Through these deliberate teaching moments, the case at hand can be completed, but the resident can learn twofold or threefold from a given case.

Last, we should consider uniform adoption of preresidency "boot camps" (held in the fourth year of medical school) that bring all entering interns to the same level of skill with regard to several basic procedures. In this way, the intern year is maximally spent on development of skills and attributes unique to surgeons and the often underused fourth year of medical school can be used to better benefit.

Using simulation and more structured teaching and assessment

A third improvement in teaching can occur through the development and use of simulation in focused areas, which allows the more rapid accretion of specific skills, and the ability to objectively assess competence in these areas. The first of these to be mandated by the American Board of Surgery is Fundamentals of Laparoscopic Surgery (FLS), a course of instruction and assessment developed by the Society of Gastrointestinal and Endoscopic Surgeons (SAGES). Completion of FLS at an early stage in residency moves the resident to a standardized threshold of knowledge and skills for laparoscopy, and allows him or her to move more confidently and rapidly into the utilization of laparoscopy in a variety of operative cases. It ensures that all residents have reached approximately the same threshold, and eliminates much of the variability and uncertainty that surrounds such skills acquisition when there is no standardized teaching or testing.

A similar evolution is occurring presently with the Fundamentals of Endoscopic Surgery (FES), a parallel course developed by SAGES for the teaching of upper and lower gastrointestinal endoscopy skills. When integrated into a complete endoscopic curriculum that includes clinical rotations and experience, it ensures that residents have acquired a baseline competence in performing these. This development promises to provide an assurance that residents who complete such training will have achieved a uniform competence in endoscopic performance.

Although still not widely adopted, residents need to receive explicit instruction in basic surgical skills and techniques, which should be practiced in a simulated environment, and then tested to proficiency. Studies have shown that performance of technical skills improves most when practice to defined goals is included; these should be outlined for trainees and rigorously measured. As with FLS certification, if basic surgical skills are mastered early in training, more rapid and confident adoption of advanced techniques is possible.

Simulators directed toward the teaching of operative skills for specific operations such as cholecystectomy have been developed, but in general lack a close correspondence to the real thing. Such simulators have never been able to duplicate tissue characteristics with regard to blunt and sharp dissection, nor to simulate bleeding and the methods used for its control. As a result, simulators in this area have never achieved much success other than in teaching manual skills manipulation, which is necessary in laparoscopic surgery, intracorporeal suturing, and similar skills that do not require an accurate depiction of tissue manipulation and dissection.

It seems likely that with increasing computer power, the accurate replication of tissue characteristics may become possible, and when that occurs it should be feasible to simulate virtually all operative procedures that are done in the abdomen. Such a development would allow the full development of skills and the presentation of variant anatomy, difficult operative situations, and so forth, all before an actual encounter with patients.

An area of simulation that has been attempted by dozens of investigators, but has been of limited scope to date has been the attempt to duplicate the diagnostic workup and clinical decision making that is at the core of surgical treatment. The ability to conduct a skilled history and physical assessment, formulate a working differential diagnosis, and use testing to establish the correct diagnoses and determine the best treatment remains difficult to teach and is generally learned only through extensive real-world experience and mentorship. It is often not learned well, and the well-documented errors of commission and omission in actual practice clearly indicate the need for improvement.

Although this theoretically should be an ideal framework in which computer simulation might be of benefit, the ability to accurately mimic in computer programing the complex ways in which information is actually gathered and the processing that occurs in a skilled clinician's brain has so far eluded programmers, and the programs that exist only simulate very basic situations and conditions. Even those often have an enforced linearity and lack of logical branching for the multiple scenarios that are present in reality, and therefore are of limited value in teaching the needed skills. Improvements in this area are badly needed.

Earlier specialty focus in residency training

Three "real-world" experiments have been conducted during the past 7 to 8 years with regard to defining the preferences of medical students to undergo the classical model of training for a surgical specialty (5 years of general surgery followed by 1–3 years of specialty fellowship) or to enter instead an "integrated" specialty track directly out of medical school in which the general surgical training is incorporated into the first 3 years of training but seamlessly transitions into the specialty training that is the ultimate goal of the fellowship. Plastic surgery was the first to introduce this model, vascular surgery was the second, and thoracic surgery the third. In plastic surgery, the overall integrated model requires 6 years, the vascular surgery model requires 5 years, and the thoracic surgery model requires 6 years.

In each of these cases, the "integrated" model has proven to be the overwhelming preference of medical students, as evidenced by a dramatic increase in the number of applications for such programs in the internship match. In plastic surgery, this has resulted in a steady increase of such integrated programs and the phasing out of the classical model. In vascular surgery, the number of integrated programs is steadily increasing and now accounts for approximately half of the 120 training programs that exist. In thoracic surgery, the experience is more limited in numbers but appears to have a similar appeal.

This experience has clearly indicated that for medical students who already have a clear focus on a specialty area for future practice, the 5-year general surgical residency is seen as an unnecessary diversion before getting to their intended area of practice. Concerns remain as to their overall breadth of experience and areas of operative competence, and experience with these programs is not yet sufficiently great to know whether graduates in the new paradigms will function equivalently to those who completed the classical programs. However, such concerns are increasingly moot, as the overwhelming preference of medical students is driving these developments in an irreversible way.

In recognition of the desire of medical students to focus earlier on the specialty area they hope to practice in, the American Board of Surgery 3 years ago adopted a "flexibility" option with regard to residency training in which an individual resident could spend 12 months during the last 3 years of residency focused on a single specialty area. It was intended that beginning in the third year and extending through the fourth and fifth years a resident could accumulate 12 months of experience in a specialty before actually entering a fellowship in that specialty after residency. Such experience would allow residents to enter fellowship with significantly enhanced knowledge of the field, and to progress more rapidly during the 1 to 3 years of fellowship training.

Utilization of this option by program directors has been limited to date. However, a group of residency programs began collaborating and agreed to form a consortium in fall of 2012 to begin a deliberate study of application of the flexibility rule to surgical training. The Flexibility in Surgical Training (FIST) consortium proposes to study the outcome for the trainees in these new flexibility tracks by periodic assessments of a number of outcome measures. By using pooled data from several institutions we expect to gain better understanding of the "flexibility rule" impact. In the training paradigm proposed by participating consortium programs, residents will be able to spend additional months of training in their area of interest. Such trainees will be able to spend this focused time sooner than traditional fellowship training allows, and will streamline and improve the experiences for all trainees in a single program, as each will be afforded a more "customized" training experience. As a result, graduates will finish training with additional clinical experience in their area of intended eventual practice.

Expanded laparoscopic surgery training

In the previous discussion it was noted that overall, surgical residents have lost significant operative experience in open abdominal surgery, but that this has not been replaced with comparable experience doing more complex laparoscopic abdominal surgery, in part due to the development of laparoscopic surgery fellowships. Although the RRC for Surgery has mandated gradually increasing complexity and volume of laparoscopic surgery, the training requirements are still modest with regard to the breadth and complexity of laparoscopic procedures actually done in practice today.

There is no intrinsic reason why the requirements for breadth and volume of laparoscopic surgery during residency should not steadily increase to correct this deficiency. The initial lack of faculty with sufficient experience to teach the laparoscopic procedures has been long since corrected, and the skills of fourth-year and fifth-year surgical residents are essentially the same as the fellows 1 year senior who enter laparoscopic fellowships. Making this transition would require the coordinated efforts of department chairs and program directors, but overall it would strengthen and expand the capabilities of graduating residents.

Increasing length of residency

The time that has effectively been lost from residency due to the 80-hour workweek was noted previously to be in the range of 6 to 12 months of in-hospital experience, largely in the urgent and emergent experience that occurs at night and on weekends. The only ways to compensate for this and achieve the same level of final training is to either train more efficiently, which has already been described, or to increase the length of residency. When the question of increasing time in residency is raised, the immediate reaction is generally that this would not be possible, as the present 5-year residency is already often viewed as too long. However, this overlooks the fact that more than 80% of surgical residents already elect to take a postresidency fellowship in a specialty or subspecialty area. Although most of these fellowships are 1 year in length, several of them are 2 years (vascular surgery, pediatric surgery, surgical oncology, transplantation) and some are 3 (thoracic surgery, plastic surgery). Thus, any discussion of extending residency applies only to the 20% of residents who currently complete only general surgical residency and do not seek subspecialty training. Extending residency by 1 year to obtain more extensive training in general surgery per se would not seem to be an insurmountable issue if the benefits clearly warranted it.

The method by which training might be increased is open to considerable debate. Currently, a few of the additional fellowships are subject to accreditation by the ACGME (vascular surgery, pediatric surgery, surgical critical care, hand surgery) but most are not. The other specialty fellowships are generally overseen by surgical specialty societies, and the degree of standardization and rigor in the oversight process is variable. Nevertheless, most of these fellowships seem to function effectively in providing the expected specialty training, and complaints are almost never heard from fellows who complete them that their training was insufficient or inadequate. Because no examinations are given for these nonaccredited fellowships, nor are other assessments made, we have no objective data with regard to differences in quality of training in different fellowships, or of overall competence gained in the specific area of training.

A recent (fall 2012) initiative by the American College of Surgeons (ACS), which is still in the formative stage, involves establishment of "advanced surgery" fellowships that would be accredited and overseen by the ACS. This effort, still in early stages, could be an important step in regulating and overseeing fellowships and the experiences they provide to trainees.

A characteristic of the fellowships, which follows from the fact that the fellow is board eligible or board certified, is that he or she is legally entitled to function independently in patient care and does not need documented oversight for all clinical activities as residents do. This allows fellows to have a degree of conditional independence and to develop conditional autonomy as their skills dictate, and this has made the fellowships attractive to surgeons who find similar experience lacking in residency today. There has been no systematic study of the effect of this greater degree of autonomy, nor has there been any comparison of the performance of surgeons who have completed fellowship versus residency only in this regard, but postresidency fellowships are an effective way of obtaining a period of training in which some independence and autonomy is available.

Adding additional skills to surgical residency training

The final area in which surgical residency might be strengthened is in the addition of technical skills that are not presently taught, but that would allow surgeons to provide more unified and comprehensive treatment for the patients they already see. One such area is the use of ultrasound for better diagnosis of conditions in breast, endocrine, vascular, and trauma diseases. This is currently done in many programs, but there are no standardized requirements established by the RRC. A second is the use of interventional catheter techniques for the diagnosis or treatment of a variety of conditions. Vascular surgery has expanded their abilities in use of catheter techniques in the past 15 years in a dramatic way to increase the endovascular capabilities of their specialty. General surgery has not done this, but there are a number of conditions in which simple catheter techniques might be used for more efficient treatment of surgical disease. Consideration should be given to the more uniform teaching and testing of such targeted skills, where it would make unified disease management more effective and efficient.

SUMMARY

The practice of general surgery has undergone a marked evolution in the past 20 years, which has been inadequately recognized and minimally addressed. The changes that have occurred have been disruptive to residency training, and to date there has been inadequate compensation for these. Evidence is now emerging of significant issues in the overall performance of recent graduates from at least 3 sources: the evaluation of external agents who incorporate these graduates into their practice or group, the opinions of the residents themselves, and the performance of graduates on the oral examination of the American Board of Surgery during the past 8 years. The environmental and technological causes of the present situation represent improvements in care for patients, and are clearly irreversible. Hence, solutions to the problems must be sought in other areas.

To address the issues effectively, greater recognition and engagement are needed by the surgical community so that effective solutions can be crafted. These will need to include improvements in the efficiency of teaching, with the assumption of greater individual resident responsibility for their knowledge, the establishment of more defined standards for knowledge and skills acquisition by level of residency training, with flexible self-assessment available online, greater focus of the curriculum on current rather than historical practice, increased use of structured assessments (including those in a simulated environment), and modifications to the overall structure of the traditional 5-year residency.

References

[1] Levitt SD. Understanding why crime fell in the 1990s: four factors that explain the decline and six that do not. J Econ Perspect 2004;18:163–90.
[2] Malangoni MA, Biester TW, Jones AT, et al. Operative experience of surgery residents: trends and challenges. Presented - APDS meeting April 26, 2013. J Surg Ed 2013, in press.
[3] Philibert I, Nasca T, Brigham T, Shapire J. Duty-hour limits and patient care and resident outcomes: can high-quality studies offer insight into complex relationships? Annu Rev Med 2013;64:467–83.
[4] Fuhrman G, Orr R, Dunn E, et al. An assessment of university versus independent general surgery program graduate performance on the American Board of Surgery examinations. J Surg Educ 2007;64:346–50.
[5] Yeo H, Viola K, Berg D, et al. Attitudes, training experiences, and professional expectations of US general surgery residents. JAMA 2009;302:1301–8.
[6] Available at: www.khanacademy.com.

Advances in Surgery 47 (2013) 271–286
ADVANCES IN SURGERY

Is the Abdominal Aortic Aneurysm Rupture Rate Decreasing?

Andy M. Lee, MD[a], Elliot L. Chaikof, MD, PhD[b,*]

[a]Department of Surgery, Beth Israel Deaconess Medical Center, Harvard Medical School, 110 Francis Street, Suite 9B, Boston, MA 02215, USA; [b]Department of Surgery, Beth Israel Deaconess Medical Center, Harvard Medical School, 110 Francis Street, Suite 9F, Boston, MA 02215, USA

Keywords

• Aneurysm • Rupture • Surveillance • Smoking • Statin • Angiotensin • EVAR • Outcomes

Key points

- By understanding the natural progression of abdominal aortic aneurysm (AAA) disease, there have been improvements in predicting and determining rupture potential.
- Smoking is the strongest independent risk factor for aneurysm development, expansion, and rupture.
- Despite the inconsistencies and lack of randomized clinical trials for available medical therapies, statins have still been shown to decrease AAA-related mortality.
- Earlier detection of AAA by screening has allowed earlier surgical intervention and medical management, reducing AAA rupture–associated mortality.
- Clinical evidence from 4 randomized trials showed no long-term benefits in early AAA repair by open or endovascular surgery compared with surveillance.

Abdominal aortic aneurysm (AAA) is a common and life-threatening condition resulting from a focal enlargement of the infrarenal aorta that occurs over a time course of several years [1]. Although present in approximately 2% of the elderly population, approximately 150,000 new cases are diagnosed each year, and the incidence is steadily increasing [2,3]. Patients with AAA have a high mortality, primarily due to rupture, which is also responsible for approximately 15,000 deaths per year in the United States [4,5]. With such a dismal prognosis, most patients with rupture do not survive long enough to reach medical care [6], and for those who do survive and

*Corresponding author. *E-mail address*: echaikof@bidmc.harvard.edu

0065-3411/13/$ – see front matter
http://dx.doi.org/10.1016/j.yasu.2013.03.004

undergo traditional open repair, the reported mortality rate continues to exceed 40% [7–10].

Electing to pursue conservative or surgical management of AAA is based on weighing the relative risk of rupture against the risk of operative mortality and morbidity in the context of estimated life expectancy [11]. Based on the work of Szilagyi and colleagues [12] in the 1960s, during the past 5 decades, the primary determinant of rupture risk has been maximum aneurysm diameter [13]. Moreover, autopsy studies have indicated that aneurysm diameter is an important determinant of rupture, with larger aneurysms having the greatest risk [14,15]. Nonetheless, there remains uncertainty concerning the risk of rupture of AAAs of varying size, which compounds the difficulties of decision making, particularly for patients of marginal fitness [15,16].

Currently, there is general agreement that fusiform aneurysms smaller than 4.0 cm maximum diameter are at low risk of rupture and should be monitored under regular ultrasound surveillance. At a diameter of 5.4 cm, patients are referred for consideration of aneurysm repair [17,18]. Debate remains for patients presenting with AAAs between 4.0 and 5.4 cm regarding the most appropriate role for either immediate treatment for aneurysms that are suitable for endovascular repair or continued surveillance and selective repair should the aneurysm exceed 5.4 cm or diameter rapidly increase (>1 cm per year) [18]. Two large trials, United Kingdom Small Aneurysm Trial (UKSAT) and Aneurysm Detection and Management (ADAM) Trial, randomized patients with asymptomatic aneurysms between 4.0 and 5.5 cm to either early elective open surgery or surveillance, with surgery recommended should the diameter exceeded 5.5 cm [19]. A 2007 systematic review that included only these 2 trials concluded that there were no statistically significant differences in all-cause mortality or long-term survival between the immediate surgery and surveillance groups at 5 to 8 years [20] (See Table 1).

Table 1
Estimated rupture risk and surveillance recommendations based on aneurysm size

Aortic abdominal aneurysm, cm	Rupture risk, %/y	Surveillance recommendations
2.9	0	
3.0–3.4	0	Repeat imaging at 3 y
3.5–4.4	0	Repeat imaging at 12 mo
4.5–5.4	0.5–2	Repeat imaging at 6 mo
5.4–5.9	3–10	
6.0–6.9	10–20	
7.0–7.9	20–40	
>8.0	30–50	

Data from Chaikof EL, Brewster DC, Dalman RL, et al, Society for Vascular Surgery. The care of patients with an abdominal aortic aneurysm: the Society for Vascular Surgery practice guidelines. J Vasc Surg 2009;50(Suppl 4):S2–49; and Brewster DC, Cronenwett JL, Hallett JW Jr, et al. Guidelines for the treatment of abdominal aortic aneurysms. Report of a subcommittee of the Joint Council of the American Association for Vascular Surgery and Society for Vascular Surgery. J Vasc Surg 2003;37(5):1106–17.

However, even with watchful surveillance, some aneurysms can still rupture at an unusually small size [12,21]. In a retrospective review of autopsies, Darling and colleagues [22] reported a rupture rate of 40% for AAAs with diameters larger than 5 cm and 12.8% for AAAs with diameters smaller than 5 cm. Similarly, Hall and colleagues [23] summarized a group of studies indicating that up to 23% of AAAs rupture at a diameter smaller than 5 cm [1]. In another series, Nicholls and colleagues [24] and Brown and Powell [15] reported a ruptured rate of 10% to 24% for AAAs 5 cm or smaller in maximal diameter [16]. The diameter threshold in AAA management is not absolute and rupture is certainly not prevented by surveillance. As a consequence, efforts have been pursued to identify parameters, such as AAA expansion rate, intraluminal thickness, wall strength, stress, and tension, that can better predict patient-specific rupture risk.

During the past several decades, there has been considerable improvement in screening and cardiovascular awareness. These changes in public health measures have affected the rate of AAA rupture, as previous studies have shown that smoking and higher mean arterial blood pressures increase rupture rates, whereas statin use decreases rupture rates [25]. Several studies now show a substantial decrease of AAA prevalence to less than 2% in men older than 65 years with evidence that the incidence of aneurysm rupture and mortality from AAA is also declining [26]. Although the pathogenesis of atherosclerosis and aneurysm differ, it is likely the natural history of aneurysmal disease has been altered by greater efforts to curtail tobacco use and improved atherosclerotic risk factor management [27].

In the patient with a small aneurysm, the main therapeutic goal is to limit continued aortic expansion to a size at which the risk of rupture is high [19]. The objective of this review was to address the lifestyle modifications, factors, and current medical therapies that influence aneurysm growth, which has contributed to the decreasing trend in AAA rupture and mortality.

AAA DETERMINANTS OF RUPTURE

Rapid expansion

Expansion rate, and its influence on AAA rupture, has been implicated as an alternative predictor of rupture and indication for surgery. Across several population-based surveillance studies, the mean annual expansion rate for AAA has been calculated to be 0.3 to 0.8 cm per year [28–31]. Although rapid AAA expansion is presumed to increase rupture risk, it is difficult to separate this effect from the influence of expansion rate on absolute diameter, which alone could increase rupture risk [32]. For instance, Limet and colleagues [33] used serial measurements and determined that aneurysmal expansion rate was related to initial aortic diameter: 5.3 mm per year for diameters smaller than 40 mm, 6.9 mm per year in the 40 to 49 mm group, and 7.4 mm per year for diameters of 50 mm or more, suggesting that risk of rupture was not only related to final size but to relative change in aneurysmal size. Similarly, in a review of 476 patients, Brown and colleagues [34] demonstrated a mean expansion rate of 8.4 mm per year for aneurysms larger than 6 cm that subsequently ruptured as opposed to 3.9 mm per year in unruptured aneurysms. Rapid AAA expansion is a risk factor for rupture and an independent measure for deciding on elective repair of small AAAs.

The AAA expansion rate can vary over time and the outcome for patients with AAA seems to be influenced by factors that affect the natural history of AAA [31]. In addition to large initial AAA diameter, Chang and colleagues [35] demonstrated that rapid expansion is independently associated with advanced age, smoking, severe cardiac disease, and stroke [32]. Moreover, in a prospective study involving 1743 patients, aneurysms expanded significantly more rapidly in current smokers than in former smokers, with an observed AAA growth rate of 20% to 25% [19,35–37]. Other factors identified as predictors of rapid AAA expansion include blood pressure and intraluminal thrombus content [32,38]. Hatakeyama and colleagues [39] demonstrated that not only are expansion rate, blood pressure, and luminal thrombus content independent risk factors for aneurysmal rupture, but the combination of all 3 factors were the most predictive of aneurysm rupture.

Biomechanical wall properties

As an alternative to maximum diameter, the biomechanical properties and dynamics of the AAA wall have been considered as predictors of rupture risk. In determining wall tension from the law of Laplace from blood pressure and computed tomography (CT) scan measurements, Hall and colleagues [23] demonstrated that aortic wall tension is a contributing variable to imminent rupture. However, due to the presence of non-uniform wall thickness and shape asymmetry, the distribution of stress values are also spatially variable across the aorta. Using patient-specific finite element simulations, 3-dimensional CT scans, and geometric computerized models, the biomechanical properties of the AAA wall and the relation to risk and site of rupture can be predicted. In a large prospective study, Fillinger and colleagues [16] showed that the peak wall stress could differentiate AAAs that required urgent repair better than maximum diameter and were not simply an acute or incidental event near the time of rupture [40,41]. It was clear that aneurysm wall stress is elevated well in advance of rupture, allowing sufficient time for repair [12,41]. Stress analysis is conceptually practical and a potentially valuable tool in predicting AAA rupture risk.

In an effort to improve the prediction of rupture risk, the effect of intraluminal thrombus (ILT) content has been incorporated into more refined models. ILT is a 3-dimensional fibrin structure composed of red blood cells, platelets, proteins, and cellular debris and is present in variable degrees between the flowing blood and the aortic wall in approximately 75% of all AAAs [42,43]. The 2 responsible factors for the weakened aortic wall involve the interplay between the ILT layer and local factors, leading to an extensive degradation of the extracellular matrix and structural proteins. In a review by Vorp and Vande Geest [1], ILT-induced biomechanical stress and hypoxia stimulate endothelial, smooth muscle, and adventitial cells to produce a proteolytic and cytokine-rich environment that effectively inhibits collagen synthesis and promotes elastin degradation. Finite element analysis suggests that ILT can reduce peak wall stress by up to 30%, which can lead to significant errors in calculating both the magnitude and the distribution of AAA wall stresses [1,42–46]. Finally, Stenbaek and colleagues [47] demonstrated, in a retrospective study of 67 patients with AAA, that no patient without a thrombus experienced rupture and those that ruptured had a significantly faster growth of their thrombus.

Smoking cessation

The first clear association between smoking and aneurysm formation was attributed in the Framingham study in 1969 [48]. Substantial research has demonstrated that cigarette smoking is the risk factor most strongly associated with aneurysm development, rupture, and expansion. For example, the Whitehall study demonstrated that risk of death from AAA increased 4-fold for smokers and the risk of death from AAA increased 14-fold for those who had smoked hand-rolled cigarettes [49,50]. Similarly, in a nested control study, Wilmink and colleagues [51] reported that current smokers and ex-smokers were 7.6 times and 3.0 times more likely to have an AAA than nonsmokers, respectively. Last, the ADAM study revealed that smoking was the risk factor most strongly associated with AAAs; the odds ratio (OR) for AAAs of 4.0 cm or larger compared with normal aortas was 5.57 [39,52].

Recently, Wang and colleagues [53] provided new mechanistic insight correlating tobacco smoking and the development of AAA. By using mouse models, they found that nicotine increases aneurysm formation by stimulating the $\alpha 2$ isoform of AMP-activated protein kinase (AMPK$\alpha 2$) in vascular smooth muscle cells (VSMCs); and activation of AMPK$\alpha 2$, in turn, resulted in phosphorylation of activator protein 2α, a transcription factor that drives the expression of and smooth muscle cell release of matrix metalloproteinase 2 (MMP-2), a matrix-degrading protein that functions to weaken the artery wall, thus facilitating aneurysm formation [54].

Smoking is a specific risk factor for AAA disease prevalence, incidence, and progression. In patients with small AAAs, by using serial ultrasounds, MacSweeney and colleagues [37] found median expansion rates were higher in patients who continued to smoke. Lindholt and colleagues [55] and Baxter and colleagues [56] evaluated and prospectively followed 117 patients with AAA and found a positive correlation between continued smoking and the rate of expansion. Furthermore, in the UKSAT study of 1090 randomized trial patients, current smokers independently exhibited a higher AAA rupture rate as compared with former and nonsmokers. Specifically, cigarette smoking status was associated with an incrementally increased AAA growth rate of 0.4 mm per year, which persisted after adjustment for potential confounding variables [56].

Although there have been no reported trials of smoking cessation in patients with AAA, smoking cessation is presumed to reduce overall AAA rupture risk.

In a prospective epidemiologic study, Hammond and Garfinkel [48] illustrated in more than 1 million men and women that the death rates from aortic aneurysms were low among patients who did not smoke and increased greatly with the amount of cigarette smoking [39]. The 2009 practice guidelines from the Society for Vascular Surgery note that there is strong evidence that smoking cessation reduces the risk of AAA growth and rupture [18]. At the present time, smoking cessation should be considered one of the most important recommendations to decrease the rate of aneurysm expansion [56].

MEDICAL THERAPY

Conservative management of small aneurysms (<5.5 cm) focuses on adjusting factors with medical therapy that otherwise promote AAA expansion. The need to identify effective medical therapies, which could reduce or eliminate small AAA growth and also improve overall outcome, is a major priority [57]. Medical therapies for AAA focus on the management of modifiable risk factors for AAA and cardiovascular disease with specific goals of reducing the need for intervention from aneurysm expansion or rupture, reducing morbidity and mortality associated with repair, and reducing cardiovascular morbidity and mortality [58]. Several agents have been tested in cohort as well as randomized studies, but, unfortunately, the study methodology has been suboptimal for lack of available randomized control trials [59] (See Table 2).

Statin therapy

Statins are 3-hydroxyy-3-methylglutaryl (HMG) coenzmye A reductase inhibitors primarily prescribed for their lipid-lowering and cardioprotective effects by

Table 2
Summarization of various types of intervention affecting risk factors in AAA development, expansion and rupture

	Impact on AAA			
Types	Development	Expansion	Rupture	Risk factors
Antibiotics (macrolides, tetracyclines)	X^A	X^A, X^C		Inflammatory
ACE inhibitors/ARB	X^A	X^A, X^C	X^A, X^C	Hypertension
Beta-blockers	X^A	X^A, X^C		Hypertension
Smoking cessation	X	X	X	Tobacco use
Statins		X^A, X^C		Hypercholesterolemia, inflammatory
Screening and surveillance		X	X	AAA diameter, wall stress, intraluminal thrombus content, family history
Surgical repair (open or EVAR)			X	

Abbreviations: AAA, abdominal aortic aneurysm; ACE, angiotensin-converting enzyme; ARB, angiotensin receptor blocker; EVAR, endovascular aneurysm repair; X^A, evidence through animal models; X^C, uncertain clinical evidence from lack of appropriate randomized trials.
Data from Refs.[56–75]

limiting the progression of atherosclerosis. Although effective in reducing atherogenic lipoproteins, statins also demonstrate a pleiotropic biologic effect, including reduction of C-reactive protein levels, which may be relevant to the pathogenesis of AAA disease [60]. They are expected to prevent AAA development through anti-inflammatory effects, such as a decrease in interleukin-6, antioxidative effects, inhibition of proteases (MMPs), and upregulation of synthesis of extracellular matrix proteins [61]. In a rat elastase-induced AAA model, simvastatin suppressed aneurysmal expansion and reduced levels of MMP-9 mediated by interfering with multiple pathways, including oxidative stress, inflammation, and extracellular matrix and matrix remodeling [62].

Statins have been shown to reduce mortality in patients who survive surgery for AAAs [63]. From a prospective trial of patients undergoing elective open AAA repair, patients were randomized to receive preoperative placebo or statin. Measured directly from aortic biopsies, Evans and colleagues [64] showed that patients on statins exhibited a 40% reduction in MMP-9 levels, which is consistent with findings from animal studies. In a meta-analysis of 4 studies examining all-cause postoperative mortality, Twine and Williams [65] showed a significant improvement with statin therapy at 1, 2, and 5 years with minimal heterogeneity among the 4 included studies.

In contrast, clinical correlation between statin and AAA growth has been largely limited to retrospective studies providing insufficient evidence for statin use in rupture prevention. From a meta-analysis of 6 retrospective and 1 prospective study, 3 observed a significant reduction in AAA expansion in patients taking a statin, whereas 4 studies showed no effect [64]. In a recent retrospective study of 211 patients, Karrowni and colleagues [5] demonstrated an association between statin use and decreased growth rate of AAA. In contrast, the Trosmo study of 4345 patients found that statin therapy increased the risk of developing AAA (OR 3.8, 95% confidence interval [CI] 1.45–9.80) [57,66]. There is strong evidence for statin therapy in reducing AAA-associated mortality but insufficient data exist for its role in reducing AAA expansion.

Beta-blocker therapy

Early retrospective studies suggested that beta-blocker therapy produced a notable decrease in AAA expansion rate. For instance, Gadowski and colleagues [67] evaluated 121 patients and demonstrated that among patients with large AAA, beta-blockers reduced mean expansion rate. However, in a subsequent double-blinded trial conducted by the Propranolol Aneurysm Trial Investigators group, 548 patients with asymptomatic AAA between 3 and 5 cm in diameter were randomized to receive placebo or propranolol [68]. After 2.5 years, the annual growth rate was similar between the 2 groups. A shortcoming of this study was poor patient compliance because of depression and other side effects, with approximately 40% of patients discontinuing the drug. Similarly, Lindholt and colleagues [69] reported in a trial of 122 patients that beta-blockers did not inhibit aneurysm expansion. These results were also compromised by low compliance, with only 22% of patients continuing the medication for 2 years [56]. A meta-analysis by Guessous and colleagues [70] of pooled results from 5 prospective cohort studies (1994–2002) showed a significant reduction in growth rate in the treated groups. Despite an established role in cardioprotection, beta-blockers lack clinical evidence that support their role in AAA rupture prevention.

Angiotensin inhibitors

A number of animal experiments using different models of aneurysmal disease have suggested an important role for the angiotensin/renin axis in aneurysm development [56]. Infusion of angiotensin is a well-accepted method of inducing AAA in a number of animal models, resulting initially in aortic dilation and eventual rupture. Cassis and colleagues [71] demonstrated that infusion of angiotensin II (AngII) to hyperlipidemic mice induces AAAs and augments atherosclerosis independent of increased blood pressure. Rateri and colleagues [72] observed more aneurysmal rupture–associated deaths, increased luminal diameters, and tissue remodeling.

Unfortunately, a randomized controlled trial has not been conducted to examine the efficacy of angiotensin-converting enzyme (ACE) inhibitor or angiotensin receptor blockade in limiting AAA progression [57]. From a Canadian-based case control study of 15,326 patients with AAA, Hackam and colleagues [73] reported that patients who received ACE inhibitors before admission were significantly less likely to present with ruptured aneurysm (OR 0.82, 95% CI 0.74–0.90) than those who did not receive ACE inhibitors. In contrast, Sweeting and colleagues [74] found in a prospective cohort study of 1701 patients enrolled to UKSAT between 1991 and 1995 that aneurysm growth rates in 169 patients taking ACE inhibitors at baseline was not substantially different when compared with the remaining 1532 patients. Despite evidence from animal experiments, clinical evidence that ACE inhibition prevents AAA rupture is limited.

Antibiotic therapy

Macrolide and tetracycline antibiotics have also been implicated in preventing AAA progression. Some have proposed that AAA progression is enhanced by secondary infection within the aortic wall [56]. More recent interest is centered on doxycycline, which has an anti-inflammatory effect and inhibits MMP function in vivo and in at least 14 separate animal models [57]. In a small randomized trial of 32 patients, aneurysm expansion rate among those receiving doxycycline was significantly lower than that in the placebo group during the 6-month to 12-month and the 12-month to 18-month periods [75]. Further validation is needed before any recommendation can be made.

SCREENING

In an effort to reduce mortality from AAA rupture, screening of small aneurysms has been the subject of much review during the past 2 decades. Much of the current guidelines are reflective of available randomized trials (ie, UKSAT and ADAM). Data from the Multicentre Aneurysm Screening Study (MASS) randomized 67,800 patients, aged 65 to 74, to receiving screening serial abdominal ultrasounds over a 4-year time course and showed a 53% relative risk reduction (95% CI 30–64) for AAA-related mortality in those who attended screening [76]. In addition, Scott and colleagues [77] performed a randomized ultrasound screening study of 15,775 male and female patients, aged 65 to 80, and were followed for over 5 years. Comparison of the control population and the group invited for screening (n = 5394) show that despite including those who refused the invitation and those unfit for surgery, screening resulted in a 55% reduction in the incidence of rupture and a 42% reduction in death from rupture. In a recent meta-analysis, Takagi and colleagues [78] identified 4 randomized controlled trials of population-based AAA screening with long-term follow-up. Pooled analysis demonstrated a statistically significant reduction in AAA-related mortality, by 4 per 1000 in men older than 65 years. Screening is an effective method that can detect AAA rupture risk, thus limiting AAA-related mortality.

Screening AAA in women has been somewhat controversial, as the lack of women in many of the randomized trials presents no clear evidence for its utility. Earlier research from a randomized screening trial of 3052 women showed significantly lower AAA prevalence (1.3% vs 7.6%) compared with men and without any notable differences in AAA-related mortality [77]. Although these data would suggest no benefit for screening in women, several additional studies must be considered [79]. From the UKSAT, the rate of AAA rupture was 3 times higher in women than in men after adjustment for age, body size, and initial AAA diameter, and the mean AAA diameter preceding rupture was 6 cm in men but only 5 cm in women [15,80]. Interestingly, there was no trend toward a benefit from early repair in women [80]. Given the conflicting data but lower prevalence, further studies are needed to determine which women would benefit most from screening [79].

Screening and surveillance programs must be rigorous and have stringent quality standards. As with any screening program, it is critical to balance the benefits of screening with the potential harms. In certain populations, the benefits of early AAA identification and subsequent repair clearly outweigh the risk of unidentified aneurysm leading to rupture and death [80].

THE ROLE OF SURGICAL INTERVENTION

The decrease in AAA rupture is reflective of increasing trends favoring more elective and earlier AAA repair. The decision on when to treat and manage asymptomatic AAAs has been the subject of debate especially for patients presenting with AAAs between 4.0 cm and 5.4 cm and selective repair for those aneurysms that enlarge beyond 5.4 cm [18]. Although almost half the early deaths that occur after elective aneurysm repair are attributed to cardiac causes, the potential benefit of early surgery must be weighed against the risk of death from rupture for the nonsurgical cohort [19]. Specifically, from the UKSAT trial, the initial 30-day operative mortality was 5.4% in the immediate surgery group and led to an early disadvantage in survival, but investigators found no statistically significant difference ($P = .03$) in long-term survival between the immediate surgery (mean survival 6.7 years) and surveillance groups (mean survival 6.5 years) [18,81]. Moreover, in the ADAM trial, operative mortality in the immediate repair group was only 2.7% but after follow-up of 4.9 years, the rate of survival among patients with low surgical risk with AAAs between 4.0 and 5.4 cm in diameter was no better than those enrolled in the surveillance arm [82]. Evidence from these 2 trials indicate no survival advantage in early open surgical repair as compared with surveillance.

Most elective AAA repairs in the United States are now performed using a minimally invasive endovascular approach. The main benefits of endovascular aneurysm repair (EVAR) as compared with open repair has been studied across 3 randomized trials and the US Medicare population and clearly exhibited lower perioperative morbidity and mortality than open surgical repair [83]. However, with regard to overall long-term survival (2–8 years), there was no significant difference between these 2 groups. Interestingly, in retrospective review of 923 patients, Zarins and colleagues [84] illustrated that this outcome may be due to preoperative aneurysm size. Patients with small AAAs (<5.0 cm) are more favorable candidates for EVAR and have a lower AAA-related death rate and higher survival rate compared with intermediate (5.0–5.9 cm) and large AAAs (>6.0 cm). These findings were also confirmed by 2 other retrospective trials from the Cleveland Clinic EVAR database and EUROpean collaborators on Stent-graft Techniques for abdominal aortic Aneurysm Repair (EUROSTAR) registry, suggesting the possibility that small AAAs may portend a better overall outcome [85–87]. Reviewing the national trends from 1993 to 2005 in AAA repair since the introduction of EVAR, Giles and colleagues [88] noted a significant decrease in the annual number of deaths from both intact and ruptured AAAs, increasing numbers of intact AAA repair after introduction of EVAR, and a concomitant decrease in ruptured AAA diagnosis and repair. The introduction of EVAR combined with increased detection may be responsible for an increasing number of intact AAA repairs in the United States, which, in principle, should result in lower mortality from AAA rupture [83].

Both the CAESAR (Comparison of surveillance vs endografting for small aneurysm repair) and PIVOTAL (Positive impact of endovascular options for treating aneurysm early) trials compared immediate EVAR to ultrasound surveillance in patients with AAA diameters between 4 and 5 cm [89,90]. These trials observed that early EVAR offered no survival advantage as compared with surveillance. Moreover, from the Cochrane Database Review, Filardo and colleagues [91] conducted a meta-analysis of the UKSAT, ADAM, CAESAR, and PIVOTAL trials and confirmed no overall advantage to early surgery for small AAAs as compared with selective surveillance in participants with asymptomatic aneurysms sized 4.0 to 5.5 cm in diameter. Nonetheless, in all of these trials, there has been a high crossover rate from surveillance to treatment arms before 5.4 cm size threshold for repair due to subjective symptoms and patient preference. Moreover, approximately 20% of patients who were

Table 3
Comparative view of randomized clinical trials for open or endovascular AAA repair versus surveillance of small aneurysms

	UKSAT		ADAM		CAESAR		PIVOTAL	
	Open repair	Survey	Open repair	Survey	EVAR	Survey	EVAR	Survey
Patient no.	563	527	569	567	182	178	366	362
Age, y	60–76		61–75		50–79		68–79	
Risk factors, %								
Current smokers	39.4	34.5	94.2	94.2	57.7	52.8	90	91.9
Former smokers	54.3	59.6	41.4	36.9	NA	NA	NA	NA
HTN	38	40	57.8	54.9	74.2	76.4	79	76.5
Medications, %								
Beta-blocker	15	16	16.9	14.8	44	37	52.6	51
ACE inhibitors	NA	NA	NA	NA	70	88	76	78.3
Statins/lipid-lowering	NA	NA	NA	NA	76	72	76.1	78.3
Outcomes, %								
Follow-up	8–12 y		3.5–8 y		54 mo		0–41 mo	
AAA repair	93.4	73.8	92.6	61.6	96.2	47.8	89	30.9
Morbidity	NA	NA	52.3	56.8	13.6	16.6	25.1	22.3
Mortality	7.1	5.8	2.7	2.1	0.6	0	0.31	0.91
Aneurysm rupture	NA	3.2	0.35	0.18	1.09	0.56	0	0.27
Overall mortality	63.9[a]	67.3[a]	25.1[b]	21.5[b]	14[c]	10.1[c]	4.1[d]	4.1[d]

Abbreviations: AAA, abdominal aortic aneurysm; ACE, angiotensin converting enzyme; ADAM, Aneurysm Detection and Management Trial; CAESAR, Comparison of surveillance vs endografting for small aneurysm repair; CI, confidence interval; EVAR, endovascular aneurysm repair; HR, hazard ratio; HTN, hypertension; NA, not applicable; PIVOTAL, Positive impact of endovascular options for treating aneurysm early; UKSAT, United Kingdom Small Aneurysm Trial.

[a]HR 0.88, 95% CI 0.75–1.02.
[b]HR 1.21, 95% CI 0.95–1.84.
[c]HR 0.76, 95% CI 0.30–1.93.
[d]HR 1.01, 95% CI 0.49–2.07.
Data from Refs.[52,81,82,84–92]

initially suitable for endovascular repair during the early period of surveillance, were no longer anatomically appropriate for EVAR as the AAA enlarged. Thus, there remains clinical uncertainty in the management of small AAAs (See Table 3).

SUMMARY

Decreased smoking has likely had the most significant impact on reducing the prevalence of AAAs. In a review of public data in England and Wales, Anjum and colleagues [25] illustrated a reduction of AAA rupture from 1997 to 2009 across all ages attributed to a concurrent decrease in prevalence of smoking. This trend has also been noted in a meta-analysis from Sweeting and colleagues [17] and attributed to a reduction in the prevalence of smoking since the mid-1970s along with an enhanced awareness of cardiovascular risk factor reduction and selective aneurysm screening. Along with an effort to reduce AAA progression and rupture, tools to predict patient-specific risk of AAA rupture are evolving with refined models that incorporate both aneurysm wall stress and wall strength likely to provide the most promising approach.

Although the role of statins, ACE inhibitors, beta-blockers, and aspirin in preventing or slowing aneurysmal rupture remains unresolved, their proven benefit in reducing long-term cardiovascular mortality suggests that these medications should be considered in any patient with a small AAA.

Currently, randomized trials do not show any survival benefit for open or endovascular repair for small aneurysms in the range of 4.0 to 5.4 cm. AAA repair, whether through an endovascular or open approach, is not without potential complication. Even at centers of excellence, the 30-day mortality rate for conventional AAA surgery is 3% to 5%, with rates of major morbidity ranging from 15% to 40% [87]. The Society for Vascular Surgery guidelines recommends surveillance for patients with a fusiform AAA of 4.0 to 5.4 cm [18,91].

The risk of AAA rupture appears to be decreasing through heightened public awareness, advanced technology for AAA detection , screening and surveillance, improved understanding of biomechanics and natural progression in AAA rupture , along with the availability of a wide range of medical therapies for risk factor reduction and minimally invasive options for AAA repair.

References

[1] Vorp DA, Vande Geest JP. Biomechanical determinants of abdominal aortic aneurysm rupture. Arterioscler Thromb Vasc Biol 2005;25:1558–66.

[2] Ouriel K, Green RM, Donayre C, et al. An evaluation of new methods of expressing aortic aneurysm size: relationship to rupture. J Vasc Surg 1992;15(1):12–8.

[3] Patel MI, Hardman DT, Fisher CM, et al. Current views on the pathogenesis of abdominal aortic aneurysms. J Am Coll Surg 1995;181(4):371–82.

[4] Johnston KW, Rutherford RB, Tilson MD, et al. Suggested standards for reporting on arterial aneurysms. Subcommittee on Reporting Standards for Arterial Aneurysms. J Vasc Surg 1991;13(3):452–8.

[5] Karrowni W, Dughman S, Hajj GP, et al. Statin therapy reduces growth of abdominal aortic aneurysms. J Investig Med 2011;59(8):1239–43.

[6] Bengtsson H, Bergqvist D. Ruptured abdominal aortic aneurysm: a population-based study. J Vasc Surg 1993;18(1):74–80.

[7] McPhee J, Eslami MH, Arous EJ, et al. Endovascular treatment of ruptured abdominal aortic aneurysms in the United States (2001-2006): a significant survival benefit over open repair is independently associated with increased institutional volume. J Vasc Surg 2009;49(4): 817–26.

[8] Visser P, Akkersdijk GJ, Blankensteijn JD. In-hospital operative mortality of ruptured abdominal aortic aneurysm: a population-based analysis of 5593 patients in the Netherlands over a 10-year period. Eur J Vasc Endovasc Surg 2005;30(4):359–64.

[9] Bown MJ, Sutton AJ, Bell PR, et al. A meta-analysis of 50 years of ruptured abdominal aortic aneurysm repair [review]. Br J Surg 2002;89(6):714–30.

[10] Heller JA, Weinberg A, Arons R, et al. Two decades of abdominal aortic aneurysm repair: have we made any progress? J Vasc Surg 2000;32(6):1091–100.

[11] Sonesson B, Sandgren T, Länne T. Abdominal aortic aneurysm wall mechanics and their relation to risk of rupture. Eur J Vasc Endovasc Surg 1999;18(6):487–93.

[12] Fillinger M. Who should we operate on and how do we decide: predicting rupture and survival in patients with aortic aneurysm. Semin Vasc Surg 2007;20(2):121–7.

[13] Szilagyi DE, Smith RF, DeRusso FJ, et al. Contribution of abdominal aortic aneurysmectomy to prolongation of life. Ann Surg 1966;164:678–99.

[14] Darling RC. Ruptured arteriosclerotic abdominal aortic aneurysms. A pathologic and clinical study. Am J Surg 1970;119(4):397–401.
[15] Brown LC, Powell JT. Risk factors for aneurysm rupture in patients kept under ultrasound surveillance. UK Small Aneurysm Trial Participants. Ann Surg 1999;230(3):289–96.
[16] Fillinger MF, Raghavan ML, Marra SP, et al. In vivo analysis of mechanical wall stress and abdominal aortic aneurysm rupture risk. J Vasc Surg 2002;36(3):589–97.
[17] Sweeting MJ, Thompson SG, Brown LC, et al. Meta-analysis of individual patient data to examine factors affecting growth and rupture of small abdominal aortic aneurysms. Br J Surg 2012;99(5):655–65.
[18] Chaikof EL, Brewster DC, Dalman RL, et al, Society for Vascular Surgery. The care of patients with an abdominal aortic aneurysm: the Society for Vascular Surgery practice guidelines. J Vasc Surg 2009;50(Suppl 4):S2–49.
[19] Powell JT, Greenhalgh RM. Clinical practice. Small abdominal aortic aneurysms. N Engl J Med 2003;348(19):1895–901.
[20] Lederle FA, Kane RL, MacDonald R, et al. Systematic review: repair of unruptured abdominal aortic aneurysm. Ann Intern Med 2007;146:735.
[21] Cronenwett JL, Murphy TF, Zelenock GB, et al. Actuarial analysis of variables associated with rupture of small abdominal aortic aneurysms. Surgery 1985;98(3):472–83.
[22] Darling RC, Messina CR, Brewster DC, et al. Autopsy study of unoperated abdominal aortic aneurysms. The case for early resection. Circulation 1977;56(Suppl 3):II161–4.
[23] Hall AJ, Busse EF, McCarville DJ, et al. Aortic wall tension as a predictive factor for abdominal aortic aneurysm rupture: improving the selection of patients for abdominal aortic aneurysm repair. Ann Vasc Surg 2000;14(2):152–7.
[24] Nicholls SC, Gardner JB, Meissner MH, et al. Rupture in small abdominal aortic aneurysms. J Vasc Surg 1998;28(5):884–8.
[25] Anjum A, von Allmen R, Greenhalgh R, et al. Explaining the decrease in mortality from abdominal aortic aneurysm rupture. Br J Surg 2012;99(5):637–45.
[26] Von Allmen RS, Powell JT. The management of ruptured abdominal aortic aneurysms: screening for abdominal aortic aneurysm and incidence of rupture. J Cardiovasc Surg (Torino) 2012;53(1):69–76.
[27] Hadjibashi AA, Mirocha J, Cossman DV, et al. Decreases in diameters of treated abdominal aortic aneurysms and reduction in rupture rate. Arch Surg 2012;17:1–4.
[28] Nevitt MP, Ballard DJ, Hallett JW Jr. Prognosis of abdominal aortic aneurysms. A population-based study. N Engl J Med 1989;321(15):1009–14.
[29] Collin J, Araujo L, Walton J. How fast do very small abdominal aortic aneurysms grow? Eur J Vasc Surg 1989;3(1):15–7.
[30] Sterpetti AV, Schultz RD, Feldhaus RJ, et al. Factors influencing enlargement rate of small abdominal aortic aneurysms. J Surg Res 1987;43(3):211–9.
[31] Glimåker H, Holmberg L, Elvin A, et al. Natural history of patients with abdominal aortic aneurysm. Eur J Vasc Surg 1991;5(2):125–30.
[32] Brewster DC, Cronenwett JL, Hallett JW Jr, et al. Guidelines for the treatment of abdominal aortic aneurysms. Report of a subcommittee of the Joint Council of the American Association for Vascular Surgery and Society for Vascular Surgery. J Vasc Surg 2003;37(5):1106–17.
[33] Limet R, Sakalihassan N, Albert A. Determination of the expansion rate and incidence of rupture of abdominal aortic aneurysms. J Vasc Surg 1991;14(4):540–8.
[34] Brown PM, Zelt DT, Sobolev B. The risk of rupture in untreated aneurysms: the impact of size, gender, and expansion rate. J Vasc Surg 2003;37(2):280–4.
[35] Chang JB, Stein TA, Liu JP, et al. Risk factors associated with rapid growth of small abdominal aortic aneurysms. Surgery 1997;121(2):117–22.
[36] Brady AR, Thompson SG, Fowkes FG, et al. Abdominal aortic aneurysm expansion: risk factors and time intervals for surveillance. Circulation 2004;110(1):16–21.
[37] MacSweeney ST, Ellis M, Worrell PC, et al. Smoking and growth rate of small abdominal aortic aneurysms. Lancet 1994;344(8923):651–2.

[38] Cronenwett JL, Sargent SK, Wall MH, et al. Variables that affect the expansion rate and outcome of small abdominal aortic aneurysms. J Vasc Surg 1990;11(2):260–8.
[39] Hatakeyama T, Shigematsu H, Muto T. Risk factors for rupture of abdominal aortic aneurysm based on three-dimensional study. J Vasc Surg 2001;33(3):453–61.
[40] Georgakarakos E, Ioannou C. Pathophysiology of abdominal aortic aneurysm rupture and expansion: new insight on an old problem. In: Grundmann R, editor. Etiology, pathogenesis and pathophysiology of aortic aneurysms and aneurysm rupture. Croatia: Rijeka; 2011. InTech; ISBN: 978-953-307-523-5.
[41] Fillinger MF, Marra SP, Raghavan ML, et al. Prediction of rupture risk in abdominal aortic aneurysm during observation: wall stress versus diameter. J Vasc Surg 2003;37(4): 724–32.
[42] Harter LP, Gross BH, Callen RA, et al. Ultrasonic evaluation of abdominal aortic thrombus. J Ultrasound Med 1983;1:315–8.
[43] Wang DH, Makaroun MS, Webster MW, et al. Effect of intraluminal thrombus on wall stress in patient-specific models of abdominal aortic aneurysm. J Vasc Surg 2002;36(3): 598–604.
[44] Inzoli F, Boschetti F, Zappa M, et al. Biomechanical factors in abdominal aortic aneurysm rupture. Eur J Vasc Surg 1993;7(6):667–74.
[45] Di Martino E, Mantero S, Inzoli F, et al. Biomechanics of abdominal aortic aneurysm in the presence of endoluminal thrombus: experimental characterization and structural static computational analysis. Eur J Vasc Endovasc Surg 1998;15(4):290–9.
[46] Mower WR, Quiñones WJ, Gambhir SS. Effect of intraluminal thrombus on abdominal aortic aneurysm wall stress. J Vasc Surg 1997;26(4):602–8.
[47] Stenbaek J, Kalin B, Swedenborg J. Growth of thrombus may be a better predictor of rupture than diameter in patients with abdominal aortic aneurysms. Eur J Vasc Endovasc Surg 2000;20(5):466–9.
[48] Hammond EC, Garfinkel L. Coronary heart disease, stroke, and aortic aneurysm. Arch Environ Health 1969;19(2):167–82.
[49] Strachan DP. Predictors of death from aortic aneurysm among middle-aged men: the Whitehall study. Br J Surg 1991;78(4):401–4.
[50] Franks PJ, Edwards RJ, Greenhalgh RM, et al. Risk factors for abdominal aortic aneurysms in smokers. Eur J Vasc Endovasc Surg 1996;11(4):487–92.
[51] Wilmink TB, Quick CR, Day NE. The association between cigarette smoking and abdominal aortic aneurysms. J Vasc Surg 1999;30(6):1099–105.
[52] Lederle FA, Johnson GR, Wilson SE, et al. Prevalence and associations of abdominal aortic aneurysm detected through screening. Aneurysm Detection and Management (ADAM) Veterans Affairs Cooperative Study Group. Ann Intern Med 1997;126(6):441–9.
[53] Wang S, Zhang C, Zhang M, et al. Activation of AMP-activated protein kinase α2 by nicotine instigates formation of abdominal aortic aneurysms in mice in vivo. Nat Med 2012;18(6):902–10.
[54] Sugamura K, Keaney JF Jr. Nicotine: linking smoking to abdominal aneurysms. Nat Med 2012;18(6):856–8.
[55] Lindholt JS, Heegaard NH, Vammen S, et al. Smoking, but not lipids, lipoprotein(a) and antibodies against oxidised LDL, is correlated to the expansion of abdominal aortic aneurysms. Eur J Vasc Endovasc Surg 2001;21(1):51–6.
[56] Baxter BT, Terrin MC, Dalman RL. Medical management of small abdominal aortic aneurysms. Circulation 2008;117(14):1883–9.
[57] Golledge J, Norman PE. Current status of medical management for abdominal aortic aneurysm. Atherosclerosis 2011;217(1):57–63.
[58] Lederle FA, Johnson GR, Wilson SE, et al. The aneurysm detection and management study screening program: validation cohort and final results. Aneurysm Detection and Management Veterans Affairs Cooperative Study Investigators. Arch Intern Med 2000;160: 1425–30.

[59] Bergqvist D. Pharmacological interventions to attenuate the expansion of abdominal aortic aneurysm (AAA)—a systematic review. Eur J Vasc Endovasc Surg 2011;41(5):663–7.
[60] Gotto AM Jr. Role of C-reactive protein in coronary risk reduction: focus on primary prevention. Am J Cardiol 2007;99:718–25.
[61] Miyake T, Morishita R. Pharmacological treatment of abdominal aortic aneurysm. Cardiovasc Res 2009;83:436–43.
[62] Kalyanasundaram A, Elmore JR, Manazer JR, et al. Simvastatin suppresses experimental aortic aneurysm expansion. J Vasc Surg 2006;43(1):117–24.
[63] Kertai MD, Boersma E, Westerhout CM, et al. Association between long-term statin use and mortality after successful abdominal aortic aneurysm surgery. Am J Med 2004;116: 96–103.
[64] Evans J, Powell JT, Schwalbe E, et al. Simvastatin attenuates the activity of matrix metalloprotease-9 in aneurysmal aortic tissue. Eur J Vasc Endovasc Surg 2007;34: 302–3.
[65] Twine CP, Williams IM. Systematic review and meta-analysis of the effects of statin therapy on abdominal aortic aneurysms. Br J Surg 2011;98:346–53.
[66] Forsdahl SH, Singh K, Solberg S, et al. Risk factors for abdominal aortic aneurysms: a 7-year prospective study: the Tromsø Study, 1994-2001. Circulation 2009;119:2202–8.
[67] Gadowski GR, Pilcher DB, Ricci MA. Abdominal aortic aneurysm expansion rate: effect of size and beta-adrenergic blockade. J Vasc Surg 1994;19(4):727–31.
[68] Propanolol Aneurysm Trial Investigators. Propranolol for small abdominal aortic aneurysms: results of a randomized trial. J Vasc Surg 2002;35:72–9.
[69] Lindholt JS, Henneberg EW, Juul S, et al. Impaired results of a randomised double blinded clinical trial of propranolol versus placebo on the expansion rate of small abdominal aortic aneurysms. Int Angiol 1999;18(1):52–7.
[70] Guessous I, Periard D, Lorenzetti D, et al. The efficacy of pharmacotherapy for decreasing the expansion rate of abdominal aortic aneurysms: a systematic review and meta-analysis. PLoS One 2008;3:e1895.
[71] Cassis LA, Gupte M, Thayer S, et al. ANG II infusion promotes abdominal aortic aneurysms independent of increased blood pressure in hypercholesterolemic mice. Am J Physiol Heart Circ Physiol 2009;296:H1660–5.
[72] Rateri DL, Howatt DA, Moorleghen JJ, et al. Prolonged infusion of angiotensin II in apoE (−/−) mice promotes macrophage recruitment with continued expansion of abdominal aortic aneurysm. Am J Pathol 2011;179(3):1542–8.
[73] Hackam DG, Thiruchelvam D, Redelmeier DA. Angiotensin-converting enzyme inhibitors and aortic rupture: a population-based case-control study. Lancet 2006;368:659–65.
[74] Sweeting MJ, Thompson SG, Brown LC, et al. Use of angiotensin converting enzyme inhibitors is associated with increased growth rate of abdominal aortic aneurysms. J Vasc Surg 2010;52(1):1–4.
[75] Mosorin M, Juvonen J, Biancari F, et al. Use of doxycycline to decrease the growth rate of abdominal aortic aneurysms: a randomized, double-blind, placebo-controlled pilot study. J Vasc Surg 2001;34(4):606–10.
[76] Ashton HA, Buxton MJ, Day NE, et al. The Multicentre Aneurysm Screening Study (MASS) into the effect of abdominal aortic aneurysm screening on mortality in men: a randomised controlled trial. Lancet 2002;360:1531–9.
[77] Scott RA, Wilson NM, Ashton HA, et al. Influence of screening on the incidence of ruptured abdominal aortic aneurysm: 5-year results of a randomized controlled study. Br J Surg 1995;82:1066–70.
[78] Takagi H, Goto SN, Matsui M, et al. A further meta-analysis of population-based screening for abdominal aortic aneurysm. J Vasc Surg 2010;52:1103–8.
[79] Pande RL, Beckman JA. Abdominal aortic aneurysm: populations at risk and how to screen. J Vasc Interv Radiol 2008;19(Suppl 6):S2–8.

[80] Lederle FA. Should abdominal aortic aneurysm be managed differently in women? Scand J Surg 2008;97(2):125–7.
[81] United Kingdom Small Aneurysm Trial Participants. Long-term outcomes of immediate repair compared with surveillance of small abdominal aortic aneurysms. N Engl J Med 2002;346:1445–52.
[82] Lederle FA, Wilson SE, Johnson GR, et al. Immediate repair compared with surveillance of small abdominal aortic aneurysms. N Engl J Med 2002;346:1437–44.
[83] Schermerhorn ML, Bensley RP, Giles KA, et al. Changes in abdominal aortic aneurysm rupture and short-term mortality, 1995-2008: a retrospective observational study. Ann Surg 2012;256(4):651–8.
[84] Zarins CK, Crabtree T, Bloch DA, et al. Endovascular aneurysm repair at 5 years: does aneurysm diameter predict outcome? J Vasc Surg 2006;44:920–30.
[85] Ouriel K, Srivastava SD, Sarac TP, et al. Disparate outcome after endovascular treatment of small versus large abdominal aortic aneurysm. J Vasc Surg 2003;37:1206–12.
[86] Peppelenbosch N, Buth J, Harris PL, et al. Diameter of abdominal aortic aneurysm and outcome of endovascular aneurysm repair: does size matter? A report from EUROSTAR. J Vasc Surg 2004;39:288–97.
[87] Ouriel K. Randomized clinical trials of endovascular repair versus surveillance for treatment of small abdominal aortic aneurysms. J Endovasc Ther 2009;16(Suppl 1):I94–105.
[88] Giles KA, Hamdan AD, Pomposelli FB, et al. Population-based outcomes following endovascular and open repair of ruptured abdominal aortic aneurysms. J Endovasc Ther 2009;16(5):554–64.
[89] Lall P, Gloviczki P, Agarwal G, et al. Comparison of EVAR and open repair in patients with small abdominal aortic aneurysms: can we predict results of the PIVOTAL trial? J Vasc Surg 2009;49(1):52–9.
[90] Cao P, De Rango P, Verzini F, et al. Comparison of surveillance versus aortic endografting for small aneurysm repair (CAESAR): results from a randomised trial. Eur J Vasc Endovasc Surg 2011;41(1):13–25.
[91] Filardo G, Powell JT, Martinez MA, et al. Surgery for small asymptomatic abdominal aortic aneurysms. Cochrane Database Syst Rev 2012;(3) CD001835.
[92] Mortality results for randomised controlled trial of early elective surgery or ultrasonographic surveillance for small abdominal aortic aneurysms. The UK Small Aneurysm Trial Participants. Lancet 1998;352(9141):1649–55.

Advances in Surgery 47 (2013) 287–297

ADVANCES IN SURGERY

Stress-induced Hyperglycemia

Is It Harmful Following Trauma?

Patrick L. Bosarge, MD, Jeffrey D. Kerby, MD, PhD*

Section of Trauma, Burns, and Surgical Critical Care, Department of Surgery, The University of Alabama at Birmingham, LHRB 112, 701 19th Street South, Birmingham, AL 35294-0007, USA

Keywords

• Trauma • Hyperglycemia • Critical care • Glycemic control

Key points

- Stress-induced hyperglycemia (SIH) is common after severe trauma and results from an imbalance of glucose production and glucose clearance induced by increased circulating levels of stress hormones and cytokines.
- SIH is associated with increased morbidity and mortality in certain medical conditions and trauma patients, although no direct causative effect has been proved.
- Prospective clinical trials have provided conflicting evidence regarding the use of tight glycemic control regimens. No prospective, randomized controlled clinical trials have been performed specifically evaluating the trauma population.
- The cause of hyperglycemia may be critically important in establishing those that may benefit from tight glycemic control regimens.
- Most institutions currently use moderate glucose control protocols. Properly designed prospective clinical trials and future technology limiting glucose variability will further clarify the appropriate levels of glucose control that result in improved outcomes.

INTRODUCTION

Hyperglycemia is well recognized as a normal metabolic stress response [1]. In settings of acute illness or injury, it has been termed stress-induced hyperglycemia (SIH) and has been defined as a transient plasma glucose level higher than 200 mg/dL in patients who are normally euglycemic. Ultimately, SIH results from an overabundance of glucose production relative to glucose clearance. More specifically, the cause of SIH is secondary to a state of enhanced glucose

*Corresponding author. Section of Trauma, Burns, and Surgical Critical Care, Department of Surgery, The University of Alabama at Birmingham, LHRB 112, 701 19th Street South, Birmingham, AL 35294-0007. *E-mail address*: jkerby@uabmc.edu

0065-3411/13/$ – see front matter
http://dx.doi.org/10.1016/j.yasu.2013.03.002 Published by Elsevier Inc.

production, diminished insulin production, and insulin resistance in peripheral tissues as a result of increases in stress hormones and cytokines (Table 1) [1,2]. Therefore, the more ill or seriously injured the patient, the higher the glucose levels secondary to the increased presence of stress hormones. This state typically persists until inflammatory mediators have decreased and the catabolic state subsides. Typical risk factors for SIH in acute trauma patients include large injury burden indicated by higher injury severity score (ISS), higher base deficit, and higher lactic acidosis [3,4]. Historically, these responses were believed to be protective to patients in acute phases of inflammation. However, in the last decade, much attention has been focused on the impact of hyperglycemia and whether aggressive treatment aimed at controlling serum glucose levels improves outcomes. SIH has been associated with several conditions including myocardial infarction [5–7], stroke [8,9], and trauma [10–12]. Published studies that evaluated the association between SIH and outcomes in these patients have consistently shown higher morbidity and higher mortality rates. However, it is still unclear whether SIH has a direct causative effect leading to worse outcomes, or is merely a marker of more severe disease. Existing studies do provide some mechanistic evidence for acute glucose toxicity, particularly in the setting of ischemia-reperfusion, which may be induced by damage to mitochondria that take up glucose in direct proportion to circulating blood glucose levels [13–15]. In the search for treatment regimens to lower morbidity and mortality in patients requiring intensive care, conflicting evidence in the treatment of hyperglycemia has emerged. This article focuses on hyperglycemia in the severely

Table 1
Mechanisms of hormones and cytokines in mediating stress-induced hyperglycemia

Hormone	Mechanism
Glucagon	Increased gluconeogenesis Increased hepatic glycogenolysis
Epinephrine	Skeletal muscle insulin resistance by altering postreceptor signaling Increased gluconeogenesis Increased skeletal muscle and hepatic glycogenolysis Increased lipolysis, increased free fatty acids Direct suppression of insulin secretion
Norepinephrine	Increased lipolysis Increased gluconeogenesis but hyperglycemia not marked except at high concentrations
Growth hormone	Skeletal muscle insulin resistance Increased lipolysis Increased gluconeogenesis
Tumor necrosis factor	Skeletal muscle insulin resistance, altered postreceptor signaling Hepatic insulin resistance

Data from McCowen KC, Malhotra A, Bistrian BR. Stress-induced hyperglycemia. Crit Care Clin 2001;17(1):107–24.

injured trauma patient, and whether available evidence currently supports the use of protocols aimed at aggressive glucose control.

HYPERGLYCEMIA: IMPACT AND APPROACH TO TREATMENT

Morbidity and mortality associated with hyperglycemia

Initial interest in hyperglycemia in the trauma patient began after the realization of worse outcomes in medical patients who had developed SIH. SIH has been associated with increased mortality and a higher incidence of congestive heart failure and cardiogenic shock in patients after myocardial infarction [5–7]. Stroke victims likewise have demonstrated higher mortality associated with SIH, and having worse odds of desirable neurologic outcomes as glucose levels increased with SIH [8,9]. As one of the more common metabolic derangements in severely injured patients, multiple efforts to examine the potential harm of hyperglycemia associated with the severely injured trauma patient have been undertaken. In 2003, Yendamuri and colleagues [10] first published a retrospective study that evaluated the association of admission hyperglycemia in trauma patients with outcome. They demonstrated that an admission glucose level greater than 200 mg/dL was independently associated with an increase in mortality in trauma patients. This finding was likewise true for a mild level of hyperglycemia (glucose >135 mg/dL). Additionally, the study found that hyperglycemia was a predictor of infectious complications in the form of pneumonia, urinary tract infections, wound infections, and bacteremia. Similarly, Sung and colleagues [11] prospectively evaluated 1003 trauma patients over a 2-year period who were admitted to the intensive care unit (ICU) or intermediate care unit of their level I trauma center. Patients were stratified into two groups based on admission glucose levels greater than or less than 200 mg/dL. To eliminate confusion between diabetic hyperglycemia (DH) and SIH, patients with history of diabetes were excluded from the study. They determined that a glucose level greater than or equal to 200 mg/dL was an independent predictor of increased mortality and infection. Laird and colleagues [12] evaluated the relationship of trauma outcomes in the ICU population differentiated by increasing levels of hyperglycemia on presentation. This retrospective study excluded patients with a known history of diabetes. For the 516 patients in the study group, hyperglycemia was evaluated at three levels of admission glucose (>110, >150, and >200). They found that only glucose levels greater than 200 mg/dL were associated with higher mortality and infection rates, leading to the conclusion that glucose levels should be maintained below 200 mg/dL but potentially not to the level of less than 110 mg/dL. Vogelzang and colleagues [16,17] defined the hyperglycemic index and applied it in a retrospective evaluation of 6099 surgical patients. Hyperglycemic index was developed by these investigators as a way of reflecting the magnitude of hyperglycemia in critically ill patients over time. Various surgical patients were evaluated in the study to include vascular, gastrointestinal, liver transplant, trauma, and other miscellaneous surgical patients. Their results demonstrated the relationship between hyperglycemia and mortality depended on the reason for admission. Trauma patients with hyperglycemia had a more pronounced mortality than for any other type of critically ill surgical patients. When comparing the trauma subgroup, trauma nonsurvivors had a statistically higher glucose level that was persistently elevated throughout the ICU stay compared with trauma survivors.

Bochicchio and colleagues [18] examined the effect of persistent hyperglycemia on critically ill trauma patients over the first week of admission. Patients were stratified based on glucose levels from Days 1 to 7 into low (0–139 mg/dL), medium (140–219 mg/dL), and high ($\geq$220 mg/dL) groups. Patients were further stratified by glucose control pattern (all low, all moderate, all high, improving, worsening, and highly variable). There was no standardized protocol for glucose management with management being left at the discretion of the treating physicians. All patients that had patterns of glucose control versus the low group demonstrated a statistically significant higher odds ratio for mortality when adjusted for age and ISS. The worsening and highly variable glucose control groups were the most predictive for increased mortality and infectious morbidity suggesting persistently elevated or increasing stress hormone activity in these patients.

Treatment of hyperglycemia in critically ill patients

Defining appropriate treatment of SIH remains an area of ongoing investigation. Van den Berghe and colleagues [19] prospective randomized controlled study examining intensive insulin therapy in surgical ICU patients was provocative and has led to additional studies designed to duplicate and validate their findings. The original study enrolled 1548 patients consisting of primarily surgical patients, most of whom had undergone some form of cardiac surgery. Those patients were randomized to either an intensive insulin therapy regimen (maintenance of glucose levels between 80 and 110 mg/dL) or a conventional regimen (infusion of insulin only if the blood glucose exceeded 215 mg/dL with maintenance of glucose levels between 180 and 200 mg/dL). Intensive therapy resulted in a reduction of mortality from 8.6% to 4% (reduction of 34%) and a reduction in overall morbidity. A subsequent study by Van den Berghe and colleagues [20] in medical ICU patients showed no improvement in overall mortality using the same protocol for glucose control as the original study. However, issues with the safety of tight glycemic control have been generated because profound hypoglycemia, defined as blood glucose less than 40 mg/dL, was identified as an independent risk factor for death in the latter study. Following this, several studies and meta-analyses were performed that had mixed results. However, although not widely adopted, several professional organizations supported and recommended tight glucose control (TGC) regimens to treat hyperglycemia [21].

The prospective, randomized controlled NICE-SUGAR study was subsequently performed to further delineate the optimal target range for blood glucose level in critically ill patients [22]. This study evaluated a mix of surgical and medical ICU patients and had death from any cause up to 90 days after randomization as its primary outcome. Patients were randomized to receive either intensive glucose control (target blood glucose range, 81–108 mg/dL) or conventional control (blood glucose $\leq$180 mg/dL). The results from this trial showed mortality was higher in the intensive arm than in the conventional glucose control arm. Based on their results, the authors suggested abandoning the lower target of glycemic control. However, the NICE-SUGAR study contained a mix of medical and surgical patients. Subsequent studies have suggested that certain subgroups of patients may have benefitted from tighter glucose control. Griesdale and colleagues [23] conducted a meta-analysis of randomized published studies (NICE-SUGAR included) examining the affect of tight glycemic control versus more conventional glucose management in ICU patients. To be included, the trials had to contain mortality data. The results demonstrated that patients in medical ICUs or mixed ICUs received no benefit in mortality in the tight glycemic control arm compared with a conventional control arm, whereas the surgical ICU subgroup, which included trauma patients, seemed to benefit from TGC (Table 2).

Treatment of hyperglycemia in trauma patients

Studies focusing strictly on trauma patients have been performed. However, to date no prospective randomized studies have been completed solely evaluating this patient population. Most of the current data evaluating the effects of treatment of hyperglycemia on outcomes in trauma use historical controls to compare eras before and after implementation of a protocol aimed at hyperglycemic control. For example, Scalea and colleagues [24] evaluated outcomes before and after the implementation of a TGC regimen and showed improved outcomes. They studied patients during the first week of ICU admission and compared the preintervention 24-month period (no TGC) with the 24-month period after institution of the TGC protocol. The protocol goal was to maintain blood glucose between 100 and 150 mg/dL, as opposed to the 80 to 110 mg/dL originally suggested by Van den Berghe [19]. When controlling for ISS, age,

Table 2
Risk ratios of mortality in clinical trials comparing IIT with conventional glycemic control in surgical patients

	Number of Deaths/Total Number of Patients		
Study	IIT	Control	Risk Ratio (95% CI)
Van den Berghe et al [19]	55/765	85/783	0.66 (0.48–0.92)
Grey et al [35]	4/34	6/27	0.53 (0.17–1.69)
Bilotta et al [36]	6/40	7/38	0.81 (0.30–2.20)
He et al [37]	7/150	6/38	0.30 (0.11–0.83)
Bilotta et al [38]	5/48	6/49	0.85 (0.28–2.60)
All surgical ICU patients	77/1037	110/935	0.63 (0.44–0.91)

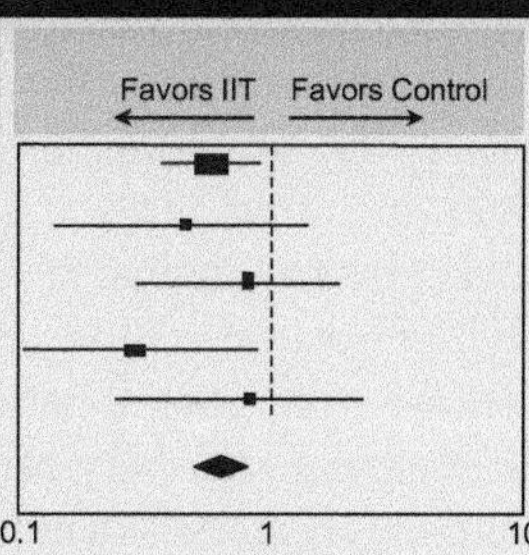

Abbreviations: CI, confidence interval; ICU, intensive care unit; IIT, intensive insulin therapy.

Adapted from Griesdale DE, de Souza RJ, van Dam RM, et al. Intensive insulin therapy and mortality among critically ill patients: a meta-analysis including NICE-SUGAR study data. CMAJ 2009;180(8):821–7.

and gender, patients with TGC experienced better outcomes in terms of morbidity, length of stay, and mortality.

These results, however, have not been duplicated in other trauma studies. Wahl and colleagues [25] evaluated results in their population of critically ill trauma patients before and after implementation of a stricter glucose control regimen. In their study, the targeted glucose level was less than 140 mg/dL. Although they showed that mean glucose levels were lower and the percentage of patients with all daily values less than the target was higher, mortality, hospital, and ICU length of stay and ventilator days did not differ between the eras compared. The incidence of severe hypoglycemia (glucose <40 mg/dL) was low and not statistically different between the two treatment approaches. Toschlog and colleagues [26] retrospectively looked at a 6-month period before and after implementation of a computerized hospital insulin protocol (CHIP) to maintain euglycemia. They evaluated glycemic control and outcome on trauma patients admitted to their ICU during this period. They demonstrated that the pre-CHIP group had a mean glucose of 130 $\pm$ 45 versus 116 $\pm$ 39 mg/dL after institution of the protocol. This modest lowering of mean glucose level was statistically significant. However, although infectious morbidity and length of stay improved in the post-CHIP group, mortality actually worsened. More recently, Kutcher and colleagues [27] reported on outcomes associated with three nonoverlapping approaches to glucose control over a 9-year period. During this time, their approach to glucose control evolved from "relaxed" (targeted blood glucose <180 mg/dL), to "aggressive" (targeted blood glucose range between 80 and 120 mg/dL), and finally to "moderate" (targeted blood glucose range of 80–140 mg/dL with institution at blood glucose $\geq$160 mg/dL). The results of their analysis revealed no difference in the incidence of multiorgan failure or mortality among the three groups.

DOES THE CAUSE OF HYPERGLYCEMIA MATTER?

The physiologic state associated with SIH is much different than that of DH, a chronic process associated with elevated glucose levels over time. This prolonged hyperglycemia subsequently leads to microvascular changes that result in diabetic disease manifestations (eg, coronary artery disease, nephropathy, and peripheral vascular disease) leading to morbidity and mortality. Because DH is the stimulus that causes the disease manifestations, effective treatment over the long term improves outcomes in these patients. In patients with DH, chronic exposure to elevated glucose levels may have led to adaptive changes at the cellular level aimed at abrogating the toxic effects of elevated glucose over time. Therefore, therapies aimed at lowering blood glucose levels in these patients may not be as beneficial. In contrast, SIH is an acute process initiated by stress hormone and cytokine release secondary to tissue damage. In this situation, because identification and initiation of treatment of hyperglycemia happen relatively soon after the initial insult, the time window for benefit of glycemic control to avoid acute glucose toxicity may not have passed. This potential differential effect may explain the disparity in results when examining tight glycemic control regimens in the surgical versus the medical ICUs [19,20]. In summary, the mechanism for potential negative impact in these two hyperglycemia states differs and their impact on outcomes after trauma likewise may not be the same.

Whether the underlying physiologic cause of the hyperglycemia, or simply the glucose level itself regardless of mechanism, has more of an impact on outcomes has not been extensively studied. Delineating whether the glucose elevation is a response to stress, secondary to poorly controlled or occult diabetes, or a mixture of both is difficult to ascertain. Most trauma studies evaluating glucose control exclude diabetic patients or make no attempt to identify patients with occult diabetes. This makes interpretation of the results of these studies difficult because the source of the hyperglycemia may determine whether a treatment regimen aimed at controlling glucose levels has an effect on outcome. This is significant given the large number of patients who present with occult diabetes. Approximately 8.3% of the United States population (25.8 million people) has diabetes, whether previously diagnosed or undiagnosed based on data from the National Center for Chronic Disease Prevention and Health Promotion of the Centers for Disease Control and Prevention [28]. It has been estimated that upward of 25% of all patients suffering from diabetes have no knowledge of their disease and thus have occult diabetes mellitus (ODM). Fortunately, new standards for the diagnosis of diabetes make it relatively easy to identify trauma patients who present with ODM. Diabetes can be diagnosed by several laboratory studies (Box 1). However, the American

Box 1: Criteria for diagnosis of diabetes

HbA_{1c} ≥6.5%: The test should be performed in a laboratory using a method that is certified by the National Glycohemoglobin Standardization Program and standardized to the Diabetes Control and Complications Trial assay[a]

or

Fasting plasma glucose ≥126 mg/dL (7 mmol/L): Fasting is defined as no caloric intake for at least 8 h[a]

or

2-h plasma glucose ≥200 mg/dL (11.1) mmol/L during an oral glucose tolerance test: The test should be performed as described by the World Health Organization, using a glucose load containing the equivalent of 75 g anhydrous glucose dissolved in water[a]

or

In a patient with classic symptoms of hyperglycemia or hyperglycemic crisis, a random plasma glucose ≥200 mg/dL (11.1 mmol/L)

[a] In the absence of unequivocal hyperglycemia, criteria 1 to 3 should be confirmed by repeat testing.

Data from American Diabetes Association. Diagnosis and classification of diabetes mellitus. Diabetes Care 2012;35(S1):8.

Diabetes Association has recently stated in its 2012 position paper that a glycosylated hemoglobin A_{1C} (HbA_{1c}) level greater than or equal to 6.5% is diagnostic for DM regardless of whether or not a history of hyperglycemia is present [29]. HbA_{1c} reflects average blood glucose levels over a 2- to 3-month period of time and is a widely used marker of chronic glycemic states.

In the trauma literature, only two studies have evaluated the true incidence of pre-existing diabetes in acutely injured patients. Kopelman and colleagues [4] prospectively evaluated trauma patients with no history of DM that presented with elevated glucose levels ($\geq$110 mg/dL) to find that nearly one-quarter of these patients had ODM. These studies are consistent with Centers for Disease Control and Prevention estimates of overall incidence of diabetes in the US population and rate of ODM in the diabetic population. Kerby and colleagues [3] retrospectively evaluated 5117 trauma patients admitted to a level 1 trauma center over a 2-year period to further define hyperglycemic populations and compare the impact of SIH versus DH on outcomes in trauma patients. HbA_{1c} levels were ascertained in addition to admission glucose and comorbidity data. In this study, approximately 8.7% of the study population (446 patients) was diagnosed with DM, of which nearly 25% (137 patients) had no prior history of DM and were newly diagnosed using HbA_{1c} values. When comparing patients with isolated SIH with those with DH (patients with hyperglycemia with known diabetes or ODM), the results showed that patients with SIH, and not those with DH, had higher mortality after trauma. This study suggests that hyperglycemia has a separate and more severe effect on mortality outcome in nondiabetic, stressed patients compared with those with hyperglycemia of diabetes. This is true even for patients who present in severe shock (defined as presenting base deficit $\geq$6). Given these results along with the underlying differences in these patient populations as outlined previously, the authors theorized that more strict glucose control protocols would most likely benefit patients with SIH as opposed to those with DH.

FUTURE DIRECTIONS

There have been no definitive prospective, randomized controlled trials evaluating glucose control regimens focused entirely on the trauma population. A properly designed, multi-institutional study of this nature will greatly add to the existing literature and clarify whether more stringent glucose control regimens lead to improved outcomes in trauma patients. Given the high prevalence of ODM in the population, these studies will preferably include prospective evaluations of stress hormones, cytokine levels, and HbA_{1c} levels to aid in determining those presenting with true SIH versus DH. The study should also be designed to either exclude patients with DH from randomization or perform an a priori subgroup analysis on patients only with true SIH. Uniform protocols for glucose monitoring that provide reasonably efficient time to glycemic control while minimizing severe hypoglycemic episodes will also be vital to any prospective evaluation. Several papers outlining various forms of CHIPs have shown them to shorten the time interval to glycemic control while reducing the frequency of hypoglycemic episodes [26,30–32]. A commercially available product is also available with proved efficacy in surgical ICUs [33,34].

SUMMARY

There is an established association between the presence of SIH and worse morbidity and mortality after trauma. However, given the limitations of existing data, no definitive statements can be made as to whether aggressive treatment of hyperglycemia actually benefits outcome. Although early studies seemed to show a clear benefit in surgical ICU patients, subsequent studies have not duplicated these results. In addition, severe hypoglycemic episodes associated with glycemic control protocols have provided further concern, because they have been associated with higher rates of mortality. These disparate outcomes in prospective, randomized trials have not allowed definitive conclusions to be drawn regarding the exact glucose levels that should be maintained. Regardless, some postinjury control of glucose levels is likely necessary. Without data to support the practice, tight glycemic control keeping glucose levels below 110 mg/dL is likely not necessary and probably detrimental to patient outcome. It seems that a more moderate level of glycemic control, aimed at providing stabilization of glucose levels while reducing hyperglycemic and hypoglycemic events, is being practiced in most institutions. Performance of prospective, randomized trials in the trauma population along with further advancement and refinement of techniques to more precisely reduce glucose variability will further clarify the level of glucose control associated with improved outcomes.

References

[1] McCowen KC, Malhotra A, Bistrian BR. Stress-induced hyperglycemia. Crit Care Clin 2001;17(1):107–24.

[2] Epstein J, Breslow MJ. The stress response of critical illness. Crit Care Clin 1999;15(1): 17–33, v.

[3] Kerby JD, Griffin RL, MacLennan P, et al. Stress-induced hyperglycemia, not diabetic hyperglycemia, is associated with higher mortality in trauma. Ann Surg 2012;256(3):446–52.

[4] Kopelman TR, O'Neill PJ, Kanneganti SR, et al. The relationship of plasma glucose and glycosylated hemoglobin A1C levels among nondiabetic trauma patients. J Trauma 2008;64(1):30–3 [discussion: 33–4].

[5] Bellodi G, Manicardi V, Malavasi V, et al. Hyperglycemia and prognosis of acute myocardial infarction in patients without diabetes mellitus. Am J Cardiol 1989;64(14):885–8.

[6] Capes SE, Hunt D, Malmberg K, et al. Stress hyperglycaemia and increased risk of death after myocardial infarction in patients with and without diabetes: a systematic overview. Lancet 2000;355(9206):773–8.

[7] Kosiborod M, Rathore SS, Inzucchi SE, et al. Admission glucose and mortality in elderly patients hospitalized with acute myocardial infarction: implications for patients with and without recognized diabetes. Circulation 2005;111(23):3078–86.

[8] Capes SE, Hunt D, Malmberg K, et al. Stress hyperglycemia and prognosis of stroke in nondiabetic and diabetic patients: a systematic overview. Stroke 2001;32(10):2426–32.

[9] Bruno A, Levine SR, Frankel MR, et al. Admission glucose level and clinical outcomes in the NINDS rt-PA Stroke Trial. Neurology 2002;59(5):669–74.

[10] Yendamuri S, Fulda GJ, Tinkoff GH. Admission hyperglycemia as a prognostic indicator in trauma. J Trauma 2003;55(1):33–8.

[11] Sung J, Bochicchio GV, Joshi M, et al. Admission hyperglycemia is predictive of outcome in critically ill trauma patients. J Trauma 2005;59(1):80–3.
[12] Laird AM, Miller PR, Kilgo PD, et al. Relationship of early hyperglycemia to mortality in trauma patients. J Trauma 2004;56(5):1058–62.
[13] Van den Berghe G. How does blood glucose control with insulin save lives in intensive care? J Clin Invest 2004;114(9):1187–95.
[14] Langouche L, Vanhorebeek I, Vlasselaers D, et al. Intensive insulin therapy protects the endothelium of critically ill patients. J Clin Invest 2005;115(8):2277–86.
[15] Vanhorebeek I, De Vos R, Mesotten D, et al. Protection of hepatocyte mitochondrial ultrastructure and function by strict blood glucose control with insulin in critically ill patients. Lancet 2005;365(9453):53–9.
[16] Vogelzang M, van der Horst IC, Nijsten MW. Hyperglycaemic index as a tool to assess glucose control: a retrospective study. Crit Care 2004;8(3):R122–7.
[17] Vogelzang M, Nijboer JM, van der Horst IC, et al. Hyperglycemia has a stronger relation with outcome in trauma patients than in other critically ill patients. J Trauma 2006;60(4): 873–7 [discussion: 878–9].
[18] Bochicchio GV, Sung J, Joshi M, et al. Persistent hyperglycemia is predictive of outcome in critically ill trauma patients. J Trauma 2005;58(5):921–4.
[19] van den Berghe G, Wouters P, Weekers F, et al. Intensive insulin therapy in critically ill patients. N Engl J Med 2001;345(19):1359–67.
[20] Van den Berghe G, Wilmer A, Hermans G, et al. Intensive insulin therapy in the medical ICU. N Engl J Med 2006;354(5):449–61.
[21] Garber AJ, Moghissi ES, Bransome ED, et al. American College of Endocrinology position statement on inpatient diabetes and metabolic control. Endocr Pract 2004;10(Suppl 2):4–9.
[22] Finfer S, Chittock DR, Su SY, et al. Intensive versus conventional glucose control in critically ill patients. N Engl J Med 2009;360(13):1283–97.
[23] Griesdale DE, de Souza RJ, van Dam RM, et al. Intensive insulin therapy and mortality among critically ill patients: a meta-analysis including NICE-SUGAR study data. CMAJ 2009;180(8):821–7.
[24] Scalea TM, Bochicchio GV, Bochicchio KM, et al. Tight glycemic control in critically injured trauma patients. Ann Surg 2007;246(4):605–10 [discussion: 610–2].
[25] Wahl WL, Taddonio M, Maggio PM, et al. Mean glucose values predict trauma patient mortality. J Trauma 2008;65(1):42–7 [discussion: 47–8].
[26] Toschlog EA, Newton C, Allen N, et al. Morbidity reduction in critically ill trauma patients through use of a computerized insulin infusion protocol: a preliminary study. J Trauma 2007;62(6):1370–5 [discussion: 1375–6].
[27] Kutcher ME, Pepper MB, Morabito D, et al. Finding the sweet spot: identification of optimal glucose levels in critically injured patients. J Trauma 2011;71(5):1108–14.
[28] National Diabetes Fact Sheet. Centers for Disease Control and Prevention 2011. Available at: www.cdc.gov/diabetes/pubs/pdf/ndfs_2011.pdf. Accessed January 9, 2013.
[29] American Diabetes Association. Diagnosis and classification of diabetes mellitus. Diabetes Care 2012;35(Suppl 1):8.
[30] Vogelzang M, Zijlstra F, Nijsten MW. Design and implementation of GRIP: a computerized glucose control system at a surgical intensive care unit. BMC Med Inform Decis Mak 2005;5:38.
[31] Dortch MJ, Mowery NT, Ozdas A, et al. A computerized insulin infusion titration protocol improves glucose control with less hypoglycemia compared to a manual titration protocol in a trauma intensive care unit. JPEN J Parenter Enteral Nutr 2008;32(1):18–27.
[32] Sood R, Zieger M, Roggy D, et al. The effectiveness of a computerized IV infusion protocol to treat hyperglycemia in burn patients. J Burn Care Res 2012;33(5):638–41.
[33] Saager L, Collins GL, Burnside B, et al. A randomized study in diabetic patients undergoing cardiac surgery comparing computer-guided glucose management with a standard sliding scale protocol. J Cardiothorac Vasc Anesth 2008;22(3):377–82.

[34] Fogel SL, Baker CC. Effects of computerized decision-support systems on blood glucose regulation in critically ill surgical patients. J Am Coll Surg 2013;216(4):828–33.
[35] Grey NJ, Perdrizet GA. Reduction of nosocomial infections in the surgical intensive-care unit by strict glycemic control. Endocr Pract 2004;10(Suppl 2):46–52.
[36] Bilotta F, Spinelli A, Giovannini F, et al. The effect of intensive insulin therapy on infection rate, vasospasm, neurologic outcome, and mortality in neurointensive care unit after intracranial aneurysm clipping in patients with acute subarachnoid hemorrhage: a randomized prospective pilot trial. J Neurosurg Anesthesiol 2007;19(3):156–60.
[37] He W, Zhang TY, Zhou H, et al. Impact of intensive insulin therapy on surgical critically ill patients. Zhonghua Wai Ke Za Zhi 2007;45(15):1052–4.
[38] Bilotta F, Caramia R, Cernak I, et al. Intensive insulin therapy after severe traumatic brain injury: a randomized clinical trial. Neurocrit Care 2008;9(2):159–66.

Advances in Surgery 47 (2013) 299–328

ADVANCES IN SURGERY

Improvement in the Diagnosis of Appendicitis

Frederick Thurston Drake, MD, MPH[a,b,*],
David Reed Flum, MD, MPH[a,b]

[a]Department of Surgery, University of Washington, 1959 NE Pacific Street, Box 356410, Seattle, WA 98195, USA; [b]Surgical Outcomes Research Center (SORCE), Department of Surgery, University of Washington, 1107 NE 45th Street, Suite 502, Seattle, WA 98105, USA

Keywords

• Appendicitis • Diagnosis • Advanced imaging • Negative appendectomy

Key points

- Although acute appendicitis is often straightforward to diagnose, clinical evaluation is susceptible to conditions that mimic the signs and symptoms of appendicitis.
- Diagnosis of appendicitis has improved over the last 25 years through the use of such strategies as clinical scoring systems, laboratory studies, diagnostic laparoscopy, and advanced imaging studies (US, CT, and MRI).
- Which strategy, or combination of strategies, clinicians choose to employ depends on practice setting, resource availability, patient population, and clinical goals.

EVIDENCE FOR IMPROVEMENT

For more than a hundred years, the diagnosis of acute appendicitis has been based on history taking, physical examination findings, and, to a lesser extent, laboratory results [1]. For experienced clinicians, an accurate diagnosis is straightforward in most patients, yet misdiagnosis stubbornly persists. There are 3 principal scenarios in which misdiagnosis occurs, and a speculative fourth:

1. appendicitis is diagnosed, the patient undergoes an operation, and non-appendiceal disease is discovered, which may or may not benefit from surgical intervention (eg, gynecologic lesions or inflammatory bowel disease of the terminal ileum); in this setting, the appendix may or may not be removed;
2. appendicitis is diagnosed, the patient undergoes an operation, and no abnormality is found; again, the appendix may or may not be removed;

*Corresponding author. *E-mail address*: ftdrake@u.washington.edu

0065-3411/13/$ – see front matter
http://dx.doi.org/10.1016/j.yasu.2013.03.003

3. appendicitis is not diagnosed but the patient does have an inflamed appendix (this would most often manifest as a patient who returned with persistent or recurrent appendicitis or with a perforation or other complication such as an abscess);
4. appendicitis is diagnosed that would have spontaneously resolved and is therefore clinically irrelevant (it has been suggested that increasing use of sensitive imaging such as computed tomography [CT] can detect mild inflammation of the appendix, which would otherwise resolve without antibiotics or surgical intervention) [2–4].

The first 2 forms of misdiagnosis, collectively referred to as negative appendectomy (NA) when the appendix is removed, are especially important to researchers interested in quality improvement, because they occur at the intersection of historical practice patterns that favor sensitivity over specificity and because appendicitis, straightforward to diagnose in most, is also closely mimicked by other pelvic diseases, particularly in reproductive-aged women. The third form of misdiagnosis (missed cases of appendicitis) is undoubtedly important, but its clinical significance is complicated to define: some cases may resolve without therapy; some early cases may progress over a period of observation, allowing for detection on repeat evaluation (but without adverse impact on patients' outcomes); or, in some instances, patients with missed diagnoses may progress to perforation and re-present with complicated appendicitis. Concern for the third scenario tended to drive clinical practice toward the first 2 forms of misdiagnosis: a high number of negative explorations for suspected appendicitis were tolerated as surgeons endeavored to miss no cases, thereby averting perforation. This strategy is exemplified by Cantrell and Stafford's 1955 admonition that

> every effort should be made to establish an exact diagnosis. If, however, this is impossible and a suspicion of appendicitis exists, exploration is mandatory. ... It is far better to subject a moderate number of patients to a theoretically unnecessary operation than to let one patient suffer perforation [5].

Based on these beliefs, frequency of NA as high as 15% to 25% was common in surgical practice until recently. A nearly 50% NA rate was considered acceptable among pregnant women given the risks of perforation during pregnancy [6–9].

However, in the 1990s, investigators began to publish the results of studies in which CT scanning was used in the evaluation of suspected appendicitis. Rao and his colleagues in Boston focused their investigations specifically on the safe reduction of NA. Although multiple follow-up studies showed that CT for appendicitis was accurate and reliable, reducing NA was not without controversy: many surgeons still feared that attempts to reduce NA would lead to an increase in the frequency of perforation [10]. As CT became nearly ubiquitous in appendicitis, the perception persisted that it was overhyped and overused: 74% of the respondents to a large survey of the American College of Surgeons

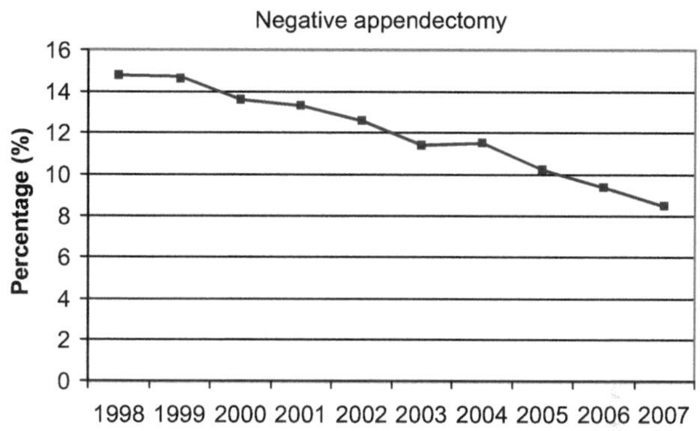

Fig. 1. Decrease in negative appendectomies (1998–2007). (*Reprinted from* Seetahal SA, Bolorunduro OB, Sookdeo TC, et al. Negative appendectomy: a 10-year review of a nationally representative sample. Am J Surg 2011;201(4):435; with permission.)

believed that the accuracy of CT scans was less than that reported in the literature and 62% believed that CT was overused in the workup for suspected appendicitis [11]. Some early reports suggested that advanced imaging was not influential in reducing NA [8,12–15]. However, evidence began to accumulate that the frequency of NA was steadily decreasing (Fig. 1) and that this relationship was associated with increased use of advanced diagnostic imaging. Moreover, these studies found no associated increase in the frequency of perforation (Fig. 2) [16–22]. There is now clear evidence that previously

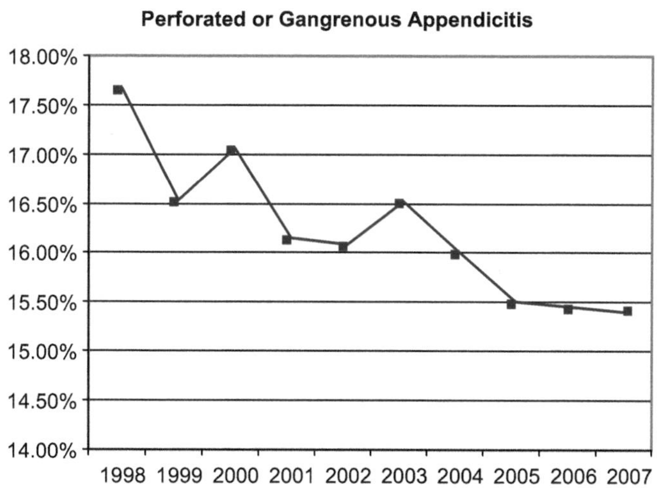

Fig. 2. Incidence of perforated or gangrenous appendicitis (1998–2007). (*Reprinted from* Seetahal SA, Bolorunduro OB, Sookdeo TC, et al. Negative appendectomy: a 10-year review of a nationally representative sample. Am J Surg 2011;201(4):436; with permission.)

common NA rates of 15% to 25% should no longer be considered acceptable. In our view, this new standard has been accomplished by integrating high-quality advanced radiographic imaging into diagnostic algorithms for suspected appendicitis.

The data behind this assertion are mostly drawn from retrospective investigations with study populations of patients who had appendectomies. In terms of causal inferences, studies with this design present some challenges: there may be uncontrolled biases in terms of why certain patients were imaged, or, in longitudinal studies over time, other changes in the diagnosis of appendicitis may have accounted for, or at least contributed to, the reductions seen in NA. All of these cautions notwithstanding, a multitude of studies over the past 25 years have evaluated the relationship between imaging and NA and have shown that the use of imaging is associated with a reduction in NA [7,16–20,22–41]. This association has not been universally shown, and there are several studies of appendectomy patients that have not found a relationship between imaging use and NA (Table 1) [8,12–15,42–46]. Several of these articles deserve mention. The 2001 article by Lee and colleagues [42], perhaps because of its unequivocal title, is frequently cited by those who argue against routine imaging in suspected appendicitis. The chief findings were that clinical examination and CT scan have equivalent sensitivity (83% vs 83.8%, respectively) and positive predictive value (PPV) (86.7% vs 83.8%) and that ultrasonography (US) performed inferiorly to both (sensitivity 35.5% and PPV 81.3%). However, these findings are limited because only 47 patients underwent CT in this group of 766 patients. Furthermore, their calculations of specificity and negative predictive value (NPV) are not reliable because such calculations cannot be based solely on patients who had an appendectomy; all patients undergoing a test are required for accurate computation of specificity and NPV.

Regarding the 2001 article by our group, the data presented were from 1987 to 1998 and showed no chronologic change in NA in Washington State, either as a percentage of all appendectomies performed (overall NA 15.5%) or as a population-based incidence. These data were based on diagnoses and procedure codes, and it was not possible to determine whether patients were being imaged more frequently (although it was clear that more imaging services were available), nor could comparisons be made between those who were and were not imaged. However, these data did clearly show, whether from lack of use or lack of effectiveness, that the purported benefits of advanced imaging were not being seen at the population level or across diverse hospital settings [8]. This population-based analysis was reinforced by a follow-up 2005 study in a large, statewide managed-health system (data from 1980–1999). The overall frequency of NA was also 15.5%, and there was no correlation between increasing use of CT and the relatively stable frequency of NA [15]. However, since these earlier studies, 2 recent analyses by our group using data abstracted directly from patient records have shown dramatic changes in the frequency of NA across Washington State: both studies demonstrated a clear reduction in NA, and both studies demonstrated a benefit for advanced imaging [22,36]. The

Table 1
Selected studies of NA from 1999 to 2012, including retrospective reviews, large database analyses, prospective observational studies, and randomized trials

Reference	Study design, population, and size	Findings
Rao et al [7], 1999	Retrospective review of pediatric and adult appendectomy patients. Patients from pre-CT era (n = 493) compared with those of CT era (n = 209). Only 59% of patients in CT era underwent CT scanning.	All patients: for pre-CT era, NA = 20%, and for CT era, NA = 7%. For female patients, 31% vs 11%, $P<.001$, for male patients, 10% vs 5%, $P = .057$, and for pediatric patients, 13% vs 7%, $P = .22$.
Walker et al [47], 2000	RCT of mandatory CT scan vs standard management in adults with suspected appendicitis (n = 108).	Mandatory CT scan: NA = 5%. Standard management: NA = 19%.
Applegate et al [26], 2001	Retrospective review of surgical database for appendectomy patients (age <21 y) at large children's hospital (n = 299).	Overall NA = 13%. For CT alone, NA = 2%, for US, NA = 17%, for CT with or without US, NA = 7% and for no imaging, NA = 14%.
Dilley et al [27], 2001	Retrospective review of pediatric appendectomy patients comparing those with and without US at a large children's hospital (n = 1007).	With US, NA = 15.6%; without US, NA = 18.3% ($P<.05$).
Flum et al [8], 2001	Retrospective cohort of appendectomy patients from a statewide discharge database (n = 85,790). No direct data on imaging use. NA determined by ICD-9 coding. 1987 to 1998.	Overall NA was 15.5% with no change seen over time. Among RA women, NA was 26.4%.
McDonald et al [12], 2001	Retrospective, before-and-after study of appendectomy patients (age ≥12 y) in selective CT era vs routine CT era (n = 226).	For selective CT era, NA = 15%, and for routine CT era, NA = 13% ($P = .7$). With CT, NA = 6.7% and without CT, NA = 16.9% ($P = .05$).
Wilson et al [48], 2001	Prospective, single-arm study. Adults and children with suspected appendicitis. Clinical decision made, then all patients had CT and US. Based on imaging results, original plan reevaluated (n = 99).	Overall: NA = 10%. For females, imaging reduced NA from potential 50%–17%. For males, NA = 8% and imaging did not change management.
Naoum et al [29], 2002	Retrospective chart review of adult appendectomy patients (n = 194). Comparison made before and after a guideline encouraging CT use.	CT scan use increased from 32% to 84%. NA before guideline = 25% and NA after guideline was 6%.

(continued on next page)

Table 1
(continued)

Reference	Study design, population, and size	Findings
DeArmond et al [32], 2003	Retrospective review of children and adult appendectomy patients. 1995 compared with 1998 (n = 778) Selective CT strategy in place over both periods.	1995: for CT, NA = 19% and for no CT, NA = 13% (P = NS). 1998: for CT, NA = 6% and for no CT, NA = 7% (P = NS).
Partrick et al [13], 2003	Retrospective review of pediatric appendectomy patients at a single large children's hospital (n = 616). Comparison made for CT, US, or no imaging. NA based on pathology report. 1997 to 2001.	CT used increased substantially and US use decreased substantially over the study period, but no trend in NA. For no imaging, NA = 8%, for CT, NA = 7% and for US, NA = 11%.
Perez et al [14], 2003	Retrospective review of children and adult appendectomy patients. 1994 (n = 100) compared with 1999–2000 (n = 118).	1994: NA = 12%; 1999–2000: NA = 17.8% (P = .32). They report a 4-fold increase in the use of CT scan.
Jones et al [16], 2004	Retrospective review of appendectomy patients, age 14–84 y (n = 389); time-based analysis of NA as CT use increased.	Progressive decrease in NA from 17% (2000) to 9% (2001) to 2% (2002). NA was 12% without CT and 7% with CT scan.
Kaiser et al [33], 2004	Retrospective review of consecutive pediatric appendectomy patients for 1991, 1994, 1997 and 2000. Large children's hospital (n = 600).	CT and US use increased steadily, and NA decreased: 23% (1991), 8.7% (1994), 8.0% (1997), and 4.0% (2000).
Lee et al [50], 2007	RCT of adult patients presenting with suspected appendicitis, randomized to mandatory or selective CT scan (n = 152).	Mandatory CT group, NA = 2.6% vs 13.9% in selective CT group. (P = NS).
Huynh et al [45], 2007	Retrospective chart review of appendicitis patients at a community hospital; adults and children, age 2 to 89 (n = 550).	For CT, NA = 11%. For no CT, NA = 13% (P = NS).
Morse et al [35], 2007	Retrospective chart review of appendectomy patients age >16 y (n = 439). Single institution.	For CT, NA = 9%; for no CT, NA = 24%. Among RA women: for CT, NA = 17% and for no CT, NA = 42%. Among men: for CT, NA = 5% and for no CT, NA = 15%.
Cuschieri et al [36], 2008	Review of multi-institution, prospectively collected data from consecutive appendectomy patients (children and adults) from 2006 to 2007 (n = 3540). NA defined by pathology report findings.	Overall NA = 5.6%. With no imaging, NA = 10%, with US, NA = 8%, and with CT, NA = 4.5%. Accuracy of imaging (based on pathology-radiology report concordance) correlated with frequency of NA.

Guss et al [37], 2008	Retrospective chart review of adult appendectomy patients. Single institution. Period A, 1990–1994 (n = 316) and Period B, 2001–2004 (n = 477).	Period A: 12% had nonhelical CT, NA = 15.5%. Period B: 82% had helical CT, NA = 7.9%.
Piper et al [38], 2008	Retrospective review of appendectomy patients (age 5–86 y) at 2 community hospitals (n = 134).	Overall NA = 9%. With imaging, NA = 3%, without imaging, NA = 10% (no *P* value reported).
Wagner et al [17], 2008	Retrospective review of appendectomy patients (pediatric and adult) at a university hospital (n = 1425); time-based methodology as well as comparison of those with and without CT.	In 2000, NA = 10.6% and in 2006, NA = 5.0%. With CT, NA = 7.2%. Without CT, NA = 14.0%. Major reduction in NA for women; less impact among men, pediatric patients.
Coursey et al [18], 2010	Retrospective chart review of adult appendectomy patients from 1998 to 2007 (n = 925). University hospital setting.	NA declined, 16.7%–8.7%. Large decrease for RA women (43% vs 7%) but not for men. CT use increased from 18.5% to 94.2%.
Raja et al [19], 2010	Retrospective chart review of adult appendectomy patients from 1990 to 1994 (n = 971) and 2003 to 2008 (n = 637). University hospital setting.	In 1990, NA = 23.0% and in 2007, NA = 1.7%. Large decrease in NA for both male and female patients. CT scan use increased from 1% in 1990 to 97.5% in 2007.
Seetahal et al [21], 2011	Retrospective review of adult appendectomy patients in the NIS from 1998 to 2007 (n = 475,651). Determination of NA based on ICD-9 coding. No data on imaging use available.	NA = 14.7% in 1998 and decreased steadily to 8.5%. Women accounted for most NA over entire period (71.3%).
Bachur et al [40], 2012	Retrospective evaluation of nationwide pediatric hospital database (PHIS). For calculation of NA, records obtained for appendectomy patients. Data from 2005 to 2009. (n = 52,426).	From 2005 to 2009, frequency of NA decreased significantly from 4.4% to 3.1%. No relationship between CT use and NA, but inverse relationship between US or US + CT use and frequency of NA.
Drake et al [22], 2012	Review of prospectively collected data on consecutive appendectomy patients (age ≥15 y) from 2006–2011 (n = 19,327). Multi-institution.	Overall: if imaged, NA = 4.5%, if not imaged, NA = 15.4%. RA women: if imaged, NA = 6.9%, if not imaged, NA = 24.7%. Males: if imaged, NA = 3%, if not imaged, NA = 10%.

Statistical significance may be assumed unless otherwise noted in the table.

Abbreviations: ICD-9, International Classification of Diseases, Ninth Revision; NIS, National Inpatient Sample; PHIS, Pediatric Health Information System; RA, reproductive age; RCT, randomized controlled trial.

statewide frequency of NA, estimated most recently for 2011, was 4.3%. Perhaps most striking were the reductions observed among reproductive-aged women. For these patients, the original 2001 study found that the average frequency of NA was 26.4% over the entire decade studied (1987–1998) [8]. This number decreased to 8.1% in the cohort of patients from 2006 to 2011, and large differences related to imaging use were evident: 24.7% of reproductive-aged women who did not receive advanced imaging underwent NA (essentially the same frequency of NA as in the 1990s) versus 6.9% of those women who did undergo imaging. After adjusting for age, white blood cell (WBC) count, and institution in a multivariate regression model, the odds of NA for reproductive-aged women without imaging were 3.5 times the odds of NA for those who were imaged [22].

Not all of the data on imaging and NA come from retrospective studies. We know of 6 studies published since 2000 that evaluated the relationship between imaging use and NA using prospective methodologies. In 3 of these studies, patients were randomized to a particular evaluation protocol [47–52]. All of these studies were strengthened by a design that focuses on patients suspected of having appendicitis, not retrospective evaluation of patients who underwent appendectomy.

In the most recent of these studies, 100 patients were evaluated by surgeons and assigned to a high, indeterminate, or low probability of having appendicitis. After allocation, CT scans were reviewed (if already ordered) or ordered if desired by the consulting surgeon. Seventy patients underwent appendectomy, and overall frequency of NA was 5.7%. Only 23 of the 63 highly suspicious patients had a CT scan, but in 2 of these patients, appendicitis was ruled out. Of the 27 indeterminate patients, 26 had CT scans; 11 were positive and 9 of these had appendicitis at appendectomy. Seven of the 10 patients in the low-suspicion group had CT, and 2 patients were found to have appendicitis. The investigators concluded that CT rarely changes management in patients highly suspicious for appendicitis (although it did assist surgeons in avoiding 2 unnecessary operations) but frequently changes management when the clinical diagnosis is less certain [52].

In 1 of the randomized investigations, 152 adult patients suspected of having appendicitis were randomized to a mandatory CT scan group or to a selective CT scan group, in which the emergency department (ED) physicians and consulting surgeons could order CT as dictated by their clinical certainty. The results were striking. CT scans were performed in 54 of 80 patients in the selective group and 70 of the 72 patients in the mandatory group. Frequency of NA in the mandatory group was 2.6% versus 13.9% in the selective group. The investigators did not find statistical significance in this difference (the article does not indicate which statistical tests were used to generate confidence intervals [CIs]), but they raised concern in their discussion for a type II error, noting that an 11% reduction in NA would certainly be clinically significant. The percentage of patients with appendicitis in each arm of the study was different (54.2% in the mandatory arm and 47.5% in the selective arm), and frequency of perforation differed as well (10.3% in the mandatory arm and 18.4% in the selective arm) [50]. Although these differences were not significant by the published CIs, perforation may have influenced diagnostic performance of clinical examination or CT. This finding likely represents insufficient sample size for adequate randomization, but may reflect the increased sensitivity of CT scan for mild appendicitis compared with clinical evaluation. (Some have argued, and the results of this study seem to support this argument, that routine CT scanning detects more cases of mild, possibly self-limiting cases of appendicitis, increasing the denominator in percentage calculations of perforation, which misleadingly reduces the number of perforations compared with populations in which CT scan is used less frequently and in which mild cases go undetected. For this reason, they argue that population-based incidences of perforation are a more reliable comparative metric [2–4,53]).

In another randomized study with a similar design and similar results, investigators found that NA was dramatically reduced by mandatory CT scanning (19% in the selective CT group vs 5% in the mandatory CT group) and that clinical management was altered in 26% of patients who underwent CT. In this study, CT scanning benefited both young men and reproductive-age women. Sensitivity of CT among patients in the mandatory CT arm was 94%, specificity was 100%, and accuracy was 96%. For those patients in the standard management arm (which could include US, observation, surgical exploration, or CT scan if requested by the consulting surgeon), sensitivity of standard management was 100%, but specificity was 67% and accuracy was 85% [47].

There is 1 randomized trial that did not show a benefit to the use of advanced imaging over clinical examination alone. In this 2003 study, adult patients were randomized to clinical evaluation alone versus clinical evaluation and CT scan. (Patients with an Alvarado score [see later discussion for detailed explanation of the Alvarado score] >8 were taken directly to the operating room (OR), but those with a score from 2 to 8 were randomized.) More than 20% of patients in both arms did not follow the study protocol, and there were substantially more men in the clinical evaluation arm than in the CT arm, a clear advantage for clinical examination. Frequency of NA is not reported, but the investigators found that accuracy was equivalent for the 2 evaluation protocols and concluded that routine CT was not useful in reducing misdiagnosis, even among patients with equivocal clinical findings [49]. Given the methodological weaknesses and the protocol violations of the study, this conclusion seems unwarranted.

A preponderance of observational and experimental data over the last 25 years support the assertion that NA has been reduced safely and without an associated increase in perforation; most studies find an association between reduced NA and the use of advanced imaging. Although most studies are based on observational data, the randomized trials highlighted suggest that the associations found in observational studies represent causal relationships. The experience in Washington State is instructive: in 2006, the Surgical Care and

Outcomes Assessment Program (SCOAP), a statewide, voluntary collaboration of surgeons and hospitals, made a commitment to safely reduce NA among its member hospitals. The strategy for this reduction was a commitment to the routine use of high-quality, benchmarked imaging before appendectomy, especially for reproductive-aged women. (In SCOAP, "benchmark" means a performance standard that is based on the outcome and process results achieved by high-performing member institutions. When quarterly, de-identified reports are issued, member hospitals can measure and monitor their own performance relative to their peers). As the use of imaging increased over the subsequent 6 years, we observed a significant decline in the number of NA, with no change in the frequency of perforation (Fig. 3) [22]. Given earlier findings that implicated suboptimal accuracy of imaging in the persistent levels of NA [15,36], SCOAP began to monitor and benchmark diagnostic performance of imaging among member hospitals. Observational data cannot prove causality, but given the temporal relationship, the size of the association, and the numerous additional studies with similar findings (including some randomized trials), we believe that there is strong evidence to support SCOAP's emphasis on high-quality imaging and that this emphasis has driven much of the observed decline in unnecessary operations.

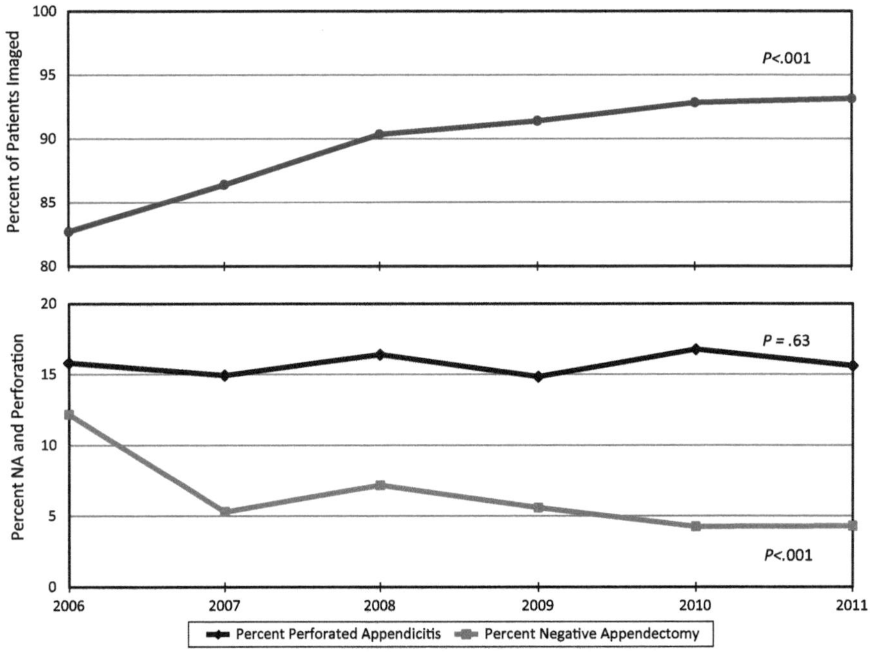

Fig. 3. Frequency of imaging use, NA, and perforation in SCOAP hospitals, 2006–2011. Use of imaging, NA, and perforation are expressed as annual percentages. The Cochran-Armitage test was used to evaluate for trends over time.

STRATEGIES FOR IMPROVEMENT

There are numerous tools that clinicians may use in evaluating patients with suspected appendicitis. How these tools are combined into practice depends heavily on the setting, resource availability, and clinical goals. For instance, in rural Kenya, accurate clinical assessment remains the cornerstone of diagnosis for everyone. In Washington State, diagnostic goals may vary depending on the patient: for children, minimizing exposure to ionizing radiation may mitigate the desire for superior diagnostic information; for women age 18 to 35 years, accurately ruling out nonappendiceal disease may be a priority; for elderly patients, in whom radiation is less of a risk, the clarity and amount of information provided by CT scan may warrant its routine use. Although we advocate for the routine use of advanced imaging in our setting, because we know that this reduces misdiagnosis and unnecessary operations, in other settings and other populations, alternate strategies may be warranted. Clinicians can use the information presented below and in Tables 1–4 to formulate their own best practices. In addition to detailing some of the history of research into the diagnosis of appendicitis, the tables present diverse study designs, settings, and populations, which may be applicable to a variety of clinical scenarios.

Clinical evaluation

Surgical textbooks describe a classic presentation of appendicitis in which an initially diffuse or periumbilical abdominal pain migrates to the right iliac fossa. Symptoms frequently include nausea, vomiting, anorexia, and, less consistently, a history of fevers or chills. Examination findings include tenderness over McBurney's point (especially rebound tenderness), Rovsing sign (pain in the right lower quadrant (RLQ) when the left lower quadrant is palpated), and the psoas sign (an exacerbation of pain in the RLQ with flexion or extension of the right hip joint), all of which indicate focal peritoneal irritation. Expected laboratory findings include a leukocytosis with a left shift and an increased C-reactive protein (CRP) level [54–56].

Several clinical scoring systems have been proposed to facilitate the accurate clinical diagnosis of appendicitis. The most well-known of these is the Alvarado score (Box 1) [57]. Introduced in 1986, the score is based on 3 symptoms, 3 signs, and 2 laboratory findings. Each of these factors equals 1 point except for tenderness in the RLQ and leukocytosis, both of which earn 2 points. Alvarado recommended taking patients to surgery for a score of 7 or greater.

Since publication of the Alvarado score, several investigators have attempted to quantify the diagnostic accuracy of clinical evaluation as well as the individual prognostic value of various signs, symptoms, and laboratory results. One study of 766 adult and pediatric appendectomy patients found that clinical assessment was overall 75% accurate in detecting and ruling out appendicitis; sensitivity was estimated at 83% and PPV 86.7%. (As noted earlier, this study is limited in that patients who were not taken to the OR were not included in the calculations of diagnostic performance.) Individual findings identified as

Table 2
Selected studies evaluating diagnostic performance of US, from 1994 to 2009

Reference	Study design	N	Sensitivity (%)	Specificity (%)
Balthazar et al [60], 1994	Prospective. Consecutive patients, age 15–82 y, with "suggestive but not typical clinical and laboratory findings of appendicitis" evaluated by both CT and US. Clinical follow-up for nonsurgical patients.	100	76	91
Horton et al [25], 2000	Prospective. Patients, age 18–65 y, with possible appendicitis but missing 1 or more classic clinical findings. Subjects randomized to CT or US. No description of follow-up protocol for nonsurgical patients.	40 (US)	76	90
Dilley et al [27], 2001	Retrospective review of all rule-out appendicitis US cross-referenced to surgical and pathology reports. Pediatric patients. Study includes repeat US. No description of follow-up protocol for nonsurgical patients.	2056	89[a] 93[b]	95[a] 95[b]
Lowe et al [89], 2001	Retrospective. Consecutive children with suspected appendicitis underwent CT and compared with a historical cohort of consecutive children who underwent US. 12 children with negative imaging studies lost to follow-up and excluded.	78 (US)	100	88
Rettenbacher et al [66], 2002	Prospective. Patients, age 5–92 y, with suspected appendicitis. All underwent US. Clinical follow-up for nonsurgical patients.	350	98[c] 97[d]	98[c] 100[d]
Poortman et al [64], 2003	Prospective. Adult and pediatric patients with suspected appendicitis. Subjects underwent both US and CT. For nonsurgical patients median follow-up was 13 mo.	226	79	78

Kessler et al [68], 2004	Prospective. Patients, age 15–83 y, with suspected appendicitis. Follow-up in nonsurgical patients was chart review and telephone call at least 6 mo from discharge. Specific US findings were evaluated for diagnostic performance. Appendiceal diameter ≥6 mm was most sensitive and specific finding for appendicitis; sensitivity and specificity for this finding reported here.	125	98	98
Keyzer et al [62], 2005	Prospective. Patients, age 16–81 y, referred for CT for suspected appendicitis; all patients underwent both CT and US. Follow-up obtained from medical record and telephone call at 1 mo.	94	77	87
Doria et al [61], 2006	Meta-analysis (adults): study design described in text.	N/A	83[e]	93[e]
Doria et al [61], 2006	Meta-analysis (children): study design described in text.	N/A	88[f]	94[f]
Gaitini et al [65], 2008	Retrospective. Adult patients with suspected appendicitis. 132 patients also underwent CT. Clinical follow-up (inpatient only) for nonsurgical patients; indeterminate results excluded from analysis (n = 17).	420	74	97
Poortman et al [63], 2009	Prospective. Adult patients with symptoms of appendicitis underwent US followed by CT for negative or indeterminate US. Clinical follow-up and inpatient observation for nonsurgical patients.	151 (US)	77	86

In the Dilley article, sensitivity and specificity were calculated for all (initial and repeat) US examinations performed during the study[a] and recalculated[b] based only on final US findings (ie, the initial US if the findings were conclusive, or the definitive US in those patients who had multiple studies). In the study by Rettenbacher and colleagues, sensitivity and specificity were calculated for appendicitis[c] and for appendicitis + alternative diagnosis.[d] Doria and colleagues calculated 95% CIs for their performance metrics: [e]sensitivity 95% CI 78%–87%, specificity 95% CI 90%–96%, [f]sensitivity 95% CI 86%–90%, specificity 95% CI 92%–95%.

Abbreviation: N/A, not applicable.

Table 3
Selected studies evaluating diagnostic performance of CT, from 1991 to 2011

Reference	Study design	N	Sensitivity (%)	Specificity (%)
Balthazar et al [90], 1991	Prospective. Patients with suspected appendicitis. CT scan with oral and IV contrast.	100	98	83
Malone et al [91], 1993	Prospective. Patients, age 4–91 y, with RLQ pain. Unenhanced CT scan from L3 to symphysis pubis.	211	87	97
Balthazar et al [60], 1994	Prospective. Consecutive patients, age 15–82 y, with "suggestive but not typical clinical and laboratory findings of appendicitis" evaluated by both CT and US. Clinical follow-up for nonsurgical patients.	100	96	89
Lane et al [92], 1997	Prospective. Adult patients with suspected appendicitis. Unenhanced helical CT from T12 to symphysis pubis. Clinical follow-up for nonsurgical patients.	109	90	97
Rao et al [93], 1997	Prospective. Patients, age 6–75 y, with suspected appendicitis. Focused, helical CT (appendiceal CT) with rectal contrast only. Follow-up for nonsurgical patients was review of outpatient records and telephone calls at 1 wk and 2 mo.	100	98	98
Lane et al [94], 1999	Prospective. Patients, age 8–86 y, with suspected appendicitis. Unenhanced, thin-slice helical CT scan. Clinical follow-up for nonsurgical patients.	300	96	99
Stroman et al [24], 1999	Prospective. Patients, age 13–89 y, with equivocal clinical findings for appendicitis. IV and oral contrast CT scan. Nonsurgical patients followed up by chart review.	107	92	85
Horton et al [25], 2000	Prospective. Patients, age 18–65 y, with possible appendicitis but missing 1 or more classic clinical finding; subjects randomized to CT or US. Focused, noncontrast CT from L3 to cecum. No description of follow-up protocol for nonsurgical patients.	49 (CT)	97	100
Walker et al [47], 2000	Randomized controlled trial of CT vs standard management. Adult patients with suspected appendicitis. Focused, helical CT scan with rectal contrast only. Telephone follow-up for nonsurgical patients.	128	94	100
Lowe et al [89], 2001	Retrospective. Consecutive children with suspected appendicitis underwent CT and compared with a historical cohort of consecutive children who underwent US. Unenhanced CT scan from inferior liver edge to symphysis pubis. 12 children with negative imaging studies lost to follow-up and excluded.	72	97	100

Wijetunga et al [95], 2001	Prospective. Patients, age 14–81 y, with suspected appendicitis but equivocal clinical findings. Focused, helical thin-slice CT scan of RLQ with oral contrast only. Follow-up for nonsurgical patients was telephone call and chart review over a period of 1–8 mo.	100	93	97
Wilson et al [48], 2001	Prospective. Patients, age 4–81 y, with suspected appendicitis. All subjects underwent limited pelvic CT with rectal contrast only and RLQ US. Nonsurgical patients followed up at 1 and 7 d.	99	94[a] 66[b]	92[a] 67[b]
Christopher et al [96], 2002	Prospective. Patients, age 5–77 y, with suspected appendicitis (those with obvious need for surgery excluded). Unenhanced helical CT. Telephone follow-up at 6–8 wk for nonsurgical patients.	101	77	94
Ege et al [97], 2002	Prospective. Patients, age 16–69 y, with RLQ pain but an equivocal clinical impression for appendicitis. Unenhanced thin-slice CT scan from L3 to symphysis pubis; clinical follow-up for nonsurgical patients.	296	96	98
Hershko et al [98], 2002	Prospective. Patients, age 15–83 y, with equivocal clinical impression for appendicitis. Helical CT scan with IV and oral contrast.	198	91	92
Poortman et al [64], 2003	Prospective. Patients (children and adults) with suspected appendicitis underwent both US and single-detector, helical, unenhanced CT scan. For nonsurgical patients, median follow-up was 13 mo.	226	76	83
in't Hof et al [99], 2004	Prospective. Adults with suspected appendicitis. All subjects underwent unenhanced helical CT from T11 to symphysis pubis followed by a diagnostic/therapeutic laparoscopy. Patients followed to 6 wk.	113	95	100
Keyzer et al [62], 2005	Prospective. Patients, age 16–81 y, referred for CT for suspected appendicitis; all patients underwent unenhanced 4-MDCT and US. Follow-up obtained from medical record and telephone call at 1 mo.	94	87	92
Doria et al [61], 2006	Meta-analysis (adults): study design described in text.	N/A	94[c]	94[c]
Doria et al [61], 2006	Meta-analysis (children): study design described in text.	N/A	94%[d]	95%[d]
Mun et al [100], 2006	Retrospective. Patients, age >17 y, referred for CT for acute abdominal pain or suspected appendicitis. Helical CT scan with IV contrast only. Patients with equivoca CT studies excluded from analysis (n = 4). No in-person follow-up; patients excludec if no documented clinical evaluation within 1 wk (35 of original 271 patients thus lost to follow-up).	173	100	97

(*continued on next page*)

Table 3
(continued)

Reference	Study design	N	Sensitivity (%)	Specificity (%)
Dearing et al [101], 2008	Retrospective. Patients, age 2–78 y, with suspected appendicitis but equivocal clinical findings. 16-MDCT scan with various contrast regimens (no rectal contrast). No description of follow-up protocol.	254	90	98
Gaitini et al [65], 2008	Retrospective. Consecutive adult patients referred for US for suspected appendicitis with 132 patients also undergoing follow-up 16-MDCT (oral and IV contrast). Clinical follow-up (inpatient only) for nonsurgical patients; indeterminate CT results not included in analysis (n = 1).	132 (CT)	100	99
Kim et al [51], 2008	Prospective. Patients, age >15 y, with suspected appendicitis. 16-MDCT with IV contrast only; there were no indeterminate CT scans. Telephone follow-up at 3 mo for nonsurgical patients.	157	98	96
Platon et al [71], 2009	Prospective. Adult patients with suspected appendicitis. Low-dose CT with oral contrast only followed by standard-dose CT and IV contrast (4-MDCT). Discharge diagnosis used for nonsurgical patients.	86	100[e] 95[f]	96[e] 96[f]
Poortman et al [63], 2009	Prospective. Adult patients with suspected appendicitis. US was followed by IV-enhanced 8-MDCT if US negative or indeterminate. Clinical follow-up and inpatient observation for nonsurgical patients.	60 (CT)	100	100
Van Randen et al [70], 2010	Prospective. Adult patients with suspected appendicitis. Subjects underwent both US and IV-enhanced abdominal CT. Diagnostic performance reflects presence of 2 or more essential CT findings.	942	96	95
Pickhardt et al [69], 2011	Retrospective. Consecutive adult patients referred for CT for suspected appendicitis or for signs/symptoms of appendicitis (ie, RLQ pain). Most patients received IV and oral contrast. Initially, 4-MDCT and 8-MDCT used; by end of study 8-MDCT, 16-MDCT, and 64-MDCT used. For nonsurgical patients, 12-mo clinical follow-up.	2871	99	98

Unless otherwise noted, CT scans were obtained of the entire abdomen and pelvis (ie, nonfocused). In the study by Wilson and colleagues, sensitivity and specificity were calculated with equivalent scans excluded[a] and with equivalent scans included,[b] Doria and colleagues calculated 95% CIs for their performance metrics: for adults,[c] sensitivity 95% CI 92%–95% and specificity 95% CI 94%–96%; for children,[d] sensitivity 95% CI 92%–97% and specificity 95% CI 94%–97%. Platon and colleagues calculated performance metrics for standard radiation dose CT[e] and for low radiation dose CT.[f]

Abbreviations: IV, intravenous; MDCT, multidetector CT; N/A, not applicable; RLQ, right lower quadrant.

Table 4
Selected studies evaluating diagnostic performance of magnetic resonance imaging, from 2009 to 2012

Reference	Study design	N	Sensitivity	Specificity
Cobben et al [74], 2009	Prospective. Patients, age 6–80 y, with clinically suspected appendicitis. Breath hold, unenhanced MRI with T1, T2, and T2 fat-suppressed sequences. Nonsurgical patients followed up in clinic at 1 wk and followed as outpatient for at least 2 y.	138	100	98
Barger and Nandalur [73], 2010	Meta-analysis. 8 prospective and retrospective articles included; studies included if the absolute numbers of true-positive, true-negative, false-positive, and false-negative results were reported.	363	97[a]	95[a]
Chabanova et al [102], 2011	Prospective. Adult patients with clinically diagnosed appendicitis. Unenhanced MRI with T1, T2, and fat-suppressed sequences. All patients underwent surgery.	48	87[b]	61
Inci et al [72], 2011	Prospective. Patients, age 14–72 y, with clinically suspected appendicitis. Unenhanced MRI with T1, T2, and fat-suppressed sequences. Clinical follow-up for 1–3 mo for nonsurgical patients.	85	96.5	66.7[c]
Johnson et al [103], 2012	Prospective. Pediatric patients, age 4–17 y, with acute abdominal pain suspicious for appendicitis. All subjects underwent MRI as well as CT or US. (MR sequences = single-shot turbo spin-echo T2 in 3 planes and T2 fat-suppressed axial sequence.) No specific mention of follow-up protocol for nonsurgical patients.	42	100	99
Moore et al [104], 2012	Retrospective. Pediatric patients, age 3–17 y, with suspected appendicitis. Unenhanced MRI with single-shot turbo spin-echo coronal T2, axial T2, and axial fat saturation T2, as well as a coronal SPAIR. Follow-up for nonsurgical patients based on chart review and discharge diagnosis.	208	97.6	97.0

Barger and colleagues calculated 95% CIs for their meta-analysis; for sensitivity,[a] 95% CI is 92%–99% and for specificity,[c] it is 94%–99%. In the study by Chabanova and colleagues, although MRI was 87% sensitive for appendicitis,[b] it was 100% sensitive in detecting pelvic abnormalities (ie, the radiologist called appendicitis but other disease found in the operating room). Of the 4 patients with no pathologic abnormalities, 3 were correctly identified by MRI, yielding a specificity of 75%. In the study by Inci and colleagues, by our calculation, specificity[c] is 89.3% (true negatives/[true negatives + false positives]); the investigators report 25 true-negative, 2 false-negative, 55 true-positive, and 3 false-positive cases ("probable appendicitis" was treated as a positive result in this study). Sensitivity of 96.5% is consistent with the raw numbers reported.
Abbreviation: SPAIR, spectral adiabatic inversion recovery.

Box 1: A practical score for the diagnosis of appendicitis (Alvarado score)

Symptoms	Migration of abdominal pain to the RLQ	1
	Anorexia (or acetone in the urine)	1
	Nausea/vomiting	1
Signs	Tenderness in the RLQ	2
	Rebound pain	1
	Increase of temperature (≥37.3 °C)	1
Laboratory	Leukocytosis (>10,000)	2
	Shift to the left (in a differentiated WBC count) (eg, neutrophilia >75%)	1

Cumulative score
5–6 compatible with acute appendicitis
7–8 probable for acute appendicitis
9–10 very probable for acute appendicitis.
A score of 5 or 6 may be observed. A score of 7 or higher should proceed to appendectomy. In the original 1986 monograph, MANTRELS was the mnemonic proposed by Dr Alvarado for use of the score.

Adapted from Alvarado A. A practical score for the early diagnosis of acute appendicitis. Ann Emerg Med 1986;15(5):557–64.

important included abdominal pain (99% of patients reported pain), nausea (81.7%), anorexia (72.4%), and emesis (67.7%). Findings with the greatest PPV were leukocytosis (PPV = 90.1%) and migration of abdominal pain (PPV = 91%) [42].

A more recent study prospectively examined the diagnostic performance of clinical impression, the Alvarado score, and CT scan in patients (age >15 years) who presented to the ED with suspected appendicitis. Sensitivity of clinical impression was 57.7% and was 42.2% for an Alvarado score of 8 or greater. Specificity was 71.6% and 79.1%, respectively. In this particular cohort of patients with suspected appendicitis, the 5 most common findings among those diagnosed with appendicitis were tenderness in the RLQ (92.2%), leukocytosis (75.6%), neutrophilia (73.3%), rebound tenderness (72.2%), and migratory pain (62.2%). Just more than half of the patients reported anorexia, nausea, or vomiting, and about a quarter were febrile [51].

Using 2 different methodologies (meta-analysis and a large cohort study), Andersson [1] examined the individual importance of specific clinical findings in suspected appendicitis. In the meta-analysis, receiver-operator curves (ROC) and likelihood ratios (LR) were generated from pooled data. Area under the ROC (AROC) was calculated (an AROC = 0.5 indicates that a test has no discriminatory ability). Anorexia (AROC = 0.58) and nausea (AROC = 0.56) had low discriminatory power. Migration of pain (AROC = 0.68) was the most valuable history finding. In terms of examination, tenderness alone had an AROC of 0.62, but signs of peritoneal irritation were stronger predictors of appendicitis: rebound tenderness had an AROC of 0.70 and guarding had an AROC of 0.68. Among laboratory tests, and also overall, WBC count, granulocyte count, and CRP level were the strongest discriminants of appendicitis (AROC = 0.77, 0.78, and 0.75, respectively). Combining 2 laboratory markers of inflammation had even stronger discriminatory and predictive power. The best performing combination was a WBC count greater than 10,000/L and CRP greater than 12 mg/L, with an AROC of 0.96 and LR of 23.3. These same investigators subsequently used a cohort of patients with suspected appendicitis to develop a clinical prediction tool that was validated in a separate prospective cohort (Box 2) [58]. In terms of sensitivity and specificity, this new tool performed similarly to Alvarado score; however, the Andersson score showed modest improvement in reducing the number of indeterminate results and in overall AROC. For the Andersson score, AROC was 0.93, and for the Alvarado score, AROC was 0.88 [58,59].

Ultrasound

US (see Table 2) has advantages over CT scanning, especially in terms of radiation exposure, but most studies have found that it performs inferiorly in terms of accuracy [25,26,28,48,60–63]. In 1 large prospective trial of US versus CT (n = 199 patients), the 2 modalities performed similarly, but completely unenhanced CT was used (ie, no oral, rectal, or intravenous [IV] contrast) and accuracy of CT in this study was inferior to most other published studies [64]. Consistently, sensitivity of US has been found inferior to its specificity [25,27,60–62,65].

To our knowledge, US has not been thoroughly evaluated in a nonacademic setting. In the 2012 SCOAP study, across a diverse group of hospitals, cumulative sensitivity of US was 47.8% [22]. Because we did not study those with

Box 2: The appendicitis inflammatory response score (Andersson score)

Variable	Level	Score
Pain or tenderness in RLQ		+1
Vomiting		+1
Rebound tenderness or muscular defense	Slight	+1
	Moderate	+2
	Strong	+3
WBC count	10–14.9 × 10^9/L	+1
	≥15.0 × 10^9/L	+2
Proportion neutrophils	70%–84%	+1
	≥85%	+2
CRP concentration	10–49 mg/L	+1
	≥50	+2
Body temperature	≥38.5 °C	+1

Summation of points

0–4 = low probability for appendicitis; outpatient follow-up if unaltered general condition

5–8 = indeterminate; in-hospital active observation with rescoring, imaging, or diagnostic laparoscopy according to local practice

9–12 = high probability for appendicitis; surgical exploration recommended

Adapted from Andersson M, Andersson R. The appendicitis inflammatory response score: a tool for the diagnosis of acute appendicitis that outperforms the Alvarado score. World J Surg 2008;32(8):1843–9; with permission.

suspected appendicitis (only appendectomies), our capture of true-negative results was limited, which prevented a calculation of specificity. Because we had access to information directly from patient charts, we were able to ascertain that the low sensitivity we observed resulted primarily from a large number of indeterminate US reports. (It is notable that many investigators exclude inconclusive results from their calculations of sensitivity, specificity, PPV, or NPV [48].) Two prospective trials of CT versus US in suspected appendicitis had similar findings: indeterminate imaging results were significantly more frequent with US than with CT [48,62]. In 1 of these, nearly 75% of US studies were equivocal, and US did not rule out a single patient without appendicitis [48].

However, in clinical investigations, US often performs better than 47.8% sensitivity. Of the 12 studies presented in Table 2, all of which obtained data from patients suspected of having appendicitis (ie, not surgical patients only), sensitivity for appendicitis ranged from 76% to 98%. A rigorous 2006 meta-analysis of CT and US included 57 studies (both retrospective and prospective) and more than 13,000 patients. Studies were included only if absolute numbers of true-positive, true-negative, false-positive, and false-negative results were available, and the data were stratified by age so that adults and children could be considered separately. In children, sensitivity for US was 88% and specificity was 94%. For adults, sensitivity was 83% and specificity was 93% [61].

A well-designed Austrian study prospectively followed 350 patients evaluated by US for suspected appendicitis and determined that sensitivity was 98%, specificity was 98%, PPV was 96%, and NPV 99%. Of the 144 patients with a high clinical suspicion for appendicitis (assessment made by experienced surgeons before US), 34.8% did not have appendicitis. Among these 144 patients, US was inconclusive in only 4 patients, missed 1 case of appendicitis, and missed 2 other nonappendicitis conditions [66]. These are impressive findings, and the investigators note that their results are possible only because of long-standing close cooperation between the diagnostic imaging and surgical teams. These results exemplify what Bachur and colleagues [40] found in a recent study of US using a large, nationwide pediatric database: although there is a significant negative association, overall, between US use and NA in pediatric hospitals, among institutions that use US infrequently, there is dramatic variability in frequency of NA. The investigators attributed this finding to varying experience levels of sonographers and those interpreting the images.

When the appendix can be visualized, US performs well [66,67]. Furthermore, in specialized centers in which US for suspected appendicitis is emphasized, high-quality results are possible. Observational data suggest that performance of US in some community settings lags behind the results achieved in clinical studies.

Computed Tomography

CT is more widely used in the workup of suspected appendicitis and there is extensive literature on the subject (see Table 3). In addition to their assessment of US, Doria and colleagues [61] also performed a meta-analysis for CT scan. The results showed a notable improvement in sensitivity for CT over US. For adults, pooled sensitivity and specificity of CT were both 94%. For children, sensitivity was 94% and specificity 95%. In a systematic review of CT scan in adults, Neumayer and Kennedy [9] found that sensitivity ranged from 77% to 100% and that specificity ranged from 83% to 100%. The results reported in this systematic review were derived from studies with diverse patient populations and in which different CT protocols were used (for instance, without enteral contrast, completely unenhanced, or with both enteral and IV contrast). Some studies considered only patients in whom clinical findings were not convincing enough to warrant immediate appendectomy (so-called atypical patients). It is likely that this variability in study population and imaging protocols (which is also reflected in Table 3) at least partially explains the wide differences in results. CT technology has also become more advanced over the last 20 years (for example 4-detector or single-detector scanners common in the early days of CT for appendicitis have given way to 64-multidetector helical scanners), leading some to suggest an association between improved technology and improved diagnostic performance [68]. Indeed, several studies of CT published since the Neumayer review and Doria meta-analysis have reported superior diagnostic performance [51,65,69,70], including 1 study that used low-dose radiation protocols [71]. One of these studies evaluated a large number of patients with suspected appendicitis (2871 consecutive adults) and followed those who did not undergo surgery with a rigorous follow-up protocol. CT scan sensitivity was 98.5%, specificity was 98%, NPV was 99.5%, and PPV was 93.9% [69]. As CT technology has improved, and as radiologists and surgeons have grown more comfortable and skillful in interpreting scans for appendicitis, many of the sensitivities and specificities reported from earlier in the era of CT for suspected appendicitis should be considered obsolete.

CT scan is also adept at revealing alternative diagnoses when appendicitis is not the cause of patients' RLQ pain. Of the 23 studies cited in the Neumayer review article, 13 articles reported the percentage of patients for whom an alternative diagnosis was uncovered by CT scan; this ranged from 6% to 36%, with a median of 21% [9]. In the large recent trial by Pickhardt and colleagues [69], alternative diagnoses were identified or suggested by CT in 42.1% of the patients who did not undergo appendectomy and who did not have CT findings suggestive of appendicitis. These CT findings represented a wide variety of clinical conditions, including other gastrointestinal conditions, gynecologic diseases, and urinary tract diseases.

Magnetic resonance imaging

Innovation in the use of magnetic resonance imaging (MRI) in the diagnosis of appendicitis has been primarily focused on its use in pregnant patients and in children (2 populations at particular risk from exposure to ionizing radiation) [72]. However, there are also studies on the use of MRI in general patients presenting with acute RLQ pain or suspected appendicitis (see Table 4). A recent meta-analysis combined the results of 8 previous studies (for a total of 363 patients). Studies were included only if the total number of true-positive, true-negative, false-positive, and false-negative results were available or derivable. Of the 363 patients included, the appendix could not be identified in only 8 patients. The investigators reported a sensitivity of 97% (95% CI 92%–99%) and specificity of 95% (95% CI 94%–99%). This meta-analysis included both enhanced and unenhanced scans [73].

In a prospective study by Cobben and colleagues [74], US was followed by MRI in all enrolled patients (n = 138). In 36 of these patients, US showed no abnormalities and did not visualize the appendix. Of these 36 patients, MRI showed that 8 had acute appendicitis and uncovered an alternative diagnosis in 4 patients. Even among patients who were clinically believed likely to have appendicitis (patients were stratified before imaging), MRI ruled out appendicitis in 22 patients, preventing 22 unnecessary operations. In 12 patients, the MRI was equivocal (ie, the appendix was not visualized), but the appendix had been visualized and noted to be normal on US in 10 of these patients. The investigators speculated that the MRI could not visualize the appendix in these 12 patients because they were thin and had little intra-abdominal fat. Although MRI is a relatively expensive imaging modality, the investigators estimated a substantial cost savings from reductions in unnecessary operations and inpatient observation. According to the investigators, 1 of the benefits of the protocol used in this study (T1, T2, and T2 fat-suppression breath-hold sequences) is that the sequences are "easy to use and learn and are quick," which has the advantage of making "MRI more user-friendly [and may] lead to its more frequent use out of hours."

Diagnostic laparoscopy

In the early 1990s, diagnostic laparoscopy arose as a tool in the diagnosis of appendicitis. This was a time in which advanced imaging was not yet routinely used (investigation into imaging was happening roughly concomitantly with the trials involving diagnostic laparoscopy). A Cochrane review updated in 2010 evaluated both the therapeutic and diagnostic benefits of laparoscopy in appendicitis. In this analysis of diagnostic laparoscopy, studies were included only if the laparoscopic procedure was explicitly designed to address diagnosis and that (at least in cases where another diagnosis was evident on laparoscopy) the macroscopically normal appendix was left in situ. In this meta-analysis, which included 14 studies, the weighted relative risk (RR) of having a normal appendix removed for patients who received diagnostic laparoscopy versus patients who proceeded directly to therapeutic appendectomy was 0.37 (however, the 95% CI was 0.13–1.01). Among reproductive-aged women, the reduction in NA was more impressive, with an RR of 0.20 (95% CI 0.11–0.34). The RR of not having a diagnosis made was also significantly reduced by diagnostic laparoscopy (0.27, 95% CI 0.17–0.44) [75].

Special populations

Pregnant patients

Appendectomy is the most common nonobstetric surgical procedure performed in pregnant women [76]. Diagnosis of appendicitis in pregnant women is challenging, because many of the typical findings of appendicitis (eg, nausea, vomiting, abdominal discomfort, increased WBC count) are also present in a normal pregnancy; furthermore, the appendix may be displaced by the developing fetus and enlarging uterus [77]. Accurate and timely diagnosis is crucial, because perforation is associated with increased fetal and maternal complications, including fetal demise [78]. This risk is why the surgical literature once indicated that NA rates of 50% were acceptable in pregnant women [9]. However, the risks to a fetus of an operation and exposure to general anesthesia are not trivial. Avoiding NA when possible is important [79], and efforts have been focused on improving the accuracy with which appendicitis is diagnosed in pregnant patients.

CT is used when appendicitis is suspected in pregnant women, but, because of the risks of ionizing radiation, many clinicians prefer to use CT only when US or MRI is inconclusive [80,81]. Estimates of fetal radiation exposure from CT scans for appendicitis range from 19.9 to 43.6 mGy depending on the trimester. A radiation dose less than 50 mGy is considered safe from deterministic effects (threshold-dependent and dose-dependent effects), and it is the point at which there is a less than 1% risk of stochastic effects (dose-independent effects without a threshold). However, malignancies are generally considered related to the stochastic effects of radiation, and Long and colleagues [81] state "there is an estimated doubling in the overall risk for childhood cancer in a fetus exposed to 30.0 mGy of radiation during an MDCT appendix protocol examination," citing RR data from the International Commission on Radiologic Protection. Because of the potential for teratogenicity and carcinogenicity, the 2007 American College of Radiology Appropriateness Criteria guidelines recommend MRI and US over CT in the evaluation of RLQ pain in pregnant patients.

US, using the graded compression technique, is the most frequently used modality for evaluating suspected appendicitis in pregnant women. Many studies report poor performance for US, related in most cases to nonvisualization of the appendix [78]. In a recent study of 99 women in the second or third trimester, US failed to locate the appendix in 97% of patients. Overall, 7 of the 99 patients had appendicitis, and only 2 of these patients had a positive US [78]. Other recent studies have reported equally dismal results for US in pregnant patients: nonvisualization ranged from 88% to 96% [82,83].

Because of this problem, MRI has emerged as a compelling option to evaluate suspected appendicitis in pregnant patients [84]. In a systematic review, Basaran and Basaran [81] compared CT scan with MRI and showed equivalent performance for both modalities in the second and third trimester of pregnancy (for both modalities, studies included mostly patients with a previous normal or inconclusive US because, in many instances, patients with conclusive US are taken directly to the OR without proceeding to CT or MRI). For CT, pooled sensitivity was 85.7% and specificity was 97.4%. For MRI, pooled sensitivity was 80% and specificity was 99% [85]. In a 2011 meta-analysis of MRI that includes 2 additional large studies not included in the Basaran review, pooled sensitivity for MRI was 91%, specificity 98%, PPV 86%, and NPV 99%. In this meta-analysis, as in most of the articles that provided data, scans in which the appendix was not seen but there was no evidence of RLQ inflammation were included as negative results for the purposes of calculating performance characteristics.

Pediatric patients

The use of imaging in pediatric patients to reduce NA has shown some variability (see Table 1). Some studies have shown improvements with increased imaging [7,26,27,33,40,41] and others have shown no reduction in NA [13,28,43]. A recent nationwide study of 52,426 pediatric patients (all after appendectomy) found that there was no association between CT scan use and NA but that the increasing use of US or US and CT (at the institutional level) was inversely associated with the frequency of NA [40]. Other studies have shown improved performance for CT over US in pediatric patients [26,33,61].

As with pregnant patients, ionizing radiation is an important concern in children. Although US may not perform as well as CT, studies based in centers that emphasize sonographic evaluation of suspected appendicitis have generated impressive results [66]. A 2001 study of US in children reported 93% sensitivity, 94.5% specificity, 86% PPV, and 97% NPV (of 2056 US evaluations for suspected appendicitis). These investigators concluded that US could improve accuracy of diagnosing appendicitis in children, especially when repeat US is used for initially indeterminate studies [27].

Recognizing the benefits of US in terms of radiation exposure and the benefits of CT in diagnostic accuracy, several high-quality studies have prospectively assessed an imaging protocol in which US is the first modality used followed by CT scan only for equivocal US. All showed acceptable sensitivity and specificity [63,65,67,86–88]. Three of these studies were performed specifically in pediatric populations: in the first study, from 1999, the algorithm achieved 94% sensitivity, 94% specificity, a PPV of 90%, and an NPV of 97% [86]. The 2 more recent studies are both from the same center [67,87]. The 2011 article reported sensitivity of 98.6%, specificity of 90.6%, a PPV of 84.6%, and an NPV of 93.3%. Frequency of NA was 8.1%. Of the 631 children who followed the imaging protocol, 52.6% were spared a CT scan and exposure to radiation. There was 1 (0.16%) missed case of appendicitis overall, (although there were 3 false-negative results from the overall protocol; 2 of these patients were taken to the OR based on clinical suspicion). Notably, nearly half of the patients who presented with possible appendicitis did not follow the imaging protocol. However, a strength of the study is the detailed description of outcomes for these noncompliant patients. In that group, there were no missed cases of appendicitis and 7.6% NA [87].

SUMMARY

Our attempts to systematically improve accuracy in the evaluation of patients with suspected appendicitis are, in some ways, hindered by the fact that the condition is so frequently straightforward to diagnose. Careful history-taking and physical examination are reliable in most patients. However, establishing the diagnosis with these skills alone remains vulnerable to conditions that masquerade as acute appendicitis. A substantial body of clinical research over the last quarter-century has shown that improved accuracy is possible. Strategies for improvement include the use of diagnostic scoring systems, laboratory makers such as CRP, diagnostic laparoscopy, and advanced imaging modalities such as CT, MRI, and US. How clinicians use these strategies depends on many factors related to practice setting, the population served, and clinical goals. In children, for instance, the desire to limit exposure to ionizing radiation competes with the greater anatomic detail that a CT scan can provide; at the same time, many hospitals that treat children do not have the resources to maintain the sort of full-time, highly sophisticated abdominal US programs that achieve the highest rates of diagnostic accuracy in clinical studies.

Trade-offs have to be made, but improvement is possible in almost all groups of patients: the clinical community should no longer settle for a 15% NA rate when 5% is clearly possible without adverse consequences. Many clinicians will be faced with the task of evaluating patients suspected of having acute appendicitis. A deliberate, proactive, and, ideally, benchmarked strategy for improving diagnosis should be the standard to which we hold ourselves and the promise we deliver to our patients.

References

[1] Andersson RE. Meta-analysis of the clinical and laboratory diagnosis of appendicitis. Br J Surg 2004;91(1):28–37.

[2] Andersson R, Hugander A, Thulin A, et al. Indications for operation in suspected appendicitis and incidence of perforation. BMJ 1994;308(6921):107–10.

[3] Andersson RE. The natural history and traditional management of appendicitis revisited: spontaneous resolution and predominance of prehospital perforations imply that a correct diagnosis is more important than an early diagnosis. World J Surg 2007;31(1):86–92.

[4] Livingston EH, Woodward WA, Sarosi GA, et al. Disconnect between incidence of nonperforated and perforated appendicitis: implications for pathophysiology and management. Ann Surg 2007;245(6):886–92.

[5] Cantrell JR, Stafford ES. The diminishing mortality from appendicitis. Ann Surg 1955;141(6):749–58.

[6] Rao PM, Feltmate CM, Rhea JT, et al. Helical computed tomography in differentiating appendicitis and acute gynecologic conditions. Obstet Gynecol 1999;93(3):417–21.

[7] Rao PM, Rhea JT, Rattner DW, et al. Introduction of appendiceal CT: impact on negative appendectomy and appendiceal perforation rates. Ann Surg 1999;229(3):344–9.

[8] Flum DR, Morris A, Koepsell T, et al. Has misdiagnosis of appendicitis decreased over time? A population-based analysis. JAMA 2001;286(14):1748–53.

[9] Neumayer L, Kennedy A. Imaging in appendicitis: a review with special emphasis on the treatment of women. Obstet Gynecol 2003;102(6):1404–9.

[10] Aanning HL. Negative appendectomy and perforation rates in the SCOAP trial. Ann Surg 2009;249(4):699 [author reply: 699–700].

[11] Sarkaria IS, Eachempati SR, Weyant MJ, et al. Current surgical opinion of computed tomography for acute appendicitis. Surg Infect (Larchmt) 2004;5(3):243–52.

[12] McDonald GP, Pendarvis DP, Wilmoth R, et al. Influence of preoperative computed tomography on patients undergoing appendectomy. Am Surg 2001;67(11):1017–21.

[13] Partrick DA, Janik JE, Janik JS, et al. Increased CT scan utilization does not improve the diagnostic accuracy of appendicitis in children. J Pediatr Surg 2003;38(5):659–62.

[14] Perez J, Barone JE, Wilbanks TO, et al. Liberal use of computed tomography scanning does not improve diagnostic accuracy in appendicitis. Am J Surg 2003;185(3):194–7.
[15] Flum DR, McClure TD, Morris A, et al. Misdiagnosis of appendicitis and the use of diagnostic imaging. J Am Coll Surg 2005;201(6):933–9.
[16] Jones K, Pena AA, Dunn EL, et al. Are negative appendectomies still acceptable? Am J Surg 2004;188(6):748–54.
[17] Wagner PL, Eachempati SR, Soe K, et al. Defining the current negative appendectomy rate: for whom is preoperative computed tomography making an impact? Surgery 2008;144(2): 276–82.
[18] Coursey CA, Nelson RC, Patel MB, et al. Making the diagnosis of acute appendicitis: do more preoperative CT scans mean fewer negative appendectomies? A 10-year study. Radiology 2010;254(2):460–8.
[19] Raja AS, Wright C, Sodickson AD, et al. Negative appendectomy rate in the era of CT: an 18-year perspective. Radiology 2010;256(2):460–5.
[20] Guller U, Rosella L, McCall J, et al. Negative appendicectomy and perforation rates in patients undergoing laparoscopic surgery for suspected appendicitis. Br J Surg 2011;98(4): 589–95.
[21] Seetahal SA, Bolorunduro OB, Sookdeo TC, et al. Negative appendectomy: a 10-year review of a nationally representative sample. Am J Surg 2011;201(4):433–7.
[22] Drake FT, Florence MG, Johnson MG, et al. Progress in the diagnosis of appendicitis: a report from Washington State's. Ann Surg 2012;256(4):586–94.
[23] Colson M, Skinner KA, Dunnington G. High negative appendectomy rates are no longer acceptable. Am J Surg 1997;174(6):723–6 [discussion: 726–7].
[24] Stroman DL, Bayouth CV, Kuhn JA, et al. The role of computed tomography in the diagnosis of acute appendicitis. Am J Surg 1999;178(6):485–9.
[25] Horton MD, Counter SF, Florence MG, et al. A prospective trial of computed tomography and ultrasonography for diagnosing appendicitis in the atypical patient. Am J Surg 2000;179(5):379–81.
[26] Applegate KE, Sivit CJ, Salvator AE, et al. Effect of cross-sectional imaging on negative appendectomy and perforation rates in children. Radiology 2001;220(1):103–7.
[27] Dilley A, Wesson D, Munden M, et al. The impact of ultrasound examinations on the management of children with suspected appendicitis: a 3-year analysis. J Pediatr Surg 2001;36(2):303–8.
[28] Bendeck SE, Nino-Murcia M, Berry GJ, et al. Imaging for suspected appendicitis: negative appendectomy and perforation rates. Radiology 2002;225(1):131–6.
[29] Naoum JJ, Mileski WJ, Daller JA, et al. The use of abdominal computed tomography scan decreases the frequency of misdiagnosis in cases of suspected appendicitis. Am J Surg 2002;184(6):587–9 [discussion: 589–90].
[30] Yetkin G, Basak M, Isgor A, et al. Can negative appendectomy rate be decreased by using spiral computed tomography without contrast material? Acta Chir Belg 2002;102(5): 334–7.
[31] Brandt MM, Wahl WL. Liberal use of CT scanning helps to diagnose appendicitis in adults. Am Surg 2003;69(9):727–31 [discussion: 731–2].
[32] DeArmond GM, Dent DL, Myers JG, et al. Appendicitis: selective use of abdominal CT reduces negative appendectomy rate. Surg Infect (Larchmt) 2003;4(2):213–8.
[33] Kaiser S, Mesas-Burgos C, Soderman E, et al. Appendicitis in children–impact of US and CT on the negative appendectomy rate. Eur J Pediatr Surg 2004;14(4):260–4.
[34] McGory ML, Zingmond DS, Nanayakkara D, et al. Negative appendectomy rate: influence of CT scans. Am Surg 2005;71(10):803–8.
[35] Morse BC, Roettger RH, Kalbaugh CA, et al. Abdominal CT scanning in reproductive-age women with right lower quadrant abdominal pain: does its use reduce negative appendectomy rates and healthcare costs? Am Surg 2007;73(6):580–4 [discussion: 584].

[36] Cuschieri J, Florence M, Flum DR, et al. Negative appendectomy and imaging accuracy in the Washington State Surgical Care and Outcomes Assessment Program. Ann Surg 2008;248(4):557–63.
[37] Guss DA, Behling CA, Munassi D. Impact of abdominal helical computed tomography on the rate of negative appendicitis. J Emerg Med 2008;34(1):7–11.
[38] Piper HG, Rusnak C, Orrom W, et al. Current management of appendicitis at a community center–how can we improve? Am J Surg 2008;195(5):585–8 [discussion: 588–9].
[39] Webb EM, Nguyen A, Wang ZJ, et al. The negative appendectomy rate: who benefits from preoperative CT? AJR Am J Roentgenol 2011;197(4):861–6.
[40] Bachur RG, Hennelly K, Callahan MJ, et al. Advanced radiologic imaging for pediatric appendicitis, 2005-2009: trends and outcomes. J Pediatr 2012;160(6):1034–8.
[41] Bachur RG, Hennelly K, Callahan MJ, et al. Diagnostic imaging and negative appendectomy rates in children: effects of age and gender. Pediatrics 2012;129(5):877–84.
[42] Lee SL, Walsh AJ, Ho HS. Computed tomography and ultrasonography do not improve and may delay the diagnosis and treatment of acute appendicitis. Arch Surg 2001;136(5): 556–62.
[43] Weyant MJ, Eachempati SR, Maluccio MA, et al. The use of computed tomography for the diagnosis of acute appendicitis in children does not influence the overall rate of negative appendectomy or perforation. Surg Infect (Larchmt) 2001;2(1):19–23.
[44] Vadeboncoeur TF, Heister RR, Behling CA, et al. Impact of helical computed tomography on the rate of negative appendicitis. Am J Emerg Med 2006;24(1):43–7.
[45] Huynh V, Lalezarzadeh F, Lawandy S, et al. Abdominal computed tomography in the evaluation of acute and perforated appendicitis in the community setting. Am Surg 2007;73(10):1002–5.
[46] Frei SP, Bond WF, Bazuro RK, et al. Appendicitis outcomes with increasing computed tomographic scanning. Am J Emerg Med 2008;26(1):39–44.
[47] Walker S, Haun W, Clark J, et al. The value of limited computed tomography with rectal contrast in the diagnosis of acute appendicitis. Am J Surg 2000;180(6):450–4 [discussion: 454–5].
[48] Wilson EB, Cole JC, Nipper ML, et al. Computed tomography and ultrasonography in the diagnosis of appendicitis: when are they indicated? Arch Surg 2001;136(6):670–5.
[49] Hong JJ, Cohn SM, Ekeh AP, et al. A prospective randomized study of clinical assessment versus computed tomography. Surg Infect (Larchmt) 2003;4(3):231–9.
[50] Lee CC, Golub R, Singer AJ, et al. Routine versus selective abdominal computed tomography scan in the evaluation of right lower quadrant pain: a randomized controlled trial. Acad Emerg Med 2007;14(2):117–22.
[51] Kim K, Rhee JE, Lee CC, et al. Impact of helical computed tomography in clinically evident appendicitis. Emerg Med J 2008;25(8):477–81.
[52] Santos DA, Manunga J Jr, Hohman D, et al. How often does computed tomography change the management of acute appendicitis? Am Surg 2009;75(10):918–21.
[53] Andersson RE. Proportion of cases of perforated appendicitis: a bad measure of quality of care. Arch Surg 2011;146(7):885 [author reply: 885–6].
[54] Schwartz SI, Brunicardi FC. Schwartz's principles of surgery. New York: McGraw-Hill; 2010. p. 1, online resource (p. xxi, 1866).
[55] Sack U, Biereder B, Elouahidi T, et al. Diagnostic value of blood inflammatory markers for detection of acute appendicitis in children. BMC Surg 2006;6:15.
[56] Noh H, Chang SJ, Han A. The diagnostic values of preoperative laboratory markers in children with complicated appendicitis. J Korean Surg Soc 2012;83(4):237–41.
[57] Alvarado A. A practical score for the early diagnosis of acute appendicitis. Ann Emerg Med 1986;15(5):557–64.
[58] Andersson M, Andersson RE. The appendicitis inflammatory response score: a tool for the diagnosis of acute appendicitis that outperforms the Alvarado score. World J Surg 2008;32(8):1843–9.

[59] de Castro SM, Ünlü C, Steller EP, et al. Evaluation of the appendicitis inflammatory response score for patients with acute appendicitis. World J Surg 2012;36(7):1540–5.
[60] Balthazar EJ, Birnbaum BA, Yee J, et al. Acute appendicitis: CT and US correlation in 100 patients. Radiology 1994;190(1):31–5.
[61] Doria AS, Moineddin R, Kellenberger CJ, et al. US or CT for diagnosis of appendicitis in children and adults? a meta-analysis. Radiology 2006;241(1):83–94.
[62] Keyzer C, Zalcman M, De Maertelaer V, et al. Comparison of US and unenhanced multidetector row CT in patients suspected of having acute appendicitis. Radiology 2005;236(2):527–34.
[63] Poortman P, Oostvogel HJ, Bosma E, et al. Improving diagnosis of acute appendicitis: results of a diagnostic pathway with standard use of ultrasonography followed by selective use of CT. J Am Coll Surg 2009;208(3):434–41.
[64] Poortman P, Lohle PN, Schoemaker CM, et al. Comparison of CT and sonography in the diagnosis of acute appendicitis: a blinded prospective study. AJR Am J Roentgenol 2003;181(5):1355–9.
[65] Gaitini D, Beck-Razi N, Mor-Yosef D, et al. Diagnosing acute appendicitis in adults: accuracy of color Doppler sonography and MDCT compared with surgery and clinical follow-up. AJR Am J Roentgenol 2008;190(5):1300–6.
[66] Rettenbacher T, Hollerweger A, Gritzmann N, et al. Appendicitis: should diagnostic imaging be performed if the clinical presentation is highly suggestive of the disease? Gastroenterology 2002;123(4):992–8.
[67] Ramarajan N, Krishnamoorthi R, Barth R, et al. An interdisciplinary initiative to reduce radiation exposure: evaluation of appendicitis in a pediatric emergency department with clinical assessment supported by a staged ultrasound and computed tomography pathway. Acad Emerg Med 2009;16(11):1258–65.
[68] Kessler N, Cyteval C, Gallix B, et al. Appendicitis: evaluation of sensitivity, specificity, and predictive values of US, Doppler US, and laboratory findings. Radiology 2004;230(2): 472–8.
[69] Pickhardt PJ, Lawrence EM, Pooler BD, et al. Diagnostic performance of multidetector computed tomography for suspected acute appendicitis. Ann Intern Med 2011;154(12): 789–96.
[70] van Randen A, Lameris W, van Es HW, et al. Profiles of US and CT imaging features with a high probability of appendicitis. Eur Radiol 2010;20(7):1657–66.
[71] Platon A, Jlassi H, Rutschmann OT, et al. Evaluation of a low-dose CT protocol with oral contrast for assessment of acute appendicitis. Eur Radiol 2009;19(2):446–54.
[72] Inci E, Hocaoglu E, Aydin S, et al. Efficiency of unenhanced MRI in the diagnosis of acute appendicitis: comparison with Alvarado scoring system and histopathological results. Eur J Radiol 2011;80(2):253–8.
[73] Barger RL, Nandalur KR. Diagnostic performance of magnetic resonance imaging in the detection of appendicitis in adults: a meta-analysis. Acad Radiol 2010;17(10): 1211–6.
[74] Cobben L, Groot I, Kingma L, et al. A simple MRI protocol in patients with clinically suspected appendicitis: results in 138 patients and effect on outcome of appendectomy. Eur Radiol 2009;19(5):1175–83.
[75] Sauerland S, Jaschinski T, Neugebauer EA. Laparoscopic versus open surgery for suspected appendicitis. Cochrane Database Syst Rev 2010;(10) CD001546.
[76] Wei PL, Keller JJ, Liang HH, et al. Acute appendicitis and adverse pregnancy outcomes: a nationwide population-based study. J Gastrointest Surg 2012;16(6):1204–11.
[77] Wang PI, Chong ST, Kielar AZ, et al. Imaging of pregnant and lactating patients: part 2, evidence-based review and recommendations. AJR Am J Roentgenol 2012;198(4): 785–92.
[78] Lehnert BE, Gross JA, Linnau KF, et al. Utility of ultrasound for evaluating the appendix during the second and third trimester of pregnancy. Emerg Radiol 2012;19(4):293–9.

[79] Ito K, Ito H, Whang EE, et al. Appendectomy in pregnancy: evaluation of the risks of a negative appendectomy. Am J Surg 2012;203(2):145–50.
[80] Patel SJ, Reede DL, Katz DS, et al. Imaging the pregnant patient for nonobstetric conditions: algorithms and radiation dose considerations. Radiographics 2007;27(6):1705–22.
[81] Long SS, Long C, Lai H, et al. Imaging strategies for right lower quadrant pain in pregnancy. AJR Am J Roentgenol 2011;196(1):4–12.
[82] Israel GM, Malguria N, McCarthy S, et al. MRI vs. ultrasound for suspected appendicitis during pregnancy. J Magn Reson Imaging 2008;28(2):428–33.
[83] Cobben LP, Groot I, Haans L, et al. MRI for clinically suspected appendicitis during pregnancy. AJR Am J Roentgenol 2004;183(3):671–5.
[84] Pedrosa I, Zeikus EA, Levine D, et al. MR imaging of acute right lower quadrant pain in pregnant and nonpregnant patients. Radiographics 2007;27(3):721–43 [discussion: 743–53].
[85] Basaran A, Basaran M. Diagnosis of acute appendicitis during pregnancy: a systematic review. Obstet Gynecol Surv 2009;64(7):481–8 [quiz: 499].
[86] Garcia Pena BM, Mandl KD, Kraus SJ, et al. Ultrasonography and limited computed tomography in the diagnosis and management of appendicitis in children. JAMA 1999;282(11):1041–6.
[87] Krishnamoorthi R, Ramarajan N, Wang NE, et al. Effectiveness of a staged US and CT protocol for the diagnosis of pediatric appendicitis: reducing radiation exposure in the age of ALARA. Radiology 2011;259(1):231–9.
[88] Poletti PA, Platon A, De Perrot T, et al. Acute appendicitis: prospective evaluation of a diagnostic algorithm integrating ultrasound and low-dose CT to reduce the need of standard CT. Eur Radiol 2011;21(12):2558–66.
[89] Lowe LH, Penney MW, Stein SM, et al. Unenhanced limited CT of the abdomen in the diagnosis of appendicitis in children: comparison with sonography. AJR Am J Roentgenol 2001;176(1):31–5.
[90] Balthazar EJ, Megibow AJ, Siegel SE, et al. Appendicitis: prospective evaluation with high-resolution CT. Radiology 1991;180(1):21–4.
[91] Malone AJ Jr, Wolf CR, Malmed AS, et al. Diagnosis of acute appendicitis: value of unenhanced CT. AJR Am J Roentgenol 1993;160(4):763–6.
[92] Lane MJ, Katz DS, Ross BA, et al. Unenhanced helical CT for suspected acute appendicitis. AJR Am J Roentgenol 1997;168(2):405–9.
[93] Rao PM, Rhea JT, Novelline RA, et al. Helical CT combined with contrast material administered only through the colon. AJR Am J Roentgenol 1997;169(5):1275–80.
[94] Lane MJ, Liu DM, Huynh MD, et al. Suspected acute appendicitis: nonenhanced helical CT in 300 consecutive patients. Radiology 1999;213(2):341–6.
[95] Wijetunga R, Tan BS, Rouse JC, et al. Diagnostic accuracy of focused appendiceal CT in clinically equivocal cases of acute appendicitis. Radiology 2001;221(3):747–53.
[96] Christopher FL, Lane MJ, Ward JA, et al. Unenhanced helical CT scanning of the abdomen and pelvis changes disposition of patients presenting to the emergency department with possible acute appendicitis. J Emerg Med 2002;23(1):1–7.
[97] Ege G, Akman H, Sahin A, et al. Diagnostic value of unenhanced helical CT in adult patients with suspected acute appendicitis. Br J Radiol 2002;75(897):721–5.
[98] Hershko DD, Sroka G, Bahouth H, et al. The role of selective computed tomography in the diagnosis and management of suspected acute appendicitis. Am Surg 2002;68(11):1003–7.
[99] in't Hof KH, van Lankeren W, Krestin GP, et al. Surgical validation of unenhanced helical computed tomography in acute appendicitis. Br J Surg 2004;91(12):1641–5.
[100] Mun S, Ernst RD, Chen K, et al. Rapid CT diagnosis of acute appendicitis with IV contrast material. Emerg Radiol 2006;12(3):99–102.
[101] Dearing DD, Recabaren JA, Alexander M. Can computed tomography scan be performed effectively in the diagnosis of acute appendicitis without the added morbidity of rectal contrast? Am Surg 2008;74(10):917–20.

[102] Chabanova E, Balslev I, Achiam M, et al. Unenhanced MR imaging in adults with clinically suspected acute appendicitis. Eur J Radiol 2011;79(2):206–10.
[103] Johnson AK, Filippi CG, Andrews T, et al. Ultrafast 3-T MRI in the evaluation of children with acute lower abdominal pain for the detection of appendicitis. AJR Am J Roentgenol 2012;198(6):1424–30.
[104] Moore MM, Gustas CN, Choudhary AK, et al. MRI for clinically suspected pediatric appendicitis: an implemented program. Pediatr Radiol 2012;42(9):1056–63.

Advances in Surgery 47 (2013) 329–333

ADVANCES IN SURGERY

INDEX

A

Note: Page numbers of article titles are in **boldface** type.

0065-3411/13/$ – see front matter

http://dx.doi.org/10.1016/S0065-3411(13)00028-6